# PHARMACOLOGY

## *(Simplified)*



*by*

**Dr. Huzaif Shaikh, MD**

BHALANI

**Bhalani Publishers**

CLEVER
PEN PUBLISHING

**First Edition : 2021**



**Published by :**
**BHALANI PUBLISHERS and**
**Clever Pen Publishing**
(A joint venture between Bhalani Publishers and National Medical Book House)
D-2 Neelkanth Business Park Co-op. Premises Society Lt.
Nathani Road, Vidyavihar (West), Mumbai - 400 086.
**Mobile** : 09867214519
**E-mail** : bhalanipublishers@gmail.com/cleverpen9@gmail.com

**ISBN** : 978-93-83794-07-2

Printed & Bound in India.

*Dedicated to*

*My Family and My Teacher*
*For their guidance and support*

# Preface

Pharmacology is a rapidly evolving subject with variety of new drugs being researched and introduced. This book is a humble attempt to simplify the subject of Pharmacology for better understanding and creating interest to explore more in the subject. Descriptive textbooks, though good for understanding the subject, are volatile and students find it difficult to compose answers while writing exams.

This book was created to help students write answers systematically and at the same time have a better grip of the topic. The author, editor and contributors have as far as possible taken care to ensure that the information in the book is accurate and up to date.

It is not possible for the book to be entirely free from human errors, some inaccuracies, ambiguities and topographical mistakes. We would welcome feedback and suggestions from teachers and students for further improvement in the book.

# Acknowledgement

I would like to express my deepest gratitude towards our dean **Dr. Azhar Ahmed Siddiqui** for promoting academic excellence in our institute and supporting upcoming researchers and authors like us. I want to express my deepest gratitude to our *Honourable Chairman* **Maulana Ghulam Ahmed Vastanvi, Dr. A. B. Solepure** and *CEO* **Dr. Ilyas Bemat.** I would also like to thank **Dr. Imran Nawaz Khan, Dr. Deepak Bhosle, Dr. Syed Maaz, Dr. Syed Asif, Dr. Zubair Quazi, Dr. Syed Jawwad Hashmi, Dr. Mohammed Shoebuddin, Dr. Aseem Badam** and other colleagues for their support during the process of writing this book. A sincere thanks to **Mr. Rajesh Bhalani** and entire team of **Bhalani Publishers** and **Mrs. Harsha Shah** from **M/s. National Medical Book House** for editing, compiling and designing this book for its timely launch. Last but not the least; I also deeply value and acknowledge the constant love and support of my parents, wife and my children.

**Dr. Huzaif Shaikh**

# Contents



## GENERAL PHARMACOLOGY



## DRUGS ACTING ON AUTONOMIC NERVOUS SYSTEM (ANS)

## DRUGS ACTING ON PERIPHERAL NERVOUS SYSTEM (PNS)



## AUTOCOIDS AND RELATED DRUGS



## DRUGS ACTING ON RESPIRATORY SYSTEM (RS)



## HORMONES AND RELATED DRUGS



## DRUGS ACTING ON CENTRAL NERVOUS SYSTEM

## DRUGS ACTING ON CARDIOVASCULAR SYSTEM



## DRUGS ACTING ON THE KIDNEY



## DRUGS ACTING ON BLOOD AND BLOOD FORMATION



## DRUGS ACTING ON GASTROINTESTINAL TRACT (GIT)



## ANTI-MICROBIAL DRUGS

## CANCER CHEMOTHERAPY



## MISCELLANEOUS TOPICS

# GENERAL PHARMACOLOGY

# 1 IMPORTANT TERMINOLOGIES

**Pharmacology :**

The term is derived from greek word ***'Pharmakon'*** meaning drug and ***'Logos'*** meaning a science. It is a science which deals with the mechanism of action, therapeutic uses, adverse effects and fate of drugs in humans or animals.

**Drug (WHO definition) :**

Any substance or product that is used or intended to be used to modify or explore physiological systems or pathological states for the benefit of the recipient

**Pharmacokinetics :**

It deals with A-D-M-E, *i.e.* absorption, distribution, metabolism and excretion of drugs. In short it deals with what the body does to a drug.

**Pharmacodynamics :**

It deals with the effects of drugs, the site at which the drug acts, the mechanism by which a drug acts and its response and duration in relation to its plasma concentration. In short it deals with what the drug does to a body.

**Clinical pharmacology :**

It is the evaluation of a new drug in healthy volunteers as well as patients. This is also called as clinical trials.

**Pharmacotherapeutics :**

It is the application of pharmacological information along with the knowledge of various diseases for its prevention and cure.

**Chemotherapy :**

It deals with the treatment of various infections and malignancies with drugs.

**Toxicology :**

It deals with the toxicity and poisonous effects of various drugs and substances.

**Pharmacy :**

It is the art and science of compounding and dispensing of a drug to humans or animals.

**Teratogenicity :**

The ability of a drug to cause retardation of growth, congenital malformations or death in a fetus when given in a pregnant mother. *E.g.* ACE inhibitors, phenytoin, alcohol, thalidomide etc.

### Pharmacognosy :

It is the study of sources of drugs from where the drugs are derived.

### Posology :

It deals with the study of dosage of drugs.

### Pharmacogenetics :

It is the study of inherited differences in the drug metabolism or drug response.

### Pharmacogenomics :

It is the use of human genome so as to choose a specific drug therapy that best suits that patient and avoiding giving the drug to non-responders.

### Pharmacoepidemiology :

It is the study of effects of a drug in large population.

### Pharmacovigilance :

It is a science which deals with D-A-U-P, *i.e.* detection, assessment, understanding and prevention of adverse effects of a drug.

## DRUG NOMENCLATURE :

It is science of how the drugs are named.

- ***Chemical name :*** It describes the drug chemically. It is given by IUPAC (International union of pure and applied chemistry).
- ***Generic or non-proprietary name :*** It describes the approved name of the drug to be used worldwide. It is given by USAN (United States approved name council) and BAN (British approved name council). The name given by both the council may differ but the drug is same. *E.g.* epinephrine and adrenaline are the same drug but, given different names by the two councils. Hence, in some countries it is called epinephrine and in others it is called as adrenaline.
- ***Brand name or proprietary name :*** It is the name given to a drug by a pharmaceutical company for marketing and sale. It is copyrighted. It is kept as small and easy to remember or catchy.
- ***Example :***

| | |
|---|---|
| **Chemical name** | Acetylsalicylic acid |
| **Generic name** | Aspirin |
| **Brand name** | Ecosprin |

## SOURCES OF DRUG INFORMATION :

The various sources from where we can get information of drug are :

- **Pharmacopoeias :** Indian / British / U.S.

- **Martindale's extra pharmacopoeia.**
- **Formularies :** National formulary prepared by Indian medical council, British national formulary.
- **MIMS** (Monthly Index of Medical Specialities), **CIMS** (Continuing Index of Medical Specialities), **IDR** (Indian Drug Review). These give information about the brands available in India and their costs etc.
- **Drug bulletins :** WHO drug bulletin.
- **Textbooks :** Standard pharmacology textbooks like Goodman & Gillman.
- **Journals :** British medical journal, Indian journal of pharmacology, Lancet. The data arising from randomized control trials is having highest acceptability.

❑❑❑❑❑

# 2 ROUTES OF DRUG ADMINISTRATION

These are the modes through which drugs are introduced in the body.

## ROUTES OF DRUG ADMINISTRATION :

### LOCAL :

- ***Topical :*** Transdermal patch, conjunctival, vaginal, urethral.
- Intra-articular
- Intra-lesional
- Infiltration
- Inhalation
- Local oral

### SYSTEMIC :

- **Enteral :** oral, sublingual, rectal and buccal.
- **Parenteral :** Intravenous, intramuscular, subcutaneous, intradermal, intra-arterial, intra-osseous, intra-thecal and intra-cardiac.

## LOCAL ROUTES :

This refers to the application of a drug to an area of the body for direct treatment. Usually there is inefficient absorption (1-15%). High local tissue levels nevertheless achievable, often higher than by systemic route. Systemic toxicity is not a problem.

### Topical :

***Transdermal :*** (details in special drug delivery systems chapter)

- The skin is relatively more impermeable to drugs than other stratified epithelia. The skin is useful to administer drugs which are very lipophilic and active in very small amounts. Drug is present in patches which release drug at constant and predictable rate. No peaks or troughs of drug concentration are seen. Site used are-chest, abdomen, upper arm, buttocks. Transdermal drug delivery avoids problems such as gastrointestinal irritation, metabolism, variations in delivery rates and interference due to the presence of food. It is also suitable for unconscious patients. The technique is generally non-invasive and aesthetically acceptable and can be used to provide local delivery over several days.
- ***Advantages :*** Bypasses first pass metabolism. Maintains constant plasma

levels for a longer period, less side effects, easy to discontinue if toxicity appears, no GIT side effects, convenient to use, compliance improves.

- ***Disadvantages :*** Local irritation, erythema, onset of action-slower, cannot achieve high concentration in plasma, cannot deliver drugs in a pulsatile manner, development of tolerance, expensive.
- ***Examples :*** Nicotine patches-help stop smoking, estradiol-prevents menopausal symptoms, fentanyl citrate-prevents severe pain, nitrate patches-for angina.

## Intra-articular :

- To deliver drugs directly in the joints. Causes local action without much systemic side effects. Aseptic precautions should be taken. *E.g.* methyl prednisolone given in knee joint arthritis.

## Intra-lesional :

- To deliver drugs directly in the lesions or swellings. Causes local action without much systemic side effects. *E.g.* methyl prednisolone given in keloid or hypertrophic scar.

## Infiltration :

- Here, the drug is infiltrated around the nerve fibers. *E.g.* local anesthetic lignocaine infiltrated before giving stitches.

## Inhalation :

- Drugs given by inhalational route are mainly used to treat diseases of respiratory system. Action of these drugs is either on bronchial tree or systemic due to absorption through lungs, *e.g.* Salbutamol and Beclomethasone in bronchial asthma. Drugs are delivered to bronchial musculature in asthma. Aerosols are formed as drug solution or microionised drug powder is converted into mist/dust respectively. Particle size which is absorbed in between 3 and 5 mm. If size < 3 mm-particles are not retained, they come out with expiration. If size > 5 mm particles are not absorbed. Preparations used for inhalation route are :

  1. ***Dry powder inhalers.***
  2. ***Metered dose aerosol (MDI) :*** drug is delivered through pressurised canister equipped with a valve through which only metered dose is discharged. Drug is most commonly stored in solution in a pressurised canister. The canister is attached to a plastic, hand operated pump. The standard metered dose inhaler on activating releases a fixed dose of medicine in aerosol form.
  3. ***Nebuliser :*** used in children and patients who cannot inspire forcefully while coordinating with inhaler opening. The air pressure required for aerosol formation is generated by an electric pump.
  4. ***Rotahalers :*** the device is loaded with rotacapsules and then drug is inhaled with forceful inspiration. Only capsules specifically made for

rotahalers are used with rotahalers. Only a small portion of drug (10%) reaches respiratory tract-a small fraction of this amount penetrates mucosa.

- *Advantages :* Systemic effects including toxicity are less, targeted delivery of drug, easy to use, less amount of drug is needed, onset of action is fast
- *Disadvantages :* Reflex bronchospasm, candida growth in oral cavity, patient has to learn the technique.

### Local-oral (Gargles and Mouthwashes) :

- They are aqueous solutions used for throat infections and hygienic purpose.
- *Advantages :* Local soothing and antiseptic action.
- *Disadvantages :* May cause staining and irritation
- *Example :* Saline gargles, Potassium permanganate solution, povidone iodine, betahexidine.

## DOSAGE FORMS USED FOR TOPICAL ROUTES :

### Eye drops :

- They are aqueous or oily solutions for instilling into conjunctival sac. They are used as anesthetics, anti infective or anti inflammatory agents, miotics, mydriatics and artificial tears.
- *Advantages :* Local effect at required place, easy to apply.
- *Disadvantages :* Requires repeated application, systemic effects occur sometimes, may cause irritation, once seal is broken, should be used within 1 month.
- *Example :* Atropine (mydriatic), Pilocarpine (Miotic), Timolol (beta blocker).

### Ear drops :

- They are aqueous or oily solutions instilled in the ear.
- *Advantages :* Avoid systemic side effect due to its local action.
- *Disadvantages :* Local irritation can occur.
- *Example :* Wax softeners, Sodium bicarbonate, Ciprofloxacin, Lignocaine.

### Eye ointment :

- They are semisolid preparations with a greasy base, to be applied in the eye.
- *Advantages :* They have longer duration of action, better for use in non-cooperative patients and children.
- *Disadvantages :* Due to greasy base eyes may become sticky.
- *Example :* Neomycin eye ointment, Chloramphenicol eye ointment, tetracycline eye ointment

### Nasal drops :

- They are aqueous solutions of drugs instilled into the nose with a dropper.
- *Advantages :* Local and quick action.

- ***Disadvantages :*** Absorption can occur producing systemic effect, local irritation.
- ***Example :*** Xylometazoline, Oxymetazoline, Ephedrine, Normal saline etc.

### Nasal sprays :

- These are drugs or combinations of drugs which by virtue of their high vapour pressure, can be carried by an air current into nasal passage and exert their effect
- ***Advantages :*** Easy to use, it covers large surface area so quick absorption.
- ***Disadvantages :*** Explosion may occur sometimes as the contents are under pressure.
- ***Example :*** Calcitonin, Vasopressin, Oxymetazoline, Azelastine etc.

### Suppositories :

- They are solid, uniformly medicated masses of medicaments.
- ***Advantages :*** Local application for systemic as well as local effect, especially helpful for unconscious or in a patient who cannot take orally, and children.
- ***Disadvantages :*** Inconvenient and sometimes irritant, aesthetic concerns/ embarrassing, local irritation.
- ***Example :*** Glycerin, Bisacodyl, Diclofenac.

### Vaginal Pessaries :

- It is the term applied to suppository shaped medications for vaginal administration. This is a topical treatment and it is important that the drug coats all the vaginal mucosa. Vaginal medications whether in pessaries or cream come with applicators which are designed to reach the upper parts of the vaginal canal. Vaginal preparations which are left in situ are best used at night because the vagina has no means of retention like sphincters and the medication can run out
- ***Advantages :*** Local application, avoid systemic effect
- ***Disadvantages :*** It may cause staining and irritation.
- ***Example :*** Nystatin, Clotrimazole.

### Ointments :

- These are lipid based. They have a greasy appearance and feel. The drug is trapped under the dressing and, the layer of the skin is softened from sweating, enabling the drug to penetrate deeply into the tissues.

### Pastes :

- They have very high powder content. They are useful in protecting areas of skin from moisture, being water repellent

### Gel and Lotions :

- They are used on the hairy areas of the body. Alcoholic gels or lotion are less messy than ointments or creams, but the evaporation of carrier is rapid, therefore, there is little penetration of the drug.

**Jellies :**

- Usually for topical, urethral, rectal application.
- ***Example :*** lignocaine jelly.

**Dusting Powder :**

- They are free flowing very fine powders having particle size < 150 mm for external use. They are used to treat superficial skin conditions. They are sterilised by dry heat and supplied in airtight glass or plastic jars with reclosable perforated lid or sprinkler holes at top.
- ***Advantages :*** Systemic side effects of drugs are avoided because of local application; it provides greater stability.
- ***Disadvantages :*** It requires repeated applications.
- ***Example :*** Clotrimazole, Neomycin powder, Sulfacetamide powder.

**Lotions :**

- They are liquid preparations meant for local application to the skin or mucous membrane without rubbing for providing soothing or antiseptic effects. These medications are preferably supplied in amber or blue coloured bottles to protect them from sunlight.
- ***Advantages :*** Systemic side effects of drugs are avoided due to local use.
- ***Disadvantages :*** Patient may experience a gritty feeling
- ***Example :*** Potassium permanganate lotion (0.1%), Cetrimide lotion (1%), Calamine lotion, Clotrimazole lotion.

**Liniments :**

- They are liquid or semiliquid preparations intended for external application by rubbing and may contain substances possessing analgesic, rubefacient, soothing or stimulating properties. They may be either emulsions or solutions.
- ***Advantages :*** Systemic side effects of drugs are avoided because of local application.
- ***Disadvantages :*** Patient may experience a burning sensation.
- ***Example :*** Turpentine liniment

**Creams :**

- They are semi solid preparations consisting of opaque emulsions for external use. Creams are used in treatment of skin conditions like eczema, pruritus as astringent, emollient, and antiseptics. They are dispensed in collapsible metal or plastic tubes, glass or plastic pots.
- ***Advantages :*** They are cosmetically more acceptable due to their less greasy nature.

- *Disadvantages :* **They are easily washed out so requires repetitive applications.**
- *Example :* **Diclofenac cream, Clobetasol cream, Neomycin cream.**

### Sprays :

- They are preparations of drugs in aqueous or alcohol containing media.
- *Advantages :* Easy to use and cover a larger surface area.
- *Disadvantages :* Explosion may occur sometimes as the contents are under pressure.
- *Example :* lignocaine spray, diclofenac spray, calcitonin nasal spray.

### Paints :

- They are simple solutions containing medicaments in semisolid solvents.
- *Advantages :* Retain the medicament in situ for longer period.
- *Disadvantages :* May cause staining and irritation
- *Example :* lignocaine mouth paint, povidone iodine paint, clotrimazole paint

## SYSTEMIC ROUTES :

### Enteral route :

#### *Oral :*

- The drug is given through mouth. It is the commonest and most favorite method of drug administration.
- ***Includes :*** Tablets, capsules, powders, spansules, syrups, mixtures, elixirs, emulsions etc.
- ***Advantages :*** Easy, convenient and cheap, non-invasive, painless and no assistance is required, no need to take aseptic precautions, both, solid and liquid dosage forms can be given.
- ***Disadvantages :*** Action is slow so it is not suitable for emergency, unpalatable drugs are difficult to administer, patients having nausea and vomiting, drugs cannot be given by this route, it may cause gastrointestinal adverse effects, it cannot be used for non cooperative and unconscious patients, certain drugs which are not present in ionised form are not absorbed if given by this route, certain drugs are destroyed by gastric juices or extensively metabolized during first pass in the liver.
- ***Example :*** paracetamol tablet, diclofenac tablet, cefixime syrup. etc.

#### *Sublingual :*

- The drug is kept below the tongue.
- ***Advantages :*** Immediate action hence can be used in emergency; action can be terminated by spitting the remaining drug, bypasses hepatic first pass metabolism.
- ***Disadvantages :*** Drug taste must be pleasant, irritant drugs cannot be given, can produce irritation in mouth.
- ***Example :*** Glyceryl trinitrate, nifedipine etc.

### *Rectal :*

- Drug is administered in the rectum via anus
- ***Advantages :*** Can be used in unconscious patient, vomiting patient, patient with swallowing problems, in case of a difficulty to find the vein for intravenous injection, in uncooperative children and for unpleasant drugs.
- ***Disadvantages :*** Anal or rectal irritation, inconvenient, aesthetic considerations, absorption is erratic, irregular and unpredictable, they are made to melt at body temperature, so needs to be kept refrigerated.
- ***Example :*** diclofenac, Bisacodyl, Sulfasalazine.

### *Buccal :*

- This is the route of administration by which drugs held or applied in the buccal area (in the cheek) diffuse through the oral mucosa and enter directly into the bloodstream. Buccal administration may provide better bioavailability of some drugs and more rapid onset of action compared to oral administration because the medication avoids first pass metabolism.
- ***Example :*** Buprenorphine, Naloxone, Glyceryl trinitrate etc.

## Parenteral Route :

Any method of drug administration that avoids the gastrointestinal tract is termed parenteral administration. Parenteral is derived from combination of 2 words : Par = beyond and Enteral = intestinal.

### *Intravenous (IV) :*

- An intravenous route means the drug is directly given into the bloodstream via superficial veins. This is one of the most commonly used route in hospitalised patients.
- ***Advantages :*** 100% bioavailability, immediate onset of action; so it can be used in emergencies, titration of dose can be done as per need, first pass metabolism bypassed, GIT adverse effects not present, can be used in unconscious, uncooperative and vomiting patients, bitter and non-palatable drugs can be given.
- ***Disadvantages :*** Aseptic precautions are mandatory, needs assistance and expertise, thrombophlebitis can occur if extravasation of drug happens during injection, expensive, invasive, painful and chances of air embolism.
- ***Example :*** Aminophylline, IV fluids, hydrocortisone etc.

### *Intramuscular (IM) :*

- Drug is injected in one of the large skeletal muscles of the body, *i.e.* deltoid, gluteus maximus and in infants in anterolateral region of the thigh in middle third region.
- ***Advantages :*** Rate of absorption is reasonably uniform, onset of action-fairly rapid, depot preparations can be given, in addition to soluble substances, mild irritants, suspensions and colloids can be injected by this route.

- ***Disadvantages :*** Aseptic precautions are mandatory, painful, danger of injecting directly into blood vessels, intramuscular absorption is not always faster than oral absorption, the volume of injection should not be more than 10 ml, pain at the site of injection, irritation, abscess formation or tissue and nerve damage may occur.
- ***Example :*** Diclofenac, tetanus toxoid, DPT etc.
- ***Note :*** Always aspirate the syringe before injecting the drug, and if blood comes in the aspiration the syringe should be withdrawn without giving the drug. This signifies that needle was in blood vessel.

### *Subcutaneous (SC) :*

- A subcutaneous injection is administered into the subcutaneous space of skin. Hyaluronidase can increase absorption, which breaks down intracellular matrix. A person with type I diabetes mellitus typically injects insulin subcutaneously. Places on the body where people can inject insulin most easily are : the outer area of the upper arm, around the umbilicus over the abdominal wall, except the area right around the navel (a 2-inch circle), the upper area of the buttock, just behind the hip bone, the front of the thigh, midway to the outer side, 4 inches below the top of the thigh to 4 inches above the knee.
- The maximum amount of medication that can be subcutaneously injected is about 2 ml.
- It can be injected with the help of insulin syringe / tuberculin syringe.
- Now, a newer pen devices needle which are of 31 gauge and are silicon coated and produces very less pain.
- ***Advantages :*** Self-administration possible, drugs in oil or implants can be given, action of the drug is sustained and uniform, less painful than IM or IV.
- ***Disadvantages :*** Onset of action is slow and prolonged action, only non-irritant substances can be injected by this route, aseptic precautions need to be taken.
- Subcutaneous drug implants can act as depot therapy, *e.g.* Medroxyprogesterone.
- ***Example :*** Insulin, heparin.

### *Intradermal :*

- Drug or substance is injected into the dermis using a fine needle. The absorption is very slow and only small quantities of the drug can be given by this route. This route is used for specific purpose only. Intradermal—the volume to be administered is 0.1 ml or less.
- ***Example :*** BCG vaccine, PPD (Mantoux test).

### *Intra-osseous :*

Here, the drug is given inside a bone, especially long bone.

***Example :*** IV fluids in neonates can be given intraosseously in tibia bone.

***Intra-thecal :***

Drugs are directly injected into the thecal sac. These drugs are given to get drugs directly into the central nervous system by avoiding the blood brain barrier commonly used for spinal anesthesia and chemotherapy.

***Example :*** opioid, Methotrexate.

***Epidural :***

Is just like intrathecal but the drug is deposited above the dura and not in the cerebrospinal fluid. Local anesthetics are often given this way during surgical procedures, especially for procedures involving the pelvis and lower extremities.

***Example :*** Lignocaine, bupivacaine.

***Intra-cardiac :***

Here, the drug is given directly in the heart.

***Example :*** Adrenaline given intra-cardiac in cardiac arrest.

# 3 SPECIAL DRUG DELIVERY SYSTEM

They are also called as targeted drug delivery systems.

**Sustained /Controlled release Tablets :**

- These formulations reduce the dosing frequency.
- They are helpful in chronic cases where patient has to take drugs for long periods.
- ***Example :*** Controlled release tablet of diclofenac.

**Implants :**

- A drug bearing device which is compatible with body is inserted or implanted either subcutaneously or in any part of the body.
- Advantage is that they deliver the drug directly to the target site in significant doses and bypass the first pass.
- ***Example :*** Norplant.

**Ocular inserts :**

- Ocular inserts are defined as sterile, thin, multilayered, drug-impregnated, solid or semisolid consistency devices placed into the conjunctival sac and whose size and shape is especially designed for delivery of drugs directly in the eye.
- ***Drugs given by ocular inserts :*** Pilocarpine, Timolol, Gentamicin, steroids.
- ***Advantages :*** Sustained release of drug over a long period, no need of frequent instillation, better compliance, accurate dosing, and no interference with vision.
- ***Disadvantages :*** Costly, foreign body sensation, difficulty of placing and removal.

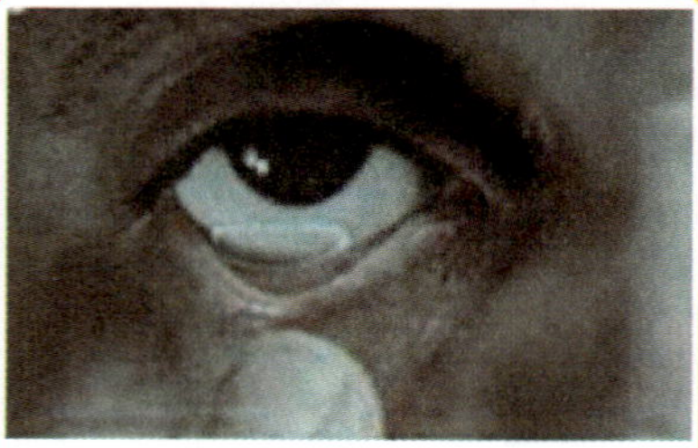

**Fig. 3.1 :** Ocular Insert

**Liposome mediated drug delivery :**

- Liposomes are a novel drug delivery system (NDDS), they are vesicular structures consisting of bilayers which form spontaneously when phospholipids are dispersed in water.
- NDDS aims to deliver the drug at a rate directly at the place of action and also reduce unwanted adverse effects.
- ***Example :*** liposomal amphotericin (antifungal drug).

### Insulin pen devices :

- Insulin pen is used to inject insulin for the treatment of diabetes mellitus.Turn the knob on the end of the pen to dial and reverse - dial the dose by selecting the number of units required by the patient.
- *Types :* Permanent or durable device with cartridges and prefilled disposable flex pens.
- *Advantages :*
  - Convenient and easier to carry than traditional vial and syringe.
  - Easy to use for blind and old patients as it is having click sound at each unit dialing.
  - More accurate dosages.
  - Less pain of injection as silicon coated needles with 31 gauge are used.
  - The body of pen acts as an insulator and maintains the temperature of insulin inside it for long period.

### Insulin pumps :

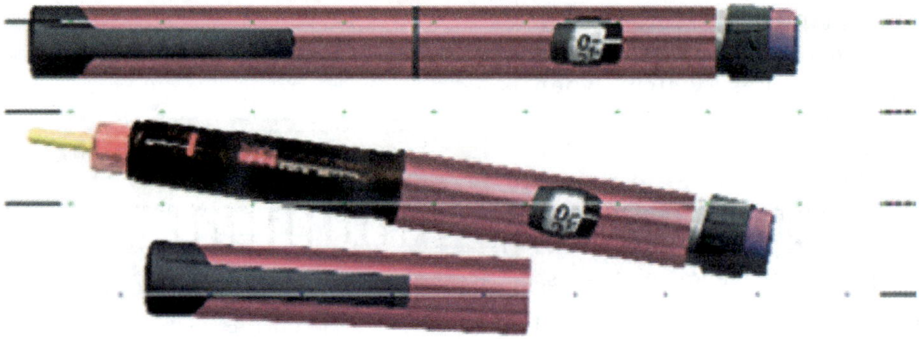

Fig. 3.2 : Insulin Pen Devices

- It is a medical device used for the administration of insulin to patients in the management of diabetes mellitus.
- It is also known as continuous subcutaneous insulin infusion therapy.
- *Components :* The pump which is battery operated, a disposable reservoir for insulin, a disposable infusion set, including a cannula for subcutaneous placement and a tubing system to connect the insulin reservoir to the cannula.

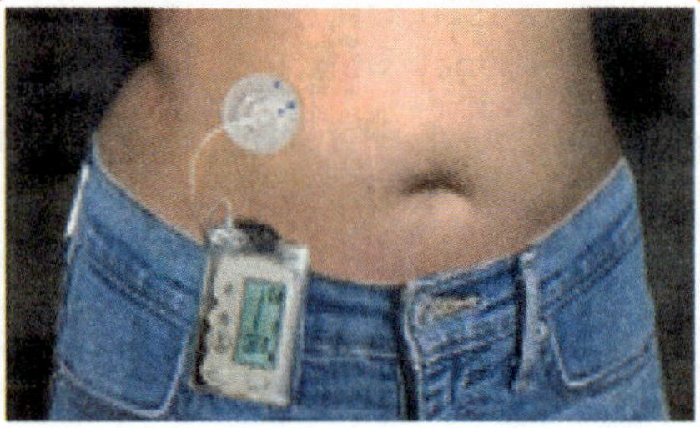

Fig. 3.3 : Insulin Pumps

- *Advantages :* Freedom from daily needle pricks, significant improvement in $HBA_{1c}$, more precise dose, continuous control of blood sugar, since the insulin pump uses only rapid acting insulin, you will not need to follow a strict schedule for eating, activity, and insulin injections.

- ***Disadvantages :*** Costly, continuous wearing of pump all the time may be uncomfortable for some patients; pump can get damaged during vigorous physical activities, scar tissue buildup around the inserted cannula, allergic reactions from the adhesive on the back of an infusion set.

**Nanoparticles :**

- Use of nanoparticles for drug delivery is gaining momentum.
- The advantages are : small doses required, target specific delivery of drugs and prevention of unwanted systemic adverse effects.
- The disadvantages are : still in nascent stages, costly, requires technical skills and acceptability can be an issue on part of patient.
- ***Example :*** Nanoparticle based doxorubicin (anti-cancer drug).

**Transdermal drug delivery system (TDDS) :**

- Transdermal Drug Delivery System is defined as self contained, discrete dosage forms which are also known as patches which when applied to the intact skin, deliver the drug through the skin at a controlled rate to the systemic circulation. It consists of both transdermal patches as well as ointments.

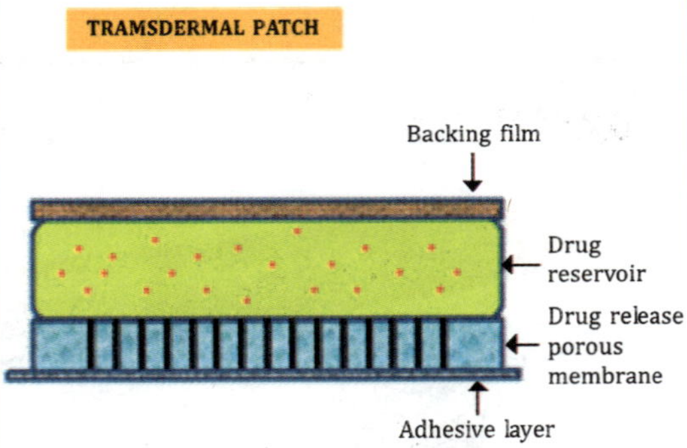


Fig. 3.4 : Tramsdermal Patch

- ***Site :*** Adhesive patch containing drug is applied to chest, upper abdomen or behind the ear.

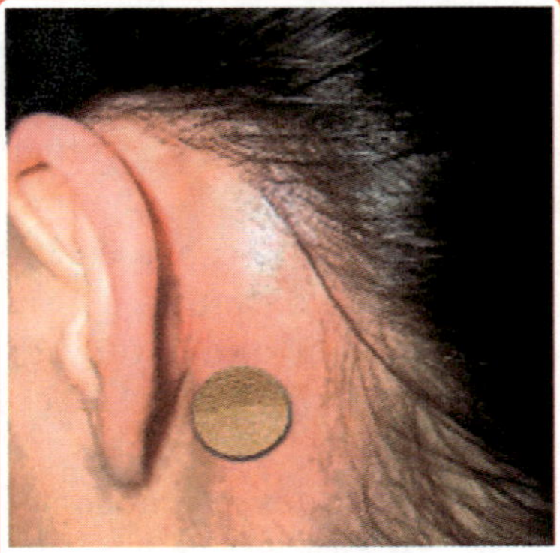

Fig. 3.5 : Adhesive Patch

- ***Advantages :*** Slow but sustained release of drug for several days and also bypasses first pass metabolism.
- ***Disadvantages :*** Local irritation at the site of application cannot be used in emergency situation.
- ***Examples :*** Hyoscine or scopolamine patch (for motion sickness), Nitroglycerin ointment (for angina pectoris), nicotine patch (for smoking cessation) and fentanyl patch (opioid analgesic).

# 4 SOURCES OF DRUGS

## DRUGS DERIVED FROM PLANT SOURCES :

| Drug | Plant |
|---|---|
| Atropine | *Atropa belladonna* |
| Quinine | *Cinchona bark* |
| Digitalis | *Digitalis lanata* |
| Morphine | *Papaver somniferum* |
| Castor oil | *Ricinus communis* |
| Pilocarpine | *Pilocarpus microphyllus* |

### Drugs derived from animal sources :

BCG vaccine, Insulin, thyroxine, anti-tetanus serum, cholera and anti-rabies vaccine.

### Drugs derived from microbial sources :

Penicillin (*penicillium notatum*) and griseofulvin (*penicillium griseofulvum*).

### Drugs derived from mineral sources :

Magnesium sulfate, ferrous sulfate, aluminium hydroxide and calcium carbonate.

### Drugs derived from recombinant technology :

Insulin, Hepatitis-B vaccine and Erythropoietin.

### Drugs derived from human sources :

Immunoglobulins, growth hormones and human chorionic gonadotropin.

### Drugs that are synthetically made in pharmaceutical company :

Paracetamol, Aspirin and fluoroquinolones.

# 5 PRESCRIPTION WRITING

"A prescription is defined as a written order given by a doctor to a pharmacist for preparing and dispensing a medicine". The word prescription has been derived from two Latin words, 'pre' meaning before and 'scriber' meaning to write.

### PARTS OF PRESCRIPTION :

- **Superscription :** This contains name and address of doctor, place of dispensing, date of prescription writing, name, age, sex and address of the patient, the prescription symbol (Rx) - an abbreviation for recipe, the latin word for 'take thou'.
- **Inscription :** This is the body of the prescription containing the names of medicinal substances, the medicinal forms, their dosage, frequency and duration of administration. Abbreviation and chemical formulae should be avoided since it leads to errors. The first letter of all the official names should be in capitals. It is always recommended to use generic drug names than brand names. In complex prescriptions containing several ingredients the order should be as follows: non-pharmacological measures, injections, capsule, tablet, liquids and topical preparations.
- **Subscription :** This contains directions to the pharmacist regarding the dosage form to be prepared and number of doses to be dispensed.
- **Transcription :** This consists of directions to the patients regarding the quantity of medicament or number or dosage units to be taken, the time and frequency of administration and the manner in which it is to be administered or applied and signature and registration number of the physician.

### COMMON ABBREVIATIONS

| Abbreviation | Full Latin Form | English Meaning |
|---|---|---|
| od | Omni die | Once a day |
| Bid | bis in die | twice a day |
| tid | ter in die | three times a day |
| qid | quater in die | four times a day |
| hs | hora somni | at bedtime |
| Stat | statim | immediately |
| Sos | si opus sit | if there is a need |
| po | per os | by mouth or orally |

| Abbreviation | Full Latin Form | English Meaning |
|---|---|---|
| IV | | intravenous |
| IM | | intramuscular |
| SC | | subcutaneous |
| ID | | intradermal |
| IP | | intraperitoneal |
| Inj | Injection | injection |
| Cap | capsula | capsule |
| Tab | tabella | tablet |
| Syr | syrupus | syrup |
| Susp | | suspension |
| Supp | suppositorium | suppository |
| Nebul | nebula | A spray / nebulisation |
| Tbsp | | Tablespoon |
| Tsp | | Teaspoon |
| mg | | Milligram |
| g | | gram |
| mcg | | microgram |
| ml | | mililiter |
| ac | ante cibum | before meals |
| pc | post cibum | after meals |
| Bol | Bolus | as a large single dose (usually intravenously) |
| dil | | dilute |
| ad lib | ad libitum | use as much as one desires |
| gtt | gutta | drop |
| sol | | solution |
| dist | | distilled |
| NPO | Nil per os | Nothing by mouth |
| lin | linimentum | liniment |
| lot | | lotion |
| NS | | Normal saline (0.9%) |
| ½ NS | | Half Normal saline (0.45%) |
| DNS | | Dextrose normal saline |
| RL | | Ringer lactate |

□□□□□

# 6 PHARMACOKINETICS

Pharmacokinetics deals with **A-D-M-E.**, *i.e.* absorption, distribution, metabolism and excretion of drugs. In short it deals with what the body does to a drug.

## TRANSPORTATION OF DRUGS :

To reach their sites of action, drugs must cross biological barriers. There are various methods by which the drugs are transported across the biological barriers or membrane :-

### Filtration :

- Free or unbound drugs of smaller molecular sizes can pass through pores or spaces between the cells.
- ***E.g.*** **:** alcohol, glucose.

### Passive diffusion :

- It is the passage of drugs across the biological membranes from higher concentration to lower concentration side (along the concentration gradient).
- The drugs that are highly lipid soluble (non-ionised drugs) can diffuse rapidly by passive diffusion.
- The drugs that are partly ionised, the diffusion would depend upon the degree of ionisation of drug and the pH of surrounding environment.
- Weakly acidic drugs like aspirin and barbiturates are non-ionised in acidic media and thus are better absorbed from places like stomach, whereas weakly basic drugs like morphine and diazepam remained non-ionised at alkaline pH and thus are better absorbed from intestine.
- Strongly acidic or strongly basic drugs remain ionised at all pH and therefore are poorly absorbed.

### Facilitated diffusion :

- It is the passage of drugs across the biological membranes from higher concentration to lower concentration side (along the concentration gradient), but requires a carrier.
- The drug forms a complex with a carrier of the biological membrane and this complex is carried through membrane, the drug is released, and the carrier molecule returns to the membrane surface.
- Does not require energy.
- It is a capacity limited process, *i.e.* the rate of diffusion depends upon the availability of carrier.

### Active transport (uphill transport) :

- It is the energy dependent, carrier mediated passage of drugs across the biological membranes from lower concentration to higher concentration side (*i.e.* against the concentration gradient and against the electrical gradient).
- The energy needed is provided by the membrane ATPase.
- It is also a capacity limited process, *i.e.* the rate of transport of drugs depends upon the availability of carrier.

### Endocytosis (pinocytosis) :

- Some water insoluble substances are engulfed by the cell membrane and are released into the cytoplasm.
- First there is formation of invaginations on the cell membrane surface which engulfs the drug, and then these invaginations are converted to a vesicle which is then pinched off from membrane.
- ***E.g. :*** Uptake of fats, starch, vitamins A, D, E, K.

## ABSORPTION :

- Absorption is the transfer of a drug from its site of administration to the systemic circulation.
- Most of the drugs are absorbed by the way of passive transport.
- Intravenous administration has no absorption.

### Factors affecting absorption of drugs are :

- Drug properties : lipid solubility, molecular weight, and polarity etc.
- Blood flow to the absorption site.
- Total surface area available for absorption.
- Contact time at the absorption surface.
- Affinity with special tissue.
- pH of the surrounding environment.
- Gastrointestinal motility and presence of food.
- Disease conditions.
- Route of drug administration.

## BIOAVAILABILITY :

Bioavailability is a measure of the fraction (F) of administered dose of a drug that reaches the systemic circulation in the unchanged form. It refers to the rate and extent of absorption of a drug from dosage form.

- For I.V. route, the bioavailability = 100%
- For oral route, the bioavailability < 100%
- For other routes, the bioavailability < 100%
- For oral route, the bioavailability is less because, the drug may be incompletely absorbed and the drug may undergo first pass metabolism in intestinal wall and/or liver or excreted in bile.

## Measurement of bioavailability :

When we compare bioavailability of two drugs, we plot a graph of plasma concentration of drug against time. We compare three characteristics from the graph :

- ***Cmax*** (Peak plasma concentration),
- ***Tmax*** (Time taken to attain peak plasma concentration) and
- ***AUC*** (The area under the curve).

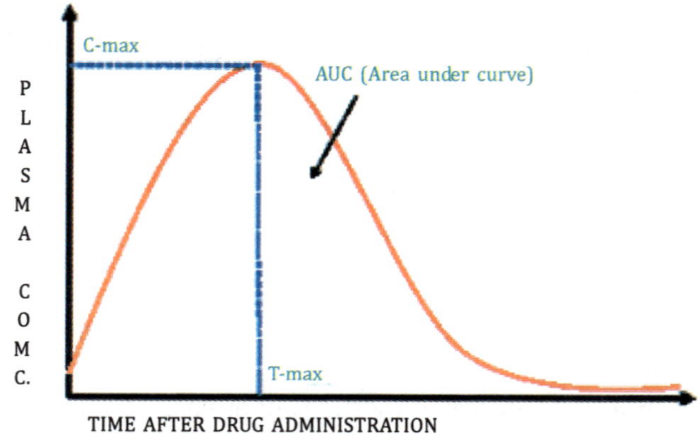


☞ The first 2 parameters are indicators of rate of absorption and the third parameter *i.e.* the AUC reflects the extent of absorption. In an ideal scenario, the Cmax, Tmax and AUC of two bioequivalent drugs should be nearly same.

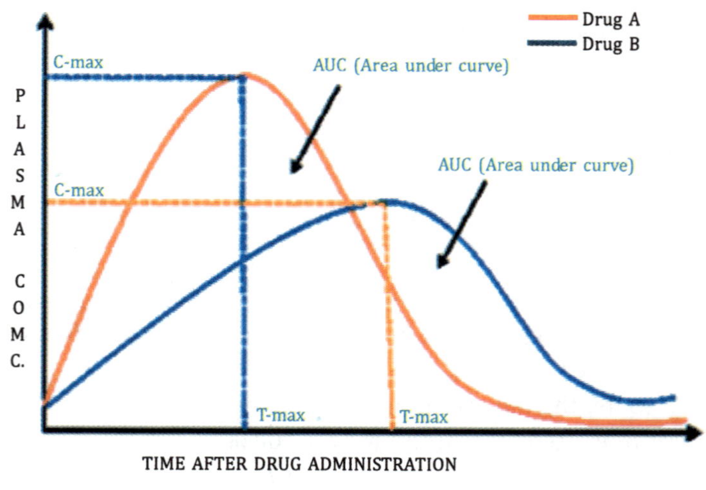


When we compare bioavailability of two drugs (drug A and drug B), as seen in the diagram, the bioavailability of drug A is more than the bioavailability of drug B. Bioavailability is measured by given formula :

$$\text{Bioavailability (F)} = \frac{\text{AUC (oral)}}{\text{AUC (IV)}} \times 100$$

### Factors affecting bioavailability :

#### *Pharmacological factors :*

- ***First pass effect :*** first pass metabolism of drugs decreases the bioavailability of orally administered drugs and also reduces plasma concentration. Therefore, certain drugs like isosorbide dinitrate are given sublingually to avoid first pass effect.
- ***Gastric emptying and motility :*** factors that increase gastric emptying allow the drugs to reach the large absorptive surface area of small intestine sooner, and increase the bioavailability.
- ***GIT diseases :*** certain gastrointestinal diseases affect the absorption and bioavailability of the drugs.
- ***Presence of food :*** generally, absorption is favored by empty stomach *e.g.* rifampicin. But, absorption of certain drugs is hampered by food *e.g.* reduced absorption of tetracyclines by milk.
- ***Route :*** bioavailability is maximum by I.V route because the drugs are directly introduced in the systemic circulation and also bypasses the first pass metabolism.
- ***Blood supply :*** the more the blood supply to the part from where the drug is absorbed, the more will be the absorption and the more will be the bioavailability.
- ***Genetic factors :*** some patients metabolise drugs very quickly and some metabolise slowly due to genetic variations. This may have variable bioavailability.

#### *Pharmaceutical factors :*

- ***Particle size :*** less the particle size, more is the bioavailability. Bioavailability of certain oral formulations may be in the following order : solution > suspension > capsule > tablet > coated tablet
- ***Degree of ionisation :*** non-ionised lipid soluble drugs are better absorbed whereas strongly acidic or basic drugs or highly ionised drugs are having lower bioavailability.
- ***Salt form :*** Salt forms of drugs are having more bioavailability. *E.g.* sodium valproate.
- ***Various excipients :*** excipients and adjuvants are the substances that are added along with the drug to the formulation for stabilisation, bulking or preservation of drug. Variable characteristics of these substances can also alter bioavailability.

### DISTRIBUTION :

- It is the passage of drug from the circulation to the tissue and site of its action.

- The extent of distribution of drug depends on its lipid solubility, ionisation at physiological pH, extent of binding to plasma and tissue proteins, differences in regional blood flow and various diseases like CCF, uremia, liver diseases.

**Volume of distribution / apparent Volume of distribution (aVd) :**

- Apparent Volume of distribution is defined as the volume that would accommodate all the drugs in the body, if the concentration was the same as in plasma.
- It is expressed in liters.

$$\text{aVd} = \frac{\text{Total amount of drug in the body (mg / kg)}}{\text{Concentration of drug in plasma (mg / L)}}$$

- For example, if total amount of drug in the body is 100 mg/kg and concentration of drug in plasma is 5 mgL, then the aVd would be (100/5) *i.e.* 20 Litres.
- ***Factors affecting aVd are :***
  - Lipid solubility of a drug.
  - pKa value of the drug.
  - Affinity for different tissues.
  - Blood supply.
  - Disease status.
  - *Plasma protein Binding :* drugs highly bound to plasma proteins have a low aVd and drugs that are less bound to plasma proteins are having high aVd.

**Redistribution :**

- Redistribution is observed in highly lipid soluble drugs. These drugs on administration are rapidly distributed to highly perfused organs like brain, liver and kidneys due to higher lipid solubility. These drugs are then redistributed to muscle, lean tissues and fat, as a result their actions gets terminated.
- ***E.g.* :** Thiopentone (ultra-short acting barbiturate) induced anesthesia.

**Plasma Protein Binding :**

- Drugs usually bind to plasma and tissue proteins in a reversible manner. The binding is always in equilibrium.

**Free drug + protein ⟺ Free drug + Protein complex**

- Acidic drugs bind to plasma albumin and basic drugs to $\alpha_1$-glycoprotein.
- ***Clinical significance of protein binding of drugs :***
  - Extent of binding depends on the individual compound. Increasing concentration of drug can progressively saturate the binding sites.
  - The protein bound drug is not available for action, metabolism and excretion.

- Extensive protein binding results in prolongation of duration of action.
- Highly protein bound drugs remain largely in vascular compartment and have a low aVd.
- Highly protein bound drugs are not easy to removed by dialysis in situations of toxicities or overdose.
- Binding of a particular drug is a capacity limited process *i.e.* it depends upon the concentration of proteins. In disease status where the plasma proteins are less, there will be higher concentration of free drug in the body.
- One dug can bind to many sites on the protein and conversely, more than one drug can bind to the same site.
- Displacement reaction : more than one drug can bind to the same site of the protein. This will result in displacement of the drug already bound to the protein by other drug. This can have significant clinical implications. *E.g.* aspirin (NSAIDs / Antiplatelet drug) can displace tolbutamide (oral antidiabetic drug) and can lead to increased free tolbutamide in the body resulting in hypoglycemia.

### What's new ?

- ***Plasma protein binding prediction softwares :***
  - Quantum plasma protein binding.
  - $S^+$ plasma protein binding.
  - Albumin binding prediction.

## METABOLISM (BIOTRANSFORMATION) :

- Biotransformation is the chemical alteration of the drug in the body so as to convert non-polar lipid soluble compounds to polar lipid insoluble compounds so that they are not reabsorbed back from the renal tubules and are excreted.
- Certain drugs are there which are excreted unchanged *e.g.* streptomycin.
- There are 3 fates of biotransformation :
  1. ***Formation of inactive metabolite from active drug :*** *E.g.* drugs like paracetamol, phenobarbitone.
  2. ***Formation of active metabolite from inactive (prodrug) drug :*** *E.g.* levodopa converted to dopamine.
  3. ***Formation of active metabolite from active drug :*** *E.g.* codeine converted to morphine.

### First pass metabolism :

- All the drugs taken orally go through the GIT. From here, they go into the intestinal wall and then through portal system before reaching the systemic circulation. First pass metabolism means that the drug undergoes metabolism in liver and intestinal wall before reaching systemic circulation. The result of this first pass effect is reduced bioavailability.
- This first pass effect may be bypassed if the drugs are given by sublingual

route (*E.g.* sublingual isosorbide dinitrate for angina pectoris) or if the drugs are given parenterally (I.V. administration of hydrocortisone).

## Process of Biotransformation :

- Biotransformation of drugs is carried out mainly in liver and also in intestine.
- The enzymes involved in biotransformation are of two types : Microsomal enzymes and non-microsomal enzymes.
- ***Microsomal enzymes :*** These are located on smooth endoplasmic reticulum, mainly in liver but also in kidneys, intestines and lungs. They are mono-oxygenases, cytrochrome P450, glucuronyl transferase. They carry out most of the oxidation, reduction, hydrolysis and glucuronide conjugation reactions.
- ***Non-microsomal enzymes :*** These are present in cytoplasm and mitochondria of liver cells and other tissues. They are oxidases, esterases, amidases and conjugates. They carry out some oxidations and reductions and all conjugation reactions except glucuronide conjugation.

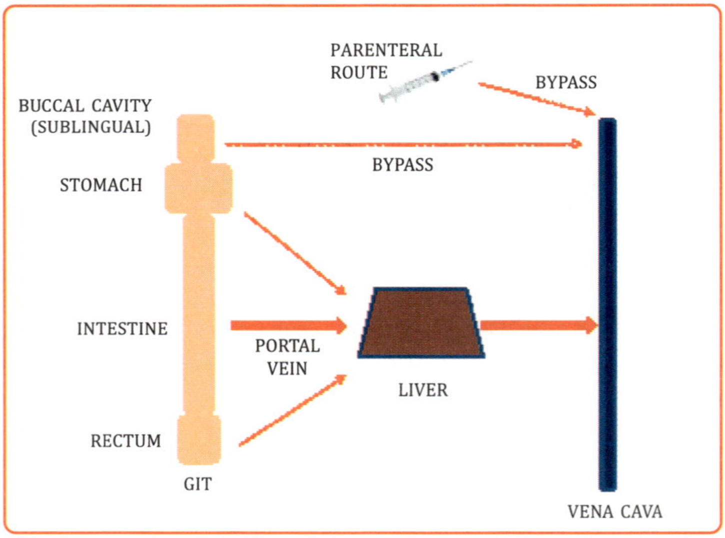


## Phases of Biotransformation :

- Biotransformation of drugs is carried out in 2 phases : Phase I and phase II.

| PHASE I (Non-synthetic reactions) | PHASE II (Synthetic reactions) |
|---|---|
| Oxidation | Glucuronide conjugation |
| Reduction | Acetylation |
| Hydrolysis | Methylation |
| Cyclisation | Sulfate conjugation |
| Decyclisation | Glycine conjugation |
| | Glutathione conjugation |
| | Ribonucleoside & ribonucleotide synthesis |

### *Phase I (Non-synthetic reactions) :*

Metabolite may be active or inactive.

#### *Oxidation :*

- One of the most important drug metabolising reactions in which there is addition of oxygen or removal of hydrogen.
- Oxidations are mainly carried out by mono-oxygenases, which later on also involves cytochrome P450, NADPH and oxygen.
- There are many types of cytochrome P450 like CYP3A4, CYP3A5, CYP3D6, CYP2C9, CYP2C19 etc. majority of the biotransformation reactions are carried out by CYP3A4 group of cytochrome P450 enzyme.
- ***E.g. :*** Barbiturates, paracetamol and corticosteroids.

#### *Reduction :*

- This reaction is opposite of oxidation and involves CYP 450 enzymes working in the opposite direction *i.e.* there is addition of hydrogen or removal of oxygen.
- ***E.g. :*** Chloramphenicol, Halothane and Warfarin.

#### *Hydrolysis :*

- Metabolism of drug molecule by taking up of water.
- Hydrolysis occurs in liver, intestines, plasma and other tissues.
- ***E.g. :*** Lidocaine, oxytocin and pethidine.

#### *Cyclisation :*

- Biotransformation of a drug by formation of ring in structure is called cyclisation.
- ***E.g. :*** Proguanil.

#### *Decyclisation :*

- Decyclisation is biotransformation of a drug by opening up of ring structure.
- ***E.g. :*** Phenytoin sodium.

### *Phase II (Synthetic reactions) :*

These involve biotransformation of a drug or its Phase I metabolite to form a lipid insoluble metabolite which is not reabsorbed back from kidneys and are easily excreted. They are also called as conjugation reactions.

| Reactions | Enzyme | Examples |
|---|---|---|
| Glucuronide conjugation | Glucuronyl transferase | Aspirin, morphine |
| Acetylation | N-acetyl transferase | Isoniazid, sulfonamides |
| Methylation | Transmethylase | Histamine, adrenaline |
| Sulfate conjugation | Sulfotransferase | Androgens, corticosteroids |
| Glycine conjugation | Glycine transferase | |

| Reactions | Enzyme | Examples |
|---|---|---|
| Glutathione conjugation | Glutathione transferase | Paracetamol |
| Ribonucleoside and ribonucleotide synthesis | — | Anti-cancer drugs |

**Factors affecting biotransformation :**

- Concurrent use of drugs : Induction and inhibition.
- Genetic polymorphism or variability.
- Pollutant exposure from environment or industry.
- Disease conditions.
- Age.
- Nutrition and diet.
- Race and species.

**Genetic variations in metabolism of drugs :**

- Not all people in the world have same metabolising capacity for the drugs. This has got significant clinical implications. *E.g.* Isoniazid which is an anti-tubercular drug is metabolized by the process of acetylation. Certain people in the world like American whites, Israelis and Scandinavians are *Slow Acetylators*. This leads to slow metabolism of isoniazid and increases its bioavailability and thus can cause isoniazid induced neuropathy. Certain people in the world like Eskimos, Japanese and Chinese are *Fast Acetylators*. This leads to fast metabolism of isoniazid and increased formation of metabolism end products in liver leading to hepatotoxicity.

**HOFMANN ELIMINATION (NON-ENZYMATIC BIOTRANSFORMATION) :**

- Certain drugs like skeletal muscle relaxant named ***Atracurium*** are metabolised in the blood spontaneously by molecular rearrangement without the action of any anzyme. This is called as Hofmann elimination.

**Enzyme induction :**

- If one drug stimulates or increases metabolism of other drug by inducing a drug metabolising enzyme, it is called as enzyme induction.
- ***Enzyme inducers :***

  **G – Griseofulvin**
  **P – Phenytoin, Phenobarbitone**
  **R – Rifampicin**
  **S – Smoking**

  **A – Alcohol**
  **C – Carbamazepine**

- ***Clinical implications :***
  - Enzyme induction can result in decreased therapeutic effect or increased activity if the metabolite of the drug is the active principle and tolerance.
  - Unwanted pregnancy can result in females using oral contraceptive pills who are prescribed enzyme inducer like rifampicin at the same time. Rifampicin induces metabolism of oral contraceptives and this can result in therapeutic failure and pregnancy.
  - Tolerance can be seen if the drug induces its own metabolism. *E.g.* carbamazepine.
  - The knowledge of enzyme induction can also be used for benefit of patients. In cases of jaundice of newborn baby, phenobarbitone can be given, which induces metabolism of bilirubin.
  - Enzyme inducers like phenytoin induces metabolism of vitamin D and can lead to vitamin D deficiency and osteomalacia.

**Enzyme inhibition :**

- A drug can inhibit metabolism of other drug which results in increased level of other drug in the body and can cause prolongation or increased effect.

- ***Enzyme inhibitors :***

  **V – Valproate**
  **I – Isoniazid**
  **C – Cimetidine**
  **E – Erythromycin**
  **K – Ketoconazole**

- ***Clinical implications :***
  - Erythromycin, if given along with theophylline will increase levels of theophylline in body due to enzyme inhibition. This leads to adverse effects of nausea and tremors.
  - Precipitation of cardiac arrhythmias with terfinadine when given along with enzyme inhibitor ketoconazole.
  - Increased bleeding tendency with Warfarin when given with cimetidine.
  - ***Beneficial effect :*** increased availability of levodopa in CNS when given with enzyme inhibitor like carbidopa.

**EXCRETION :**

Excretion of drugs out of the body occurs by various routes.

**Major Routes of Excretion :**

- Renal Excretion.
- Biliary Excretion.

### Minor Routes of Excretion :

- Pulmonary excretion.
- Salivary excretion.
- Mammary excretion via milk.
- Skin /Dermal excretion via sweat.
- Tears.

### Major Routes of Excretion :

- ***Renal excretion :***

  The principal methods involved in the urinary excretion of drugs are :

  - Glomerular filtration.
  - Passive tubular reabsorption.
  - Active tubular secretion.

  **Glomerular filtration :**

  - Depends upon the renal blood flow.
  - Normal GFR is 125 ml/min.
  - Glomerular filtration occurs to low molecular weight drugs. Only free drugs *i.e.* which are not bound to plasma proteins are filtered.

  **Passive tubular reabsorption :**

  - Occurs in distal convoluted tubules & collecting ducts.
  - It's the passive diffusion of unionised, lipophilic drugs.
  - Lipophilic drugs can be reabsorbed back into systemic circulation and excretion in urine will be low.
  - Ionised drugs are poorly reabsorbed & so urinary excretion will be high.

  **Active tubular secretion :**

  - It occurs mainly in proximal tubules which lead to active secretion of drugs in the lumen.
  - Anionic and cationic transporters mediate active secretion of anionic and cationic drugs.
  - Can transport drugs against concentration gradients.
  - Penicillin is an example of actively secreted drug.
  - Transport of drugs like penicillin is blocked by probenecid as they compete for tubular secretion in the PCT.

  Changing pH of urine by chemicals can inhibit or enhance the drug reabsorption from renal tubules back into the systemic circulation. Ion trapping is used to enhance renal clearance of drugs during toxicity. Urine is normally slightly acidic and favors excretion of basic drugs. Acidification of urine increases excretion of basic drugs such as morphine, quinine. Alkalinisation of urine increases excretion of acidic drugs as aspirin.

- ***Biliary Excretion :***
  - Occurs to few drugs that are excreted into feces.
  - Such drugs are secreted from the liver into bile and then into the duodenum.
  - **Enterohepatic circulation :** Drugs excreted in the bile in the form of glucuronides are hydrolysed in intestine by normal bacterial flora, liberating free drug. This free drug can be reabsorbed back into blood if the drugs are lipid soluble. This is enterohepatic recycling of drugs. This prolongs the duration of action of drugs *e.g.* digoxin, morphine, thyroxine.

**Minor Routes of Excretion :**

- ***Pulmonary excretion :***
  - Gases and other volatile drugs such as general anesthetic agents that enter the body primarily through the respiratory tract are excreted by this route.
  - No specialised transport systems are involved in this method, simple diffusion across cell membranes is predominant.
  - The rate of loss of gases is not constant; it depends on the rate of respiration and pulmonary blood flow.
  - The degree of solubility of a gas in blood also will affect the rate of gas loss.
  - Gases such as nitrous oxide, which are less soluble in blood, will be excreted rapidly, almost at the rate at which the blood delivers the drug to the lungs.
  - Ethanol, which has relatively high blood gas solubility, is excreted very slowly by the lungs.

- ***Salivary excretion :***
  - The pH of saliva varies from 5.8 to 8.4. Unionised lipid soluble drugs are excreted passively.
  - The bitter taste in the mouth of a patient is indication of drug excreted.
  - Some basic drugs inhibit saliva secretion and are responsible for mouth dryness.
  - Compounds excreted in saliva are Caffeine, Phenytoin, Acyclovir, Theophylline.

- ***Excretion through breast milk :***
  - pH of milk varies from 6.4 to 7.6. Free unionised and lipid soluble drugs diffuse passively.
  - Highly plasma bound drug are less secreted in milk.
  - Excretion of drug in milk is important as it gains entry in breast feeding infants and may result in adverse effects in babies.

- ***Excretion through sweat :***
  - Drugs excreted through skin via sweat follows pH partition hypothesis. Excretion of drugs through skin may lead to urticaria and dermatitis.
  - Compounds like benzoic acid, salicylic acid, alcohol and heavy metals like lead, mercury and arsenic are excreted in sweat.

## KINETICS OF DRUG ELIMINATION :

### Plasma half life of a drug :

- Is the time required for the plasma concentration of a drug to fall to 50 % of its initial concentration. It is a measure of duration of action. It also determines the dosing interval of a drug.
- Factors affecting plasma half life of a drug :
  - Decreased metabolism, as seen in liver diseases and use of microsomal enzyme inhibitors.
  - Decreased clearance, as seen in renal diseases and congestive heart failure.
  - High plasma and tissue protein binding of drugs.
  - Enterohepatic recycling of drugs.

### First order kinetics :

Majority of the drugs follow $1^{st}$ order kinetics. The characteristics of $1^{st}$ order kinetics are :

- A constant fraction of drug is eliminated at a constant interval of time.
- The elimination of drug is directly proportional to the plasma concentration.
- The plasma half life remains constant irrespective of the dose.
- After a single dose, 97% of the drug gets eliminated after 5 half lives.

### Zero order kinetics :

Hardly a few drugs follow zero order kinetic (*e.g.* ethyl alcohol). The characteristics of zero order kinetics are :

- A constant quantity of drug is eliminated per unit time.
- The elimination of drug is constant irrespective of the plasma concentration.
- The plasma half life of a drug is never constant.

### Mixed order kinetics (Michaelis-Menten kinetics) :

1. It is a dose dependent kinetics where smaller doses are handled by first order kinetics, but as the plasma concentration reaches higher levels, they follow zero order kinetics. The reason is because the drug metabolising enzymes or the elimination process gets saturated at higher concentration.
2. The plasma half lives changes with the dose. Hence, the drugs that follow mixed order kinetics require constant monitoring.
3. ***E.g. :*** phenytoin, digoxin, warfarin, tolbutamide.

### Steady state plasma concentration :

- A state at which the therapeutic plasma concentration of the drug remains constant.

### *Loading Dose :*

It is the large initial dose that is given to achieve rapid therapeutic plasma level after administration of the drug, the plasma concentration decreases due to distribution of drug to other tissues. These doses balance the drug distribution. This is important for drugs with long half lives.

### *Maintenance Dose :*

This is the dose required to maintain the therapeutic level of the drug constant or the steady state of the drug. These doses balance the amount of drug lost during metabolism and clearance.

## METHODS OF PROLONGATION OF DRUG ACTION :

In certain conditions we need to give drugs for longer durations, such as in chronic diseases. Hence, the frequent dosing can be quite inconvenience to the patients. This can reduce the patient compliance. This can also lead to variable concentration of the drugs in plasma. These problems can be overcome by prolonging the action of the drugs.

### Advantages of prolonging drug action :

- Reduced frequency of drug administration.
- Improved convenience for patients.
- Improved compliance by patients to treatment.
- Reduced fluctuations in plasma concentration of drugs.
- Can have overnight action of drug without disturbing sleep.

The various methods by which prolongation of drug action can be done are :

### By prolonging absorption :

1. ***Oral :***

   **Methods :**

   - ☞ Controlled release tablets / capsules.
   - ☞ Sustained release tablets / capsules.
   - ☞ Coating the drug with resins or other material.
   - ☞ Spansules.

2. ***Parenteral :***

   **Methods :**

   - ☞ Oily injection preparations.
   - ☞ Depot injections (*E.g.* progesterone depot injection).
   - ☞ Injections in insoluble form (*E.g.* lente insulin).
   - ☞ Combine drug with protein (*E.g.* insulin + protamine).
   - ☞ Use of pellets.

- Use of biodegradable implants with drugs.
- Use of a vasoconstrictor (*E.g.* adrenaline along with lignocaine).

3. ***Transdermal :***

**Methods :**

- Ointments (*E.g.* nitroglycerine ointment).
- Transdermal patch (*E.g.* Hyoscine patch, nicotine patch).
- Transdermal strips.

4. ***Other routes :***

**Methods :**

- Ocuserts in the eye (*E.g.* Pilocarpine ocusert)

***By increasing plasma protein binding of a drug :***

- Nowadays, drug preparations are made which makes the drug highly bound to plasma protein. It is then slowly released in free form for the action over the period of time. *E.g.* sulfonamides.

***By slowing the metabolism of a drug :***

**Methods :**

- A drug can inhibit metabolism of other drug which results in increased level of other drug in the body and can cause prolongation or increased effect (enzyme inhibition). An example is of increased accessibility of L-dopa in brain when given along with carbidopa (peripheral decarboxylase inhibitor).
- Adding a functional group to a drug : *e.g.* adding ethinyl functional group to estradiol can make estradiol to act longer.

***By slowing the excretion of a drug :***

**Methods :**

- A uricosuric drug named probenecid inhibits excretion of penicillins (*e.g.* ampicillin). This prolongs action of ampicillin.

## CALCULATION OF DRUG DOSES :

There are many formulae to calculate drug dosages in patients.

### Young's formula :

This is the formula based on age, weight and BSA (body surface area). It is used to calculate drug dose in children upto the age of 12 years.

$$\text{Child's dose} = \frac{\text{Age in years} \times \text{Adult dose}}{\text{Age} + 12}$$

### Clark's formula :

Dose calculation using Clark's formula is done by considering body weight as parameter.

$$\text{Individual dose} = \frac{\text{Body weight (Kg)} \times \text{Average adult dose}}{70}$$

**Formula based on BSA (body surface area) :**

$$\text{Individual dose} = \frac{\text{BSA (m}^2\text{)} \times \text{Adult Dose}}{1.8}$$

**Drug dosage calculation in renal diseases :**

- Firstly, we have to calculate creatinine clearance (in ml/min) by **cockroft gault formula** as given below :

  $$\text{Creatinine clearance} = \frac{\text{(140-age in years)} \times \text{(weight in kg)}}{72 \times \text{serum creatinine level}}$$

  [Note : For females, we have to multiply the value by 0.85]

- Now, the dose to be given in a renal patient is calculated as :

  $$\text{Corrected dose} = \frac{\text{Normal dose} \times \text{Patient's creatinine clearance}}{\text{Normal creatinine clearance}}$$

□□□□□

# 7 PHARMACODYNAMIC

Pharmacodynamics is the study of drug effects *i.e.* what a drug does to the body. It starts with describing what the drugs do, and goes on to explain how they do it.

## PRINCIPLES OF DRUG ACTION :

The basic types of drug action can be broadly classed as :

- **Stimulation :** It is selective enhancement of the level of activity of specialised cells or tissues. *E.g.* Adrenaline stimulates heart.
- **Depression :** It is selective diminution of activity of specialised cells or tissues. *E.g.* Pantoprazole depresses gastric acid secretion.
- **Irritation :** A nonselective and noxious effect which is particularly applied to less specialised cells like the epithelial cells. Strong irritation results in inflammation, corrosion, necrosis and morphological damage.
- **Replacement :** It is the use of natural metabolites or hormones in deficiency states. *E.g.* Levodopa in Parkinson's, Insulin in diabetes mellitus.
- **Cytotoxic action :** It is selective cytotoxic action on microbes or cancer cells without significantly affecting the host cells. *E.g.* antibiotics and anticancer drugs.

## DRUG-RECEPTOR INTERACTION :

- **Affinity :** is a measure of the tightness with which a drug binds to the receptor.
- **Intrinsic activity (IA) :** is a measure of the ability of an agonist that is bound to the receptor to generate an activating stimulus and produces a change in cellular activity.
- **Agonist :** An agent which activates a receptor to produce an effect similar to that of the physiological signal molecule. Agonists have both affinity and intrinsic activity (IA = 1). *E.g.* acetylcholine on cholinergic receptors.
- **Inverse agonist :** An agent which activates a receptor to produce an effect opposite to that of the agonist. Inverse agonists have affinity but intrinsic activity ranges between zero and minus one (IA between 0 and –1). *E.g.* β-carbolines are inverse agonist of benzodiazepine receptors.
- **Antagonist :** An agent which prevents the action of an agonist on a receptor or the subsequent response, but does not have any effect of its own. Antagonists have affinity but no intrinsic activity (IA = 0). *E.g.* atropine blocks the cholinergic muscaranic receptors.

- **Partial agonist :** An agent which activates a receptor to produce submaximal effect but antagonises the action of a full agonist. Partial agonists have affinity and low intrinsic activity (IA between 0 and 1). *E.g.* pentazocine is partial agonist at m receptors of the opioid receptor category.

## MECHANISM OF DRUG ACTION :

- Majority of drugs produce their effects by interacting with a specific target molecule, which usually is a protein. Such mechanism confers selectivity of action to the drug.
- Functional proteins that are targets of drug action can be grouped into four major categories :
  1. Enzymes
  2. Ion channels
  3. Transporters
  4. Receptors

### 1. Enzymes :

- Almost all biological reactions are carried out under catalytic influence of enzymes;
- Drugs can either increase or decrease the rate of enzymatically mediated reactions.

**Enzyme inhibition :**

- Selective inhibition of a particular enzyme is a common mode of drug action.
- Such inhibition is either competitive or noncompetitive.
- ***E.g. :***

| Enzyme | Substrate | Competitive inhibitor |
|---|---|---|
| Dopa decarboxylase | Levodopa | Carbidopa |

### 2. Ion Channels :

- Ligand gated channels (*E.g.* nicotinic receptor).
- G-proteins and are termed G-protein regulated channels (*E.g.* cardiac $\beta_1$ adrenergic receptor activated $Ca^{+2}$ channel).
- Drugs can also act on voltage operated and stretch sensitive channels by directly binding to the channel and affecting ion movement through it, *e.g.* local anesthetics which obstruct voltage sensitive $Na^+$ channels.
- Certain drugs modulate opening and closing of the channels, *e.g.* Calcium channel blocker like nifedipine blocks L-type of voltage sensitive $Ca^{+2}$ channel.
- Ethosuximide which is an anti-epileptic drug inhibits T-type of $Ca^{+2}$ channels in thalamic neurons.

### 3. Transporters :

- Various substrates are translocated across membranes by binding to specific transporters or carriers which either facilitate diffusion in the direction of the concentration gradient or against the concentration gradient using ATP.

### 4. Receptors :

- They are the binding site located on the surface or inside the effector or target cell that serves to recognize the signal molecule or the drug and initiate the response.

***GPCR (G-protein coupled receptor) :***

- These are membrane bound receptors coupled to the effector system through G-proteins like GDP (Guanosine diphosphate) or GTP (Guanosine triphosphate).
- The effector systems are : Adenylyl cyclase-cAMP and Phospholipase-C-inositol phosphate.
- The G-proteins have 3 subunits – $\alpha$, $\beta$ and $\gamma$.
- There are 3 main varieties of Ga protein subtypes – Gs, Gi and Gq.
  - Gs (stimulatory) : Adenylyl cyclase activation, $Ca^{+2}$ channel opening.
  - Gi (Inhibitory) : Adenylyl cyclase inhibition, $K^{+}$ channel opening.
  - Gq : Phospholipase C activation.
- ***E.g.*** muscaranic cholinergic receptors, adrenoreceptors.

***Ion channel receptor (Ionotropic receptor) :***

- These cell surface receptors, also called ligand gated ion channels, enclose ion selective channels (for $Na^{+}$, $K^{+}$, $Ca^{+2}$ or $Cl^{-}$) within their molecules.
- Agonist binding opens the channel and causes depolarization or hyper polarisation or changes in cytosolic ionic composition, depending on the ion that flows through.
- ***E.g.*** nicotinic cholinergic receptor, $GABA_A$ receptor.

***Kinase linked receptors :***

- Made up of a large extracellular ligand binding domain connected through a single transmembrane helical peptide chain to an intracellular subunit having enzymatic property.
- ***E.g.*** Insulin receptors, growth factor receptors.

***Intracellular receptor (Cytosolic receptors) :***

- These are intracellular (cytoplasmic or nuclear) soluble proteins which respond to lipid soluble chemical messengers that penetrate the cell.

- The liganded receptor diamer moves to the nucleus and binds other co-activator/co-repressor proteins which have a modulatory influence on its capacity to alter gene function.
- All steroidal hormones (glucocorticoids, mineralocorticoids, androgens, estrogens), thyroxine, vit D and vit A function in this manner.

***Down-regulation and Up-regulation of receptors :***

- Prolong exposure to high concentration of agonist or an endogenous neurotransmitter cause reduction in number of receptors available for activation. This is called as Down-regulation of receptors. This results due to endocytosis or internalisation of the receptors from cell surface. ***E.g.*** down-regulation of $\beta_2$ receptors is responsible for reduced effect in asthma patients to $\beta_2$ agonist like salbutamol after prolong use.
- In contrast, if there is prolong occupation of a receptor by an antagonist or blocker, it leads to increase number of receptors. This is called as Up-regulation of receptors. This results due to exocytosis or externalisation of the receptors from cell surface. ***E.g.*** there is up-regulation of $\beta_1$ receptors in thyrotoxicosis which increases cardiac sensitivity to catecholamines leading to tachycardia.

**Drug potency and efficacy :**

- ***Potency :*** is the concentration of a drug required to produce a given physiologic effect.
- ***Efficacy :*** is the maximal level of response a drug can produce.

The potency and efficacy of drugs can be detected by plotting log dose-response (LDR) curve. The closer the LDR curve towards y axis, the greater is the potency. Efficacy of a drug is denoted by the height of LDR curve of a drug. More the height, more is the efficacy.

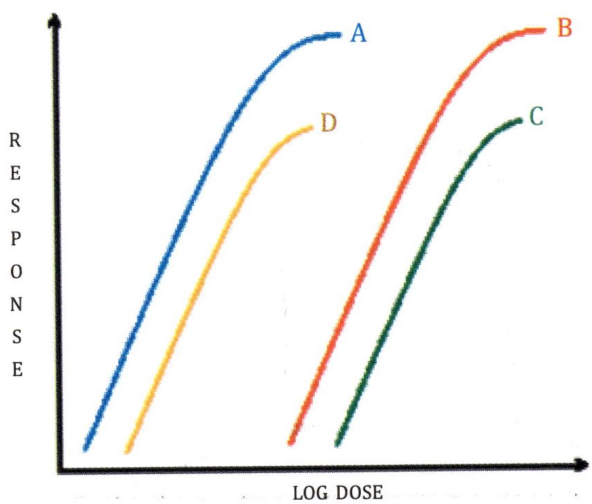

- Drug B is less potent but equally efficacious as drug A.
- Drug C is less potent and less efficacious than drug A.
- Drug D is more potent than drugs B & C, less potent than drug A but less efficacious than drugs A & B, and equally efficacious as drug C.

## THERAPEUTIC INDEX (margin of safety) :

It is measured by the following formula :

$$\textbf{Therapeutic indiex} = \frac{LD_{50}}{ED_{50}}$$

Where, Median effective dose ($ED_{50}$) is the dose which produces the specified effect in 50% individuals and median lethal dose ($LD_{50}$) is the dose which kills 50% of the recipients. For a safe drug, the therapeutic index should be more than 1.

### Therapeutic window :

It is the window of optimum therapeutic range of plasma concentration of drugs at which most of the patients experience the desired therapeutic effects. Below this range, it leads to therapeutic failure and above this range; it leads to toxicity of drugs. This is significant for the drugs whose safety margin is low (*e.g.* digoxin, lithium, phenytoin) and the drugs should be maintained in the therapeutic range. This is done by constantly monitoring the plasma levels of these drugs. This is called as TDM (Therapeutic Drug Monitoring). TDM can be done by various methods like HPLC (High performance liquid chromatography).

### Certain safety factor :

Drug safety can also be assessed by determining the certain safety factor. It is calculated by the following formula :

$$\textbf{Certain safety factor} = \frac{LD_{1}}{ED_{99}}$$

Where, $ED_{99}$ is the dose effective in 99% of subjects and $LD_1$ is the dose which is lethal to 1% of the subjects.

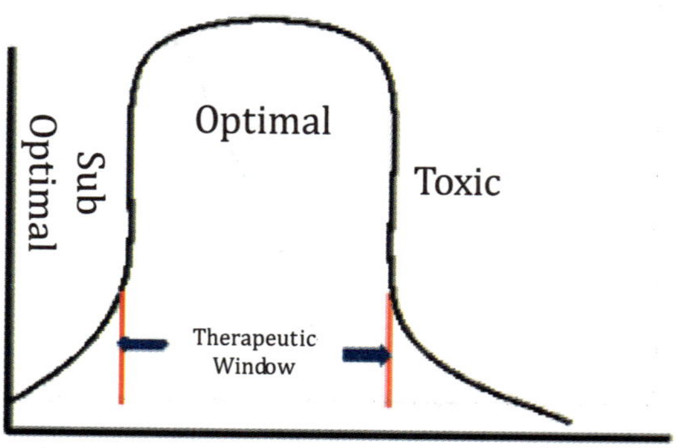

## TOLERANCE :

Increased amount of drug required to produce pharmacological response.

- Usually seen with alcohol, morphine, barbiturates, CNS active drugs
- **Reverse tolerance :** Same amount of drug produces increased pharmacological response.

### Types of tolerances :

***Innate tolerance :***

- Genetically lack of sensitivity to a drug.
- ***E.g. :*** Rabbits tolerate to atropine in large doses

***Acquired tolerance :***

- Occurs due to repeated use of drug.
- ***Types :*** Pharmacokinetic tolerances, Pharmacodynamic tolerance and acute tolerance (Tachyphylaxis).
- ***Pharmacokinetic tolerances :*** Repetitive administration causes decrease in their absorption or increases its own metabolism. ***E.g.*** : Chronic alcoholics tolerate large amount of alcohol because their thickened gastric mucosa decreases absorption of alcohol.
- ***Pharmacodynamic tolerance :*** Due to down regulation of receptors. ***E.g.*** : Morphine, caffeine, nicotine.
- ***Acute tolerance (Tachyphylaxis) :*** Acute development of tolerance after a rapid and repeated administration of a drug in shorter intervals. ***E.g.*** : Ephedrine, tyramine.

**Tachyphylaxis**

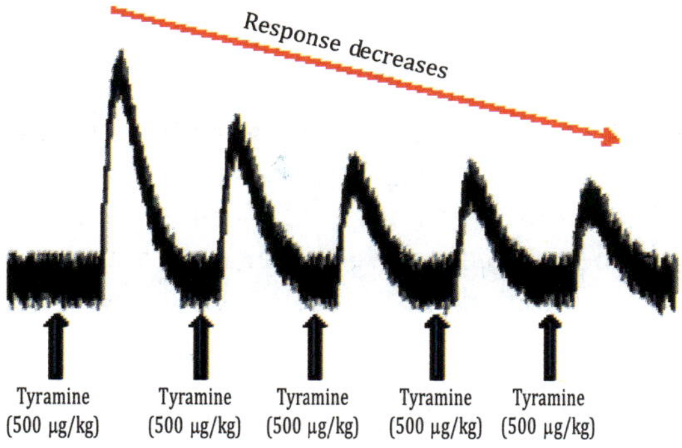


***Cross tolerance :***

- Cross tolerance among drugs belonging to same category. ***E.g.*** Morphine-Heroin.

## AGONISM :

Activation of a receptor to produce a physiological effect. Types of agonism :-

- **Summation :** Two drugs eliciting same response, but with different mechanism and their combined effect is equal to their summation. (1+1=2). ***E.g.*** aspirin (NSAIDs) and Codeine (opioid).
- **Additive :** Combined effect of two drugs acting by same mechanism. ***E.g.*** aspirin (NSAIDs) and paracetamol (NSAIDs).
- **Synergism (Supra additive) :** The combined effect of two drug effect is higher than either individual effect. (1+1=3). ***E.g.*** Sulfamethoxazole + Trimethoprim, Levodopa + Carbidopa.

## ANTAGONISM :

Effect of two drugs is less than sum of the effects of the individual drugs. Types of antagonism :

- **Chemical antagonism :** They are chemical antidotes to each other. ***E.g.*** heparin-protamine sulfate, chelating agents-heavy metals.
- **Physiological antagonism :** they have opposite effects on the same physiological system. ***E.g.*** adrenaline-histamine.
- **Pharmacokinetic antagonism :** One drug affects the absorption, metabolism or excretion of other drug and reduces their effect. ***E.g.*** Warfarin in presence of phenobarbitone, warfarin metabolism is increased, its effect is reduced.
- **Pharmacodynamic antagonism :** Pharmacodynamic antagonism between two drugs acting at same receptors. It is of 2 types :
  - Competitive (Reversible)
  - Non competitive (Irreversible)

  - ***Competitive antagonism (Reversible antagonism) :*** This inhibition is commonly observed with antagonists that bind reversibly to the same receptor site as that of an agonist. This type of inhibition can be overcome increasing the concentration of agonist. ***E.g.*** Atropine is a competitive antagonist of Ach.

  - ***Non competitive antagonism (Irreversible antagonism) :*** It occurs when the antagonist dissociates very slowly or not at all from the receptors result that no change when the agonist applied. Antagonist effect cannot be overcome even after increasing the concentration of agonist.

## DRUG INTERACTIONS :

All effective drugs have the potential for producing both benefits and risks associated with desired and undesired effects. Patients often receive several drugs at the same time. Some diseases, such as diabetes mellitus, coronary artery disease, cancer and AIDS, demand the need for polypharmacy, which works better than any one of the drugs alone. In other cases, the patient is suffering from several conditions, each of which is being treated with one or more drugs by different speciality of doctors. Drug interaction is defined as "Modification of response of body to one drug by another drug when they are administered simultaneously or in quick successions".

Drug interactions are categorised as :

1) Interactions inside the body (In-vivo interactions)
   - Pharmacokinetic Interactions
   - Pharmacodynamic Interactions
2) Interactions outside the body (In vitro interactions)

### 1) In-vivo interactions :

***Pharmacokinetic interactions :*** are those which alter/ modify the pharmacokinetics of a drug when administered simultaneously or in quick successions with another drug. Pharmacokinetics include absorption, distribution, metabolism, excretion of drug. Interaction may take place at any stage of pharmacokinetics.

- **Absorption interaction :** ***E.g.*** milk decreases the absorption of tetracyclines by forming chelates.
- **Distribution interactions :** ***E.g.*** Salicylate displaces tolbutamide and Warfarin from the protein binding sites leading to hypoglycemia and hemorrhage.
- **Metabolism interactions :** ***E.g.*** enzyme induction (rifampicin-oral contraceptives) and enzyme inhibition (metronidazole-alcohol).
- **Excretion interactions** : ***E.g.*** acidification of urine increases excretion of basic drugs like morphine and alkalisation of urine increases excretion of acidic drugs like salicylates.

***Pharmacodynamic interactions :*** are those which alter/ modify the pharmacodynamics of a drug when administered simultaneously or in quick successions with another drug without changing its concentration. This may lead to additive effect to response to a drug known as **Synergism**. These interactions are beneficial to patient as they reduce the therapeutic dose required but should be monitored. ***E.g.*** when Ampicillin is given with Probenecid, it inhibits tubular secretion of Ampicillin and hence prolong its antibiotic action. Or the interaction may result in reducing the therapeutic response of one drug known as **Antagonism.** These interactions are harmful and should be avoided. ***E.g.*** when Tetracyclines are given with Cephalosporins, bactericidal action of Cephalosporins may be antagonised by bacteriostatic action of Tetracyclines, so we should avoid concurrent use.

### 2) In vitro interactions :

These are Drug interactions taking place outside the human body *i.e.* before administration. Certain drugs react with each other when their solutions are mixed which lead to inactivation of one or both the drugs and there occur no or low therapeutic response. ***E.g.*** penicillin and gentamicin mixed in same syringe.

# 8 ADVERSE DRUG REACTIONS

## ADVERSE DRUG REACTION :

A response to a drug which is noxious and unintended, and which occurs at doses normally used in man for the prophylaxis, diagnosis or therapy of disease, or for the modifications of physiological function.

### Adverse event :

Any untoward medical occurrence that may present during treatment with medicine but which does not necessarily have relationship with treatment.

## CLASSIFICATION OF ADVERSE DRUG REACTIONS :

### Predictable reaction (Type A or Augmented) :

- These are mainly based on pharmacological properties of the drug.
- These are common, expected, reversible, dose related and preventable.
- High incidence and low mortality.
- Dose reduction is needed.
- These include :
    1. ***Side effects :*** Unavoidable, unwanted pharmacodynamics effect that occur at therapeutic doses. ***E.g.*** Atropine which is used as preanesthetic medication for its antisecretory action produces dryness of mouth.
    2. ***Secondary effects :*** These are indirect consequence of primary action of drug. ***E.g.*** Tetracycline suppresses bacterial flora.
    3. ***Toxicity :*** Overdose or prolong use of drug results in toxic effect. ***E.g.*** Streptomycin causes vestibular damage.

### Non Predictable reaction (Type B or Bizarre) :

- Mainly include allergy and idiosyncrasy.
- They are less common, non-dose related, serious.
- Sometimes requires withdrawal of drug.
- Low incidence and high mortality.
- Immunological or genetic basis for reactions.
- These include :
    1. ***Drug allergy :*** It is immunologically mediated reaction producing stereotype symptoms which are unrelated to pharmacodynamics profile of drug. This is also called as drug hypersensitivity. Different types of allergic reactions are :

- **Type I or immediate hypersensitivity** occurs within minutes. The drug causes formation of IgE antibodies which attaches to mast cells. On re-exposure to the same drug, it causes degranulation of mast cells leading to release of histamine which is chemical mediator of allergy. ***E.g.*** anaphylactic shock.
- **Type II or cytotoxic reaction** occurs within 72 hours of drug administration. Drug binds to RBC which is recognised by IgG antibody. The antigen-antibody reaction causes lysis of RBC. ***E.g.*** quinidine induced hemolysis.
- **Type III reaction or serum sickness** occurs within 1-2 weeks of drug administration. It is immune complex mediated reaction. ***E.g.*** Glomerular nephritis following NSAIDs use.
- **Type IV or delayed hypersensitivity reaction** : It usually occurs late. It is a T cell mediated reaction. ***E.g.*** contact dermatitis.

2. ***Genetically determined reactions :*** Different individual respond to drugs in different ways. This is due to genetic variations amongst them. *E.g.* Primaquine induced hemolysis if given in G6PD deficient patients.
3. ***Idiosyncratic reactions :*** Genetically determined abnormal reactivity to a drug. It is not found in majority cases. Produces uncharacteristic reaction. Type of reaction is restricted to individuals with particular genome. *E.g.* halothane induced malignant hyperthermia.

### Type C : Chronic use :

- On continuous or chronic use.
- ***E.g.*** Immunosuppression on prolong steroid use leading to fungal infection.

### Type D : Delayed :

- Delayed type reaction. ***E.g.*** carcinogenicity, mutagenicity.

### Type E : End of treatment :

- Due to abrupt withdrawal. ***E.g.*** flaring up of arthritis after abrupt withdrawal of steroids.

### Type F : Failure :

- Failure of therapy. ***E.g.*** failure of vaccines, contraceptives.

### DEPENDING UPON SEVERITY ADR are graded into :

| Severity | Description | Examples |
|---|---|---|
| **Mild** | • No antidote needed<br>• No treatment needed<br>• No hospitalisation needed | Drowsiness caused by Anti-histaminics |
| **Moderate** | • Requires change in treatment<br>• Requires prolong hospitalisation<br>• Requires specific treatment | NSAIDs induced edema & hypertension. |

| Severity | Description | Examples |
|---|---|---|
| **Severe** | • Potentially life threatening<br>• Have to discontinue the drug<br>• Requires specific treatment for ADR | ACE inhibitors induced angio-oedema. |
| **Lethal** | • May directly or indirectly contribute to patient's death | Acetaminophen overdose induced liver failure. |

## PHOTOSENSITIVITY :

It is cutaneous reaction resulting from drug induced sensitisation of skin to UV radiation.

**Two types** of reactions are there :

1. **Phototoxic reaction :** Drug or its metabolite accumulates in skin, absorbs light and undergoes a photochemical reaction followed by photo biological reaction in local tissue damage. ***E.g.*** tar products.
2. **Photoallergic reaction :** Drug or its metabolite which induces cell mediated immune response which on exposure to light of longer wave lengths produces a papular or eczematous contact dermatitis. ***E.g.*** sulfonamides, chloroquine, sulfonylurea.

## PHARMACOVIGILANCE :

It is the science and activities relating to the detection, assessment, understanding and prevention of adverse effect or any other Drug related problems.

### Activities involved in Pharmacovigilance :

- Post marketing surveillance and other methods of ADR monitoring such as voluntary reporting by Doctors.
- Dissemination of ADR data through drug alerts, medical letters, and advisories sent to Doctor by pharmaceuticals.
- Changes in the labelling by medicines indicating restriction in use or statuary warning, precaution or even withdrawal of the drug.

### Who can report :

Any healthcare professional (Doctors, nurse, dentist, pharmacist) may report the ADR. They have to fill the ADR form and that has to be submitted to nearby adverse drug monitoring center. Helpline is there (hotline 1800-180-3024), Email : pvpi.compat@gmail.com. ADR can also be reported on smartphones by pvpi app.

### Pharmacovigilance Programme of India :

The Central Drugs standard control organisation (CDSCO), New Delhi, under the control of Ministry of Health & Family welfare, Government of India started the Pharmacovigilance programme in July 2010. The National co-ordinating center (NCC) for monitoring ADR is at The Indian pharmacopoeia Commission (IPC), Ghaziabad (U.P.). ADR are reported from all over country to NCC- PvPI which works in collaboration with Global center WHO UPPSALA Monitoring center Sweden.

# 9 ESSENTIAL MEDICINES AND RATIONAL DRUG USE

## ESSENTIAL MEDICINES :

- WHO defines essential medicines as the medicines that satisfy healthcare needs of majority of the population and which should be available at all times, in adequate amount, in appropriate dosage and at a price the individual and the community can afford. WHO has published latest $19^{th}$ essential medicines list in 2015.
- This model is only a rough guideline and individual countries can modify or make their own list of essential medicines considering the healthcare needs of their citizens and presence of different diseases.
- Every country should update the essential medicine list every 2-3 years as per changing healthcare and medicine scenario.
- In India, this list is prepared by DCGI (drug controller general of India) under ministry of health and family welfare. The first list was made in 1996 and the recent was updated in 2015 which had 376 drugs in total.

## RATIONAL DRUG USE :

- Rational prescribing or use of drugs includes following 8 R : Right patient, Right drug, Right dose, Right route, Right frequency of administration, Right duration of therapy, Right cost and Right documentation.

## P-DRUGS :

Every practicing doctor should have his personalised drug (P-drug). This enables him for convenient and efficient prescribing & also saves time. It can be done in following steps :

- Achieve a definitive diagnosis.
- Set your therapeutic goals.
- Prepare a list of the drugs that can be used.
- Select few drugs comparing safety, efficacy, suitability and cost.
- Select a P-drug from this group.

# 10 NEW DRUG DEVELOPMENT

The process of development of a new drug has to go through following phases :

**NEW DRUG DISCOVERY**

↓

**PRE-CLINICAL STUDIES (ANIMAL STUDIES)**

↓

**CLINICAL TRIAL (HUMAN TRIALS)**

↓

**APPROVAL**

## NEW DRUG DISCOVERY :

Various drugs discovery methods are : random screening, molecular designing (target & compound centred approach), molecular modification and serendipity (Happy observation / by chance).

## PRE-CLINICAL STUDIES (Animal studies) :

Drugs that passed initial screening are subjected to animal tests. The various pre-clinical studies done are :

### Pharmacodyanamic studies :

- They include : Cellular level studies, receptor activity study, molecular level studies, graded & quantal assays. Used to calculate $ED_{50}$.

### Toxicity studies :

- They include : Acute Toxicity studies, sub-acute toxicity studies, chronic toxicity studies, local toxicity studies and special toxicity studies like effect on reproductive functions, teratogenicity, carcinogenicity and mutagenicity.

### Pharmacokinetic studies :

- They include : Absorption, distribution, metabolism and excretion of a drug. Used to calculate relative bioavailability and elimination half life.

### Assessment of Safety Index :

- Calculate $LD_{50}$ and $ED_{50}$, calculate therapeutic index, calculate certain safety factor, determine MTD (maximum tolerated dose), NoAEL (no adverse effect level dose), HED (human equivalent dose) and FIH (first in human dose).

## CLINICAL TRIAL (human trials) :

- A clinical trial is a scientifically and ethically designed experiment conducted in human subjects with the aim of answering well framed specific questions regarding the efficacy or safety of a drug. This is done in human subjects when the drug has shown promise in animal studies. Clinical trials are done in following phases :

### Phase 0 : (Microdosing) :

- Phase 0 is a technique for studying the behavior of drugs in humans through the administration of doses so low ("sub-therapeutic" usually less than 100 mcg) they are unlikely to produce whole body effects, but high enough to allow the cellular response to be studied.
- This allows the observation of a drug's pharmacokinetics with a low risk of side effects. This is called a "Phase 0 study" and is usually conducted before clinical Phase I to predict whether a drug is viable for the next phase of testing. Human microdosing aims to reduce the resources spent on non-viable drugs and the amount of testing done on animals.

### Phase I :

- Done to find safe dose range (safety & tolerability). It is first in man study.
- Participants are healthy volunteers.
- Not done for drugs which are too toxic (anticancer, HIV drugs).
- Sample size : 25-100 subjects.

### Phase II :

- Determines efficacy of the drug (proof of claims) and done in patients with the study disease.
- Early phase I : 100-200 subjects.
- Late phase I : 200-400 subjects.

### Phase III : (Confirmatory trials-confirm drug is safe and effective)

- It is randomised, double blinded, cross over and multicentric.
- 1000-5000 subjects.
- Phase III followed by new drug application and licensing

### Phase IV : (Post-marketing surveillance)

- Detect long term and rare side effects and is done in post licensing phase.
- New indication might also be found.

- Periodic safety update report (PSUR) is to be submitted.
- This phase is followed by free marketing of drug.

## ORPHAN DRUGS :

Sometimes, a drug is not developed because the costs required for manufacturing are more than the costs gained from the sale of drug. This is especially seen with drugs for rare diseases as number of patients are low. Such drug is called as an '**orphan drug**', the disease called as '**orphan disease**' and the patient called as an '**orphan patient**'. Such drugs are developed by government offered incentives like tax relief, exclusive marketing rights and certain perks offered.

### Examples of orphan drugs :

1. Digibind (Digitalis toxicity).
2. Fomepizole (methyl alcohol poisoning).
3. Miltefosine (kalaazar).
4. Acetyl cysteine (Paracetamol toxicity).
5. Atovaquone (AIDS associated pneumocystis carinii pneumonia).

# DRUGS ACTING ON AUTONOMIC NERVOUS SYSTEM (ANS)

# 11 INTRODUCTION TO THE AUTONOMIC NERVOUS SYSTEM (ANS)

## THE DIVISIONS OF NERVOUS SYSTEM :

- **Central nervous system :** Brain and spinal cord.
- **Peripheral nervous system :**
  - *Somatic nervous system :* Skeletal muscles.
  - *Autonomic nervous system :* Parasympathetic & Sympathetic nervous system.

## AUTONOMIC NERVOUS SYSTEM :

- The responses of ANS are not under conscious control. Hence, called as autonomic.
- The ANS consists of afferent neurons that convey information from the receptors located in the viscera to the CNS, and the efferent neurons that convey impulses from the CNS to the effector organs.
- ANS is divided into Parasympathetic (cholinergic) & Sympathetic (adrenergic) nervous system. Functionally, these two are generally antagonistic in nature.

## PARASYMPATHETIC (CHOLINERGIC) NERVOUS SYSTEM :

- Neurotransmitter : *Acetylcholine.*
- The regulatory functions of parasympathetic nervous system affect these sites : Heart rate, gastric secretions, bladder and bowel, vision, bronchial smooth muscle.

## SYMPATHETIC (ADRENERGIC) NERVOUS SYSTEM :

- Neurotransmitters : *norepinephrine (noradrenaline), epinephrine (adrenaline) and dopamine.*
- Main functions are : Regulation of cardiovascular system, regulation of body temperature and implementation of "fight or flight" reaction.

❑❑❑❑❑

# 12 DRUGS ACTING ON THE PARASYMPATHETIC NERVOUS SYSTEM : CHOLINERGIC DRUGS

*(Also management of Glaucoma, Myasthenia gravis and Organophosphate poisoning)*

- The main neurotransmitter in the parasympathetic nervous system is Acetylcholine (ACh).
- ACh is not used therapeutically because it is ultrashort acting (few seconds). and very rapidly hydrolysed by acetylcholinesterase present in the synaptic cleft and has action on both the nicotinic as well as muscarinic cholinergic receptors (non-selective).
- Considering ACh as prototype of cholinergic system, we will discuss the pharmacology of ACh before cholinergic drugs.

## ACETYLCHOLINE :

### Synthesis, storage, release and metabolism :

- ***Synthesis :*** ACh is synthesised in cholinergic nerve endings by acetylation of choline with acetylcoenzyme-A.
- ***Storage :*** It is then transported into the presynaptic vesicles where it is stored.
- ***Release :*** When an action potential is generated, there is influx of $Ca^{+2}$ ions. The vesicles get attached to the nerve ending membrane and then the ACh is released in the synaptic cleft by exocytosis of vesicles. This ACh then acts on the post-synaptic cholinergic receptors to cause cholinergic actions.
- ***Metabolism :*** The actions of ACh are terminated by metabolism of ACh. It is metabolised by enzyme *Acetylcholinesterase* (AchE) to choline and acetic acid. Choline is then recycled for ACh synthesis. Acetylcholinesterase is of two types :
  - *True acetylcholinesterase* : It is present in the synaptic cleft. It metabolises ACh and other cholinergic agents but does not metabolise butyrylcholine and succinylcholine (skeletal muscle relaxant).
  - *Pseudocholinesterase (Plasma cholinesterase/Butyryl cholinesterase)* : It is synthesised in liver and found in plasma. It metabolises succinylcholine. Genetic variations are seen with this enzyme. Some patients have atypical pseudocholinesterase which metabolises succinylcholine slowly which may lead to prolong apnea.

## CHOLINERGIC RECEPTORS (Acetylcholine receptors) :

- There are two types of receptors :
  - Nicotinic
  - Muscaranic

**NICOTINIC RECEPTORS**

| Type | Location | Function |
|---|---|---|
| $N_M$ (Muscle type) | Skeletal Muscles | Skeletal muscle contraction |
| $N_N$ (Neuronal type) | • Autonomic ganglia<br>• Adrenal medulla | • Transmission of impulse<br>• Secretion of E and NE |

**MUSCARINIC RECEPTORS**

| Type | Location | Function |
|---|---|---|
| $M_1$ (Neuronal - Gastric) | • Autonomic ganglia<br>• Gastric glands | • Transmission of impulse<br>• Gastric acid secretion |
| $M_2$ (Cardiac) | • SA node, AV node, atrium, ventricles | • Decreased heart rate and conductivity (vagal inhibition of heart) |
| $M_3$ (Glandular) | • Exocrine glands<br>• Smooth muscles | • Increased exocrine secretions<br>• Smooth muscle contractions |

## PHARMCOLOGICAL ACTIONS OF ACH :

- **Nicotinic actions :**
  - $N_M$ : Skeletal muscle contraction.
  - $N_N$ : Transmission of impulse through autonomic ganglia.
- **Muscaranic actions :**

  The major actions of ACh on muscaranic cholinergic receptors can be remembered by a mnemonic **'BUS-MILD-DHR'.**

  - **B** – Bronchoconstriction
  - **U** – Urination
  - **S** – Salivation
  - **MI** – Miosis
  - **L** – Lacrimation
  - **D** – Defecation
  - **DHR** – Decreased Heart Rate

  - ***Eye : $M_3$ receptors :***
    - Contraction of circular muscle of Iris : Miosis.
    - Contraction of ciliary muscle : opens canal of schlemm, facilitates drainage of aqueous humor and reduces intraocular pressure.
    - Lacrimal glands : Lacrimation.
  - ***Salivary glands : $M_3$ receptors***
    - Salivation.
  - ***Lungs : $M_3$ receptors***
    - Bronchoconstriction and increased bronchial secretions.

- ***GIT :***
  - *$M_1$ receptors :* Increased gastric acid secretion.
  - *$M_3$ receptors :* Increased motility of GIT, relaxation of sphincter and increased secretions. This results in defecation.
- ***Heart : $M_2$ receptors***
  - Decreased heart rate (Bradycardia), decreased conductivity and decreased force of contraction.
- ***Urinary bladder : $M_3$ receptors (Detrusor muscle and sphincter)***
  - Contraction of detrusor muscle and relaxation of sphincter - urination.
- ***Sweat glands : $M_3$ receptors***
  - Sweating.
- ***Penis : $M_3$ receptors***
  - Penile erection (Parasympathetic : position).

## CHOLINERGIC DRUGS (Parasympathomimetics / Cholinomimetics) :

- These are the drugs that mimic the action of Acetylcholine (ACh) at the cholinergic receptors.

### Classification :

*Directly acting :*

- **Choline esters :** Acetylcholine, Methacholine, Bethanechol, Carbachol.
- **Alkaloids :** Muscarine, Nicotine, Arecoline, Pilocarpine.

*Indirectly acting (Anticholinesterases) :*

- **Reversible :** Physostigmine, Neostigmine, Pyridostigmine, Rivastigmine, Edrophonium, Donepezil, Tacrine
- **Irreversible :**
  - *Organophosphates* : Dyflos (DFP), Ecothiopate, Malathion, Parathion, Diazinon
  - *Carbamates* : Propoxur.

### Pharmacological actions of Parasympathomimetics / Cholinomimetics :

- Same as that of ACh described above.

*Acetylcholine :*

- ACh is not used therapeutically because it is ultrashort acting (few seconds) and very rapidly hydrolysed by acetylcholinesterase present in the synaptic cleft and has action on both the nicotinic as well as muscarinic cholinergic receptors (non-selective).

### *Methacholine :*

- Methacholine is used for methacholine challenge test for diagnosis of bronchial asthma.
- ***Methacholine challenge test :*** methacholine is given by nebulisation in suspected patients of bronchial asthma. It causes bronchoconstriction and the degree of bronchoconstriction is assessed by spirometry. Also the reversibility of broncho-constriction after giving a bronchodilator is checked.

### *Bethanechol and Carbachol :*

- They are resistant to hydrolysis by both true AchE as well as pseudocholinesterase.
- They have affinity for muscarinic receptors especially of GIT and bladder.
- ***Uses :*** Carbachol is not used nowadays. Bethanechol is used for Postoperative and postpartum urinary retention, neurogenic bladder atony, GI atony, Postoperative and postpartum paralytic Ileus, Xerostomia (salivary gland malfunction).
- ***Dose :*** Bethanechol 2.5 mg SC injection or 10-40 mg orally.

### *Muscarine :*

- It is found in poisonous mushrooms *Amanita Muscaria* and *Innocybe species.* It is not used clinically but, toxicity can result by consuming such mushrooms.
- ***Mushroom poisoning :***
  - *Clinical features :* all muscaranic effects (BUS-MILD-DHR) and hallucinations.
  - *Treatment :* Injection Atropine (anticholinergic drug) 1-2 mg every 30 minutes and other supportive measures.

### *Nicotine :*

- It is an alkaloid found in tobacco plant namely *Nicotina tabacum* (nightshade family).
- It is having all cholinergic actions (like acetylcholine) as described above.
- It is highly addictive and abused in various forms like dried tobacco, cigarette, bidi, snuff etc.
- ***Use :*** nicotine chewing gums or patches are used to prevent withdrawal symptoms and to reduce cravings in patients who are on tobacco de-addiction programme.

### *Arecoline :*

- It is an alkaloid found in *Areca nut* (betel nut / supari).
- It has cholinergic actions.
- It is not used clinically.

### *Pilocarpine :*

- Obtained from the leaves of *Pilocrapus microphyllus.*

- It has prominent muscarinic actions.
- It causes sweating, salivation and increases other secretions also.
- ***Actions on eye :*** If it is used topically in the eye, it penetrates the cornea, causes miosis, contracts the ciliary muscle and reduces the IOP (intraocular pressure).
- ***Uses :***
  - 0.5-4% eye drops for open angle glaucoma.
  - To counteract mydriatics after refraction testing.
  - To prevent or break adhesions of iris with lens or cornea by alternating with mydriatics.
  - Other use : pilocarpine 5-10 mg orally is used to stimulate salivary secretions in xerostomia, after radiotherapy or laryngeal surgery.
- ***Adverse effects :*** stinging sensations in the eye, headache, painful spasms of accommodation.

***Anticholinesterases (anti ChEs) :***

- These are the agents which inhibit AChE enzyme, protect ACh from hydrolysis and thus indirectly produce and potentiate cholinergic effects.

***Mechanism of action :***

- The antiChEs react with AChE enzyme in the same way as ACh. There are 2 sites on the AChE enzyme namely the *anionic site* and *esteratic site*. Some antiChEs like edrophonium gets attached to anionic site and organophosphates get attached to the esteratic site and inhibit the AChE enzyme.
- *Aging of AChE enzyme :* By the loss of one of the alkyl group the phosporylated AchE enzyme may become resistant to hydrolysis and cannot be reactivated thus causing irreversibility.

***Pharmacological Actions :***

- All nicotinic and muscarinic cholinergic effects described under ACh.

**Uses of Parasympathomimetics / Cholinomimetics :**

- ***As miotics :*** Pilocarpine / Physiostigmine / Ecothiopate for Glaucoma, to counteract mydriatics after refraction testing and to prevent or break adhesions of iris with lens or cornea by alternating with mydriatics.
- ***Belladonna (Atropine) poisoning :*** It is caused by consumption of datura plants namely *Datura stramonium* and *Atropa Belladona*. The symptoms are opposite to that of cholinergic features (anticholinergic symptoms - opposite of BUS-MILD-DHR). Treatment is by physiostigmine (2 mg IV or IM) because physiostigmine can cross blood-brain-barrier and can antagonise both central as well as peripheral anticholinergic effects.
- ***Post-operative decurarisation :*** Neostigmine (0.5-1 mg IV) is used for reversal of skeletal muscle relaxation action of d-tubocurarine after surgery is over.

- ***Myasthenia Gravis :*** Edrophonium is used for diagnosis and Neostigmine / Pridostigmine are used for treatment.
- ***Alzheimer's disease :*** Rivastigmine / Donepezil / Tacrine.
- ***Cobra snake bite :*** Though antisnake venom is the main treatment, neostigmine is used to counteract curare like action of cobra venom. It is given along with atropine.
- ***Postoperative and postpartum paralytic ileus :*** Bethanechol.
- ***Postoperative and postpartum urinary retention :*** Bethanechol.
- ***Xerostomia :*** Pilocarpine / Bethanechol.

## GLAUCOMA :

Glaucoma is a chronic progressive optic nerve damage caused due to increased intraocular pressure (IOP) of > 21 mm Hg (Normal IOP is 10-20 mm of Hg).

### Drainage of aqueous humor occurs by 2 routes :

- Through the trabecular network into the canal of Schlemm (drains about 90%).
- Uveoscleral pathway (drains about 10%).

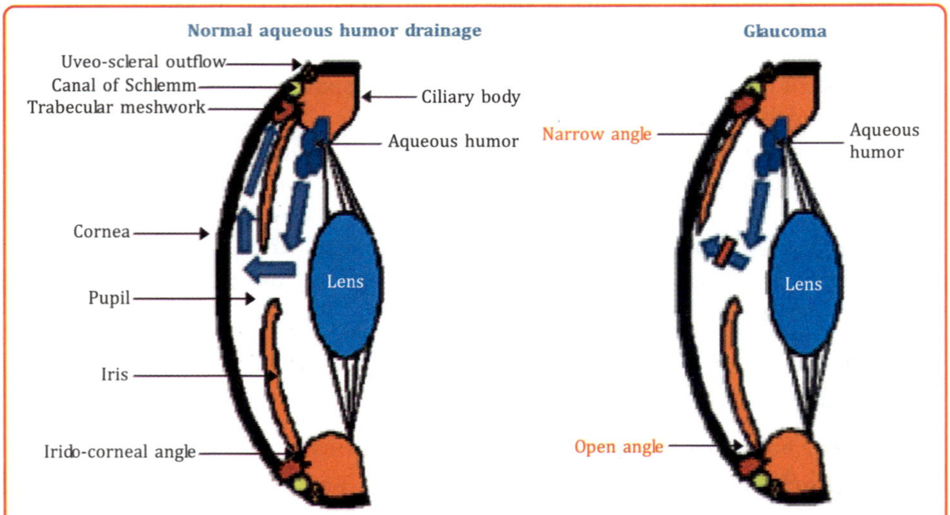


### Types of Glaucoma :

***Narrow angle glaucoma (Acute congestive glaucoma) :***

- It is an acute painful emergency condition of the eye.
- **Cause :** It is due to lack of drainage of aqueous humor through the canal of schlemm due to reduction of irido-corneal angle (narrow angle).
- **Symptoms :** Severe eye pain, nausea, vomiting, prostration, redness of eye, photophobia, lacrimation and rapid, progressive impairment of vision.
- **Treatment :** It is primarily treated by surgical or laser iridotomy along with drugs.

### *Open angle glaucoma (Chronic simple glaucoma) :*

- Genetically predisposed degenerative condition.
- **Cause :** Irido-corneal angle is normal but the patency of the trabecular meshwork is disrupted.
- **Symptoms :** Progressive, painless visual loss and if untreated, leads to blindness.
- **Treatment :** Usually chronic and is treated by drugs.

### Receptors and enzyme in relation to glaucoma :

- Aqueous humor is formed in the ciliary body and it drains through the pupil, goes through the irido-corneal angle and then into the drainage system (trabecular meshwork, canal of schlemm and uveoscleral outflow).
- There are certain receptors and enzyme responsible for the formation and secretion of aqueous humor in the eye. Most of the drugs used for treatment of glaucoma act on these receptors.

| Receptors and enzyme | Location | Function |
|---|---|---|
| **$\alpha_1$ adrenergic** | Ciliary muscle blood vessels | Vasoconstriction & reduction of aqueous humor secretion. |
| **$\alpha_2$ adrenergic** | Ciliary epithelium | Reduction of aqueous humor secretion. |
| **$\beta_2$ adrenergic** | Ciliary epithelium | Increasing aqueous humor secretion. |
| **$M_3$ Muscarinic** | Ciliary muscle | Contraction of ciliary muscle, Miosis, Increases Irido-corneal angle. |
| **Carbonic anhydrase** | Ciliary epithelium | Produces $HCO_3$ |

### Drugs used in the Treatment of Glaucoma :

#### *Drugs that reduce aqueous humor production :*

- **β-adrenergic blockers :** Timolol, Levobunolol, Carteolol, Betaxolol.
- **$\alpha_2$ adrenergic agonists :** Apraclonidine, Brimonidine.
- **Carbonic anhydrase inhibitors :** Acetazolamide, Dorzolamide, Brinzolamide.

#### *Drugs that increase aqueous outflow :*

- **$\alpha_1$-adrenergic agonists :** Epinephrine, Dipivefrin.
- **Parasympathomimetics (Miotics) :** Pilocarpine, Echothiophate, Physiostigmine.
- **Prostaglandin analogues :** Latanoprost, Bimatoprost, Travoprost.

#### *Other drugs :*

- **Osmotic agents** : Mannitol, Glycerol.

**β-adrenergic blockers :**

- ***Mechanism of action :*** They block β-receptors in ciliary body which reduces c-AMP and thus reduces aqueous humor production and IOP.
- ***Advantages over miotics :*** No change in pupil size, no headache, no fluctuations in IOP, once / twice daily administration.
- ***Dose :*** Timolol / Betaxolol 0.25-0.5% eye drops BD.
- ***Betaxolol :*** Selective $\beta_1$ – blocker therefore, less likely to cause bronchospasm, less likely to cause systemic side effects. It has also got neuroprotective effect.

**$\alpha_2$ adrenergic agonists :**

- ***Mechanism of action :*** They have agonistic action on the $\alpha_2$ adrenergic receptors on the ciliary body, thus reducing aqueous humor production and IOP.
- Apraclonidine is used topically (1%) as an adjunct.
- ***Adverse effects :*** Itching, lid dermatitis, follicular conjunctivitis, eye lid retraction and dryness of mouth & nose.

**Carbonic anhydrase inhibitors :**

- ***Oral :*** Acetazolamide
- ***Topical :*** Dorzolamide, Brinzolamide.
- ***Mechanism of action :*** These drugs inhibit carbonic anhydrase enzyme which reduces formation of $HCO^{3--}$ ions. This leads to reduction of aqueous humor production and IOP.
- ***Dosage :*** Acetazolamide 125 mg, 250 mg orally TDS or QID.
- ***Adverse effects :*** High risk of systemic effects with acetazolamide like paraesthesias, kidney stones, aplastic anemia and depression.
- ***Dorzolamide :*** 1st topical CA inhibitor launched in market. Advantage is that it is not absorbed systemically. It is available as 2% solution (applied TDS). Adverse effects are mainly local like corneal edema, allergic reaction, burning & stinging sensation.
- ***Brinzolamide :*** Available as 1% solution. Better tolerated than dorzolamide.

**$\alpha_1$-adrenergic agonists :**

- ***Mechanism of action :*** $\alpha_1$-adrenergic agonistic action on ciliary body blood vessels reducing formation of aqueous humor by vasoconstriction. But, the main action is increased uveoscleral outflow of aqueous humor thereby reducing IOP.
- ***Adverse effects :*** Irritation and pigmentation of conjunctiva.
- ***Dipivefrine :*** It is a prodrug converted into adrenaline inside the eye. The advantage is that it is better tolerated and longer acting than adrenaline.

**Parasympathomimetics (Miotics) :**

- ***Mechanism of action :*** They activate muscarinic $M_3$ receptor on ciliary body which causes contraction of ciliary muscle. This improves drainage of aqueous humor and thus, reduces IOP.

- ***Pilocarpine :*** 0.5-4% eye drops is most commonly used. The action is rapid and lasts only for 4-6 hours therefore, 6-8 hourly administration of drops is needed. Moreover IOP fluctuates in between. To counteract this problem, a longer acting sustained delivery system called '*ocusert*' has been used and also 4% gel is used for once daily bed time use.
- ***Adverse effects :*** Stinging sensations in the eye, headache, painful spasms of accommodation.
- ***Other drugs :*** Anticholinesterases like Physiostigmine and Ecothiopate can also be used.
- ***Use :*** Chronic simple glaucoma, as adjuncts in acute congestive glaucoma.

**Prostaglandin analogues :**

- ***Mechanism of action :*** Prostaglandins ($PGF_{2a}$) decreases IOP by increasing uveoscleral outflow of aqueous humor.
- ***Latanoprost :***
  - Available as 0.005% solution for topical use in eye.
  - *Used :* OD in evening.
  - *Drawback :* It requires refrigeration & protection from sunlight.
  - *Adverse effects :* conjunctival hyperemia, Iris pigmentation on long term use.
- ***Bimatoprost :***
  - It is a synthetic analogue.
  - Available as 0.03% solution for topical use in eye.
  - Used OD.
  - Does not require refrigeration.
- ***Advantages :*** Once daily administration in evening, potent IOP lowering effect, good efficacy, once daily application and absence of systemic complications.
- ***Use :*** they are used as adjunct to α-blockers in acute congestive glaucoma. PG-analogues have become the first choice drugs in some developed countries.

**Osmotic agents :**

- Mannitol and Glycerol are used.
- ***Mechanism of action :*** They reduce IOP by producing intraocular dehydration by osmotic action.
- Mannitol is given as IV and glycerol is given orally.
- ***Use :*** They are mainly used to terminate acute attack of acute congestive glaucoma.

**Surgical procedures for glaucoma :**

- Trabeculoplasty
- Iridotomy

- Iridectomy
- Filtering procedures
- Canaloplasty

## MYASTHENIA GRAVIS :

**Can you guess which bollywood superstar has Myasthenia Gravis ?**

Myasthenia Gravis is an autoimmune disease that is characterised by production of IgG antibodies to cholinergic-nicotinic $N_M$ receptors at the skeletal muscle end plates. This results in decrease in number of $N_M$ receptors.

### Mechanism :

In myasthenia gravis, the number of cholinergic-nicotinic $N_M$ receptors at the skeletal muscle end plates for binding of acetylcholine is significantly reduced due to their obliteration by $N_M$ receptor antibodies ($N_M$ – ab). Moreover, Acetylcholinesterase (AChE) molecules which are located near the end plate rapidly metabolise the ACh. This reduces ACh quantity. The overall effect is reduced skeletal muscle contraction and weakness.

### Clinical features :

- Muscle weakness, ocular motor disturbances, ptosis, diplopia, oropharyngeal muscle weakness, difficulty in chewing, swallowing, or talking, limb weakness. The thymus shows pathological changes in most of the patients of myasthenia gravis (immune nature of the disease).

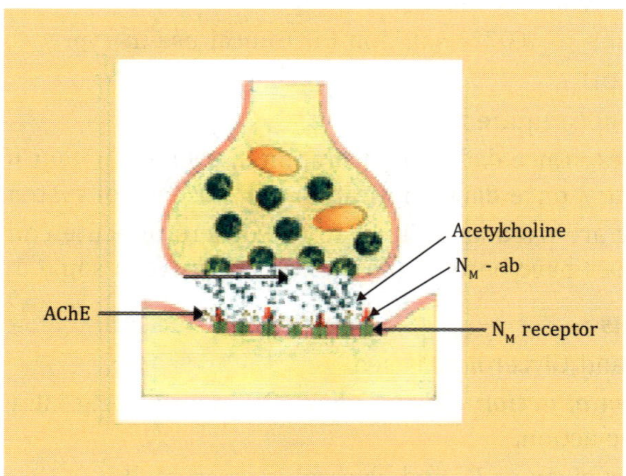


### Diagnosis :

- $N_M$ – ab titre by immunoassay, Electromyography, CT scan : to detect thymoma.
- ***Edrophonium test :*** This test is used to differentiate between cholinergic overactivity and myasthenia gravis. We give 1-2 mg IV of Edrophonium. If the

muscle weakness is due to cholinergic overactivity, patient's symptoms will worsen, but if no effects are seen, 5-8 mg is again given IV. Now, the patient of myasthenia gravis shows improvement in symptoms. Edrophonium is short acting and the actions last for only 5 minutes. Edrophonium is a reversible-anticholinesterase which inhibits AchE in the synaptic cleft. As a result ACh is not metabolised and more and more ACh is available for action at $N_M$ receptors.

**Treatment :**

- ***Reversible Anti-AChE :*** They inhibit the AChE and make more ACh available at the muscle end plate. Drugs used are :
  - Inj. Neostigmine 0.5-2.5 mg IM or SC along with Atropine (To treat muscarinic effects of neostigmine) or
  - Tablet Neostigmine 15-30 mg OD orally along with Atropine or
  - Tablet Pyridostigmine 60 mg TDS orally.
- ***Glucocorticoids :*** They act as immunosuppressants and help in reducing the formation of $N_M$ receptor antibodies. Drug used :
  - Tablet prednisolone 10 mg OD. (increased slowly to maximum of 100 mg)
- ***Immunosuppressants :*** They also help in reducing the formation of $N_M$ receptor antibodies. Drug used :
  - Azathioprine
  - Cyclosporine
- ***Plasmapheresis :*** It is used in patients who are not responding to drug therapy. It removes the $N_M$ - ab from the plasma.
- ***Thymectomy :*** When myasthenia gravis is associated with thymoma or when the disease is not controlled by drug therapy, thymectomy is done.

## ORGANOPHOSPHATE POISONING (OP Poisoning) :

- **Organophosphates :** Dyflos (DFP), Ecothiopate, Malathion, Parathion, Diazinon.
- These are irreversible inhibitors of acetylcholinesterase enzyme (anti-AChE).
- They are easily available and extensively used as pesticides and insecticides in agriculture.
- Mode of poisoning : accidental or suicidal.

**Clinical features :**

- As they are indirectly acting cholinomimetics, the symptoms seen in their poisoning or toxicity are mostly muscaranic cholinergic symptoms.
- Nausea, vomiting, lacrimation, salivation, copious tracheo-bronchial secretions, breathlessness, involuntary urination & defecation, fall in BP, bradycardia, convulsions, coma and death due to respiratory failure.

- In short : **'BUS-MILD-DHR'**
    - **B** – Bronchoconstriction
    - **U** – Urination
    - **S** – Salivation
    - **MI** – Miosis
    - **L** – Lacrimation
    - **D** – Defecation
    - **DHR** – Decreased Heart Rate

**Treatment :**

***Primary measures :***

- Remove patient away from the site of exposure.
- Remove contaminated clothes.
- Wash body parts with soap and water.
- Check for A, B, C (airway, breathing, circulation).
- Gastric lavage with potassium permanganate.

***Pharmacotherapy :***

- **Anticholinergics :**
    - To counteract muscarinic cholinergic symptoms of OP poisoning.
    - Injection Atropine 2 mg IV every 10 min till the signs of atropinisation (dilatation of pupils, tachycardia and dryness of all body secretions).
- **Acetylcholinesterase (AchE) reactivators (oximes) :**
    - Pralidoxime, Obidoxime, Diacetyl-monoxamine (DAM).
    - Inj. Pralidoxime 1-2 gm IV slowly.
    - It attaches to the anionic site of the AChE enzyme. Its oxime end reacts with phosphorus atom attached to the esteratic site. The oxime-phosphate complex thus formed diffuses away leaving reactivated AChE enzyme.
    - Oximes are not effective in carbamate poisoning because in carbamate poisoning, the anionic site is not free for attachment of oximes.
    - One more important thing here is that AchE reactivators should be given within 24 hours before the AChE enzyme undergoes aging and becomes resistant to hydrolysis.
- **Antibiotics :**
    - Inj. Ceftriaxone 1 g IV 12 hourly can be given to prevent infection like aspiration pneumonitis.
- **Inj. Furosemide** 40 mg slow IV if pulmonary edema present.
- **Inj. Diazepam** 10 mg IV slowly if convulsions. May be repeated, if needed.

# 13 DRUGS ACTING ON THE PARA-SYMPATHETIC NERVOUS SYSTEM : ANTI-CHOLINERGIC DRUGS

**ANTICHOLINERGIC DRUGS (Parasympatholytics / Anti-muscarinic drugs) :**

- Drugs that block or inhibit the actions of acetylcholine (ACh) in the parasympathetic nervous system *i.e.* on muscarinic receptors ($M_1$, $M_2$, $M_3$) are called anti-cholinergics.
- Nicotinic receptor ($N_N$, $N_M$) antagonists also block certain actions of ACh, they are generally referred to as Ganglion blockers and Neuromuscular blockers.

**Mechanism of Action :**

- They are competitive antagonists and compete with ACh. They block the ACh at the muscarinic receptors. As a result, ACh is unable to bind to the receptor site to cause a cholinergic effect

**CLASSIFICATION OF ANTI-CHOLINERGIC DRUGS :**

- ***Natural alkaloids :*** Atropine, Hyoscine (Scopolamine)
- ***Semisynthetic derivatives :*** Homatropine, Atropine methonitrate, Hyoscine butylbromide, Ipratropium bromide, Tiotropium bromide.
- ***Synthetic derivatives :***
  - ☞ **Mydriatics :** Cyclopentolate, Tropicamide.
  - ☞ **Antisecretory antispasmodic :** Glycopyrolate, Dicyclomine, Pirenzepine, Telenzepine, Drotaverine, Valethamate.
  - ☞ **Vesicoselective :** Oxybutinin, Flavoxate.
  - ☞ **Antiparkinsonian :** Trihexyphenidyl (Benzhexol), Benztropine.

  (*Other drugs having anticholinergics effects* : *Tricyclic antidepressants, Antihistaminics, Antipsychotics etc*).

**Chemistry :**

- ***Natural alkaloids :*** Atropine is derived from plants *Atropa Belladona* and *Datura Stramonium*. Hyoscine (Scopolamine) is derived from plant *Hyoscyamus niger.*
- ***Semisynthetics :*** are obtained by combining the natural organic base (tropine or scopine) with any organic acids.
- ***Synthetic :*** They don't have atropine or scoline portion in their chemical structure.

**Muscaranic cholinergic receptors :**

- Before proceeding to the pharmacological actions of anticholinergics (antimuscarinics), let us revise the muscarinic receptors.

- Here, we will see only the muscaranic receptors and not the nicotinic receptors because anticholinergics (antimuscarinics) drugs are having actions on muscaranic receptors only.

| MUSCARINIC RECEPTORS | | |
|---|---|---|
| **Type** | **Location** | **Function** |
| **$M_1$ (Neuronal - Gastric)** | • Autonomic ganglia<br>• Gastric glands | • Transmission of impulse.<br>• Gastric acid secretion. |
| **$M_2$ (Cardiac)** | • SA node, AV node, atrium, ventricles | • Decreased heart rate and conductivity (vagal inhibition of heart). |
| **$M_3$ (Glandular)** | • Exocrine glands<br>• Smooth muscles | • Increased exocrine secretions.<br>• Smooth muscle contractions. |

## Pharmacological actions (Atropine as prototype) :

- *CNS :*
  - ***Small doses :*** These effects are not appreciable.
  - ***Therapeutic doses :*** stimulates medullary centers; vagal, respiratory, vasomotor centers.
  - ***Large doses :*** stimulates higher cerebral centers; cortical excitation, drowsiness, disorientation, hallucinations, respiratory failure, coma, death.
  - ***Depresses vestibular excitation :* antimotion sickness property.**
- *CVS :*
  - ***Small doses :*** decrease heart rate.
  - ***Large doses :* increase heart rate** (Block $M_2$ receptors in heart).
  - No considerable effect on BP (Since cholinergic system not involved in maintenance of BP).
- *Eye :*
  - Dilated pupils (**mydriasis**).
  - Decreased accommodation due to paralysis of ciliary muscles (**cycloplegia**).
  - This results into long lasting blurring of vision and photophobia.
- *Body temperature :*
  - Rise in body temperature occurs at high doses (inhibition of sweating as well as stimulation of temperature centers in hypothalamus).
- *GIT :*
  - Relax smooth muscle tone of GIT (**Antispasmodic action**).
  - Decrease intestinal and gastric secretions (**Antisecretory action**).
  - Decrease motility and peristalsis (**Constipation**).

- ***Genitourinary :***
  - Relaxed detrusor muscle.
  - Increased constriction of internal sphincter.
  - ***Net result :* urinary retention.**
- ***Glandular :***
  - Decreased bronchial secretions, salivation, sweating, acid-pepsin and mucus secretions in stomach (**Dryness of mouth and decreased secretions**).
- ***Respiratory system :***
  - Decreased bronchial secretions.
  - Dilates bronchial airways **(Bronchodilation)**.

**In short :** anticholinergic actions are **'opposite of BUS-MILD-DHR'**

| | Cholinergic actions | | Anti-cholingergic actions |
|---|---|---|---|
| **B** | – Bronchoconstriction | → | Bronchodilation |
| **U** | – Urination | → | Urinary retention |
| **S** | – Salivation | → | Decreased Salivation |
| **MI** | – Miosis | → | Mydriasis |
| **L** | – Lacrimation | → | Decreased Lacrimation |
| **D** | – Defecation | → | Constipation |
| **DHR** | – Decreased Heart Rate | → | Increased heart rate |

**Uses :**

- ***As antisecretory :***
  - Preanesthetic medication (Glycopyrolate).
  - Peptic ulcers (Pirenzepine, Telenzepine).
  - GI hypersecretory states.
- ***As antispasmodic :***
  - Dicyclomine, Hyoscine butyl bromide etc.
  - Intestinal, biliary, renal colic.
  - Functional diarrhea.
  - Irritable bowel syndrome.
  - Gastritis, gastric dyspepsia.
  - Urinary frequency, urgency.
  - Dysmenorrhea.
  - Spasmodic colics in gastroenteritis.
- ***Motion sickness :***

  Nausea and vomiting associated with travelling in a bus, car or any other modes of transport.

- Tab. Scopalamine (Hyoscine) 0.2-0.4 mg or
- Scopalamine (Hyoscine) 1.5 mg transdermal patch behind the ear or
- Tab. Promethazine 25 mg (antihistaminic).
- These drugs should be used 30-60 minutes before travel (they are of no use after motion sickness sets in).

- ***Bronchial asthma, COPD :***
    - Ipratropium, Tiotropium used.
    - Exercise-induced bronchospasms.
    - Chronic bronchitis.

- ***As mydriatic and cycloplegic :***
    - **Diagnostic :** for ophthalmic examination of retina and measurement of refractive errors.
    - **Therapeutic :** alternately used with miotics to break adhesions in iritis, iridocyclitis.
    - For this purpose, instead of atropine, shorter acting derivatives like cyclopentolate and tropicamide are used nowadays.

| Drug | Strength (%) | Duration of Mydriasis | Comments |
|---|---|---|---|
| **Atropine** | 1 | 7-10 days | Produces systemic effects. |
| **Homatropine** | 1-2 | 1-3 days | Unsatisfactory cycloplegia in children. |
| **Cyclopentolate** | 0.5-1 | 24 hours | Not suitable for children. |
| **Topicamide** | 0.5-1 | 3-6 hours | Produces less cycloplegia, Less rise in IOP. Most commonly used. |

- ***As cardiac vagolytic : Increases the heart rate (Atropine)***
    - In partial AV block.
    - Myocardial infarction, digitalis toxicity.
    - Sinus bradycardia.

- ***Parkinson's Disease :***
    - Tremors and rigidity in parkinson's disease is due to cholinergic overactivity (over dopaminergic underactivity) in basal ganglia.
    - Centrally acting anticholinergics like Trihexyphenidyl (Benzhexol), Benztropine are used.
    - These centrally acting anticholinergics are also used to treat extra-pyramidal symptoms of antipsychotic drugs.

- ***Poisonings and toxicities : (Atropine)***
    - Organophosphate poisoning.

- ☞ Mushroom poisoning.
- ☞ To treat muscarinic effects of neostigmine in myasthenia gravis.

### Adverse effects (Anticholinergic side effects) :

These are nothing but extension of pharmacological actions of anticholinergics.

- Dry mouth, blurred vision, decreased visual accommodation, increased intraocular pressure, urinary retention, constipation, dryness of eyes, tachycardia, **CNS :** excitation, restlessness, irritability, disorientation, hallucinations, delirium, dry and hot skin (decreased sweating and increased body temperature).

### Contraindications :

- Benign prostatic hyperplasia (urinary retention).
- Glaucoma (increases IOP).

## ATROPINE SUBSTITUTES :

These are the semisynthetic and synthetic derivatives of atropine that are used in place of atropine for various conditions.

### Why there is need for Atropine substitutes ?

- Atropine is having non-selective action, whereas atropine substitutes are highly selective with respect to receptor and organs.
- Atropine's actions last for longer period (*e.g.* cycloplegia and mydriasis), while that of substitutes are for shorter period.
- With Atropine, there are higher incidence of anti-cholinergic side effects which are less with substitutes.
- Some substitutes (*e.g.* Glycopyrrolate) are not having central actions as that of Atropine.

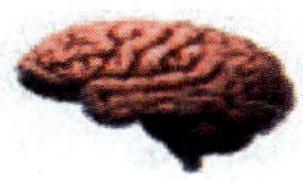
**Benztropine, Benzhexol**

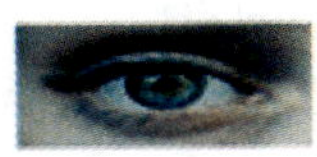
**Homatropine, Cyclopentolate, Tropicamide**

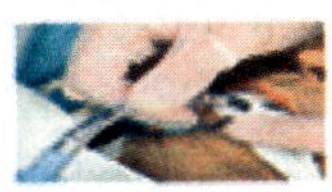
**Glycopyrrolate**

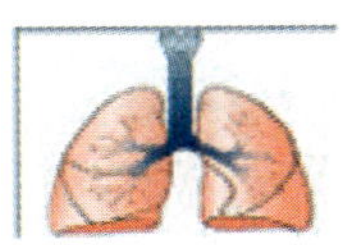
**Ipratropium, Tiotropium**

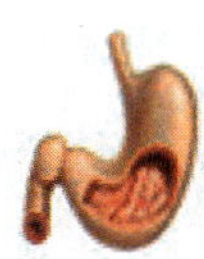
**Pirenzepine, Telenzepine**

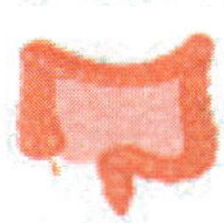
**Dicyclomine, Hyoscine butyobromice**

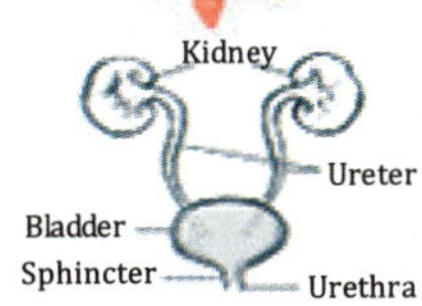

**Oxybutinin, Flavuxate**

### Atropine substitutes used :

- ***Hyoscine butyl bromide :***
  - ☞ **Use :** Gastrointestinal spastic conditions, Motion sickness.
  - ☞ **Dose :** 20-40 mg oral, IM.

- ***Atropine methonitrate :***
  - **Use :** Abdominal colic, hyperacidity.
  - **Dose :** 2.5-10 mg orally, IM.
- ***Ipratropium bromide :***
  - Selectively acts on the muscarinic $M_3$ receptors on bronchial smooth muscles and causes bronchodilation.
  - **Use :** COPD, Bronchial asthma.
  - **Dose :** 40-80 microgram inhalational via nebulisation / inhaler.
- ***Tiotropium bromide :***
  - A longer acting congener of Ipratropium.
  - **Use :** COPD, Bronchial asthma.
- ***Glycopyrrolate :***
  - **Use :** For preanesthetic medication and during anesthesia.
  - **Reason :** It does not have any central action, potent and rapidly acting antimuscarinic.
  - **Dose :** 0.1-0.3 mg IM or 1-2 mg oral.
- ***Pirenzepine, Telenzepine :***
  - Inhibits gastric secretion without causing systemic anticholinergic side effects (selective blockade of gastric $M_1$ receptors).
  - **Use :** Peptic ulcer, Gastritis.
- ***Dicyclomine :***
  - It has direct smooth muscle relaxant action, antispasmodic action, and antiemetic action and has fewer anticholinergic side effects.
  - **Use :** Dysmenorrhea, abdominal colic, renal colic, irritable bowel syndrome.
  - **Dose :** 20 mg oral / IM.
- ***Drotaverine :***
  - A new non-cholinergic smooth muscle antispasmodic which acts by inhibiting PDE-4 enzyme which increases cAMP and causes smooth muscle relaxation.
  - **Use :** Dysmenorrhea, abdominal colic, renal colic, irritable bowel syndrome.
  - **Dose :** 40-80 mg TDS.
- ***Valethamate :***
  - It is another antisecretory-antispasmodic drug which is used as atropine substitute.
  - **Use :** especially used in delayed dilatation of cervix during delivery.
  - **Dose :** 10 mg BD orally.

- ***Oxybutinin and Flavoxate :***
  - They have high affinity for receptors of urinary bladder (vesicoselective).
  - **Uses :** For treating urinary incontinence, urgency, frequency, dysuria associated with neurogenic bladder, spina bifida, nocturnal enuresis, overactive bladder.

- ***Mydriatics :***
  - **Atropine :**
    - Undesirable for refraction testing.
    - Pupils dilate in 30-40 min, cycloplegia in 1-3 hrs and last for a week.
  - **Homatropine :**
    - 10 times less potent than atropine.
    - Pupils dilate in 45-60 min, last for 1-3 days.
    - It can be used in adults, but produces unsatisfactory cycloplegia in children.
  - **Cyclopentonate :**
    - Potent and fast acting (dilatation 30-60 min and last for 1 day).
    - Preferred for cycloplegic for refraction, uveitis, iritis.
  - **Tropicamide :**
    - Quickest (onset 20-40 min, brief duration for 3-6 hrs).
    - Used for refraction testing in adults and for fundoscopy, but is unreliable for cycloplegia.

## ATROPINE TOXICITY (Belladona Poisoning) :

- Belladona poisoning occurs due to accidental or suicidal consumption of seeds and fruits of plants *Atropa Belladona* and *Datura Stramonium*. It can also occur due to overdose or accidental consumption of Atropine.

### Clinical features : (anticholinergic symptoms)

- Dry mouth, blurred vision, decreased visual accommodation, increased intraocular pressure, urinary retention, constipation, dryness of eyes, dry and hot skin, tachycardia, excitation, restlessness, irritability, disorientation, hallucinations, delirium, hypotension, cardiovascular collapse, respiratory failure, convulsions, coma and death.

### Diagnosis :

- History of consumption of Atropa belladonna or Datura stramonium.
- ***Clinical diagnosis :*** Anticholinergic manifestations.
- Methacholine or Neostigmine fails to induce cholinergic muscarinic effects.

### Treatment :

- Maintain vitals.

- Patient kept in dark quiet room.
- Gastric lavage with tannic acid.
- Cold sponging or ice bags to reduce body temperature.
- ***Specific antidote :*** Physiostigmine (1-3 mg) IV antagonises both central and peripheral effects. It can be repeated 6 hourly.
- ***Diazepam :*** for convulsions (IV).

# 14 DRUGS ACTING ON THE SYMPATHETIC NERVOUS SYSTEM : ADRENERGIC DRUGS

## ADRENERGIC / SYMPATHETIC NERVOUS SYSTEM :

- **Neurotransmitters :**
  - E : Epinephrine (Adrenaline)
  - NE : Norepinephrine (Noradrenaline)
  - DA : Dopamine.
- They are called as catecholamines.
- E and NE are mainly synthesized in adrenal medulla.
- Main functions are : Regulation of cardiovascular system, regulation of body temperature and implementation of "fight or flight" reaction.

## SYNTHESIS, STORAGE, RELEASE AND METABOLISM OF CATECHOLAMINES :

**Synthesis :**

**Phenylalanine**

↓

**Tyrosine**

↓

**DOPA**

↓

**Dopamine**

↓

**Norepinephrine**

↓

**Epinephrine**

**Storage :** They are then transported into the presynaptic vesicles where it is stored.

**Release :** When an action potential is generated, there is influx of $Ca^{+2}$ ions. The vesicles get disrupted and then the catecholamines are released in the synaptic cleft. These catecholamines then act on the post-synaptic adrenergic receptors to cause sympathetic actions.

**Reuptake :** It is the uptake of the catecholamines in the presynaptic neuron from the synaptic cleft. They are then again transported to the presynaptic vesicles. This re-uptake along with metabolism of catecholamines results in termination of their action.

**Metabolism :**

- The catecholamines are metabolised by 2 main enzymes :
  - MAO (monoamine oxidase) : MAO-A and MAO-B.
  - COMT (Catachol-O-methyltransferase).
- MAO-A metabolises Epinephrine and Nor-epinephrine, whereas MAO-B metabolises Dopamine.
- The end product of catecholamine metabolism is VMA (Vanillyl mandelic acid). The 24 hours VMA estimation in urine is used in diagnosis of adrenal tumors like pheochromocytoma where there is increased production of E and NE in adrenal medulla.

## ADRENERGIC RECEPTORS (Sympathetic receptors) AND THEIR ACTIONS :

- They are divided into :
  - $\alpha$ adrenergic receptors : $\alpha_1$ and $\alpha_2$.
  - $\beta$ adrenergic receptors : $\beta_1$, $\beta_2$ and $\beta_3$.
  - Dopamine DA receptors : $D_1$ and $D_2$.

**ALPHA RECEPTORS**

| | $\alpha_1$ | $\alpha_2$ |
|---|---|---|
| **Location** | • Blood vessels<br>• Genitourinary system<br>• Eye (Radial muscle of iris) | • Pre-synaptic nerve terminals. |
| **Function** | • Vasoconstriction,<br>• Constriction of bladder sphincter<br>• Mydriasis<br>• Gland secretion<br>• Ejaculation | • Inhibition of neurotransmitter release.<br>• Decreased central sympathetic outflow. |
| **Agonist** | Phenylephrine | Clonidine |
| **Antagonist** | Prazosin | Yohimbine |

**BETA RECEPTORS**

| | $\beta_1$ | $\beta_2$ | $\beta_3$ |
|---|---|---|---|
| **Location** | • Heart<br>• JG cells of kidney | • Bronchi<br>• Uterus | Adipose tissue |

| | $\beta_1$ | $\beta_2$ | $\beta_3$ |
|---|---|---|---|
| | | • Blood vessels of skeletal muscles.<br>• Eye (ciliary epithelium). | |
| **Function** | • ↑ Heart rate<br>• ↑ Force of contraction<br>• ↑ Renin release | • Bronchodilation<br>• Uterine relaxation<br>• Vasodilation of skeletal blood vessel<br>• ↑ aqueous humor secretion | • Lipolysis<br>• Thermogenesis |
| **Agonist** | Dobutamine | Salbutamol | — |
| **Antagonist** | Metoprolol, Atenolol (β-blockers) | — | — |

| DOPAMINE RECEPTORS | | |
|---|---|---|
| | $D_1$ | $D_2$ |
| **Location** | • Renal and mesenteric blood vessels & CNS | • Presynaptic |
| **Function** | • Vasodilation of Renal & mesenteric blood vessels | • ↓ NE release<br>• Modulates dopamine release |

## SYMPATHOMIMETICS :

- Drugs that mimic the action of catecholamines.

### Classification :

*Directly acting Sympathomimetics :*

- **Catecholamines :**
  - ***Endogenous :*** Adrenaline, Nor-adrenaline, Dopamine.
  - ***Synthetic :*** Isoprenaline, Dipivefrine, Dobutamine, Fenoldopam.
- **Non-catecholamines :**
  - ***Selective $\alpha_1$ agonists :*** Phenylephrine, Naphazoline, Oxymetazoline, Xylometazoline.
  - ***Selective $\alpha_2$ agonists :*** Clonidine, α-Methyldopa, Apraclonidine, Brimonidine.
  - ***Selective $\beta_1$ agonists :*** Dobutamine (synthetic catecholamine).
  - ***Selective $\beta_2$ agonists :*** Salbutamol, Terbutaline, Salmeterol, Formeterol, Isoxuprine, Ritodrine.
  - ***Selective $\beta_3$ agonists :*** Mirabegron.

*Indirectly acting Sympathomimetics :*

- Tyramine, Amphetamines, Methamphetamine, Methylphenidate, Modafinil.

### Sympathomimetics having mixed action :

- Ephedrine, Pseudoephedrine.

### Therapeutic classification :

- ***Pressor agents :*** Nor-adrenaline, Phenylephrine, Ephedrine, Dopamine.
- ***Cardiac Stimulants :*** Adrenaline, Dobutamine, Isoprenaline.
- ***Nasal Decongestants :*** Phenylephrine, Naphazoline, Xylometazoline, Oxymetazoline, Ephedrine, Pseudoephedrine.
- ***Bronchodilators :*** Salbutamol, Salmeterol, Terbutaline, Formeterol.
- ***Uterine Relaxants :*** Salbutamol, Terbutaline, Ritodrine, Isoxsuprine.
- ***CNS Stimulants :*** Amphetamine, Methamphetamine, Methylphenidate, *Modafinil.*
- ***Anorectics :*** Fenfluramine, dexfenfluramine and sibutramine.

### ADRENALINE :

- Has $\alpha_{1,}$ $\alpha_{2,}$ $\beta_1$, $\beta_2$ effect and weak $\beta_3$ action.

### Actions :

- ***CVS :***
    - **Heart :** Increases heart rate and force of contraction ($\beta_1$ effect). Rhythm is altered, cardiac output is enhanced and oxygen consumption is increased.
    - **BP :** It causes '**Biphasic response'** where rise in systolic blood pressure is due to $\beta_1$ and $\beta_1$ action followed by fall in diastolic blood pressure

Biphasic response

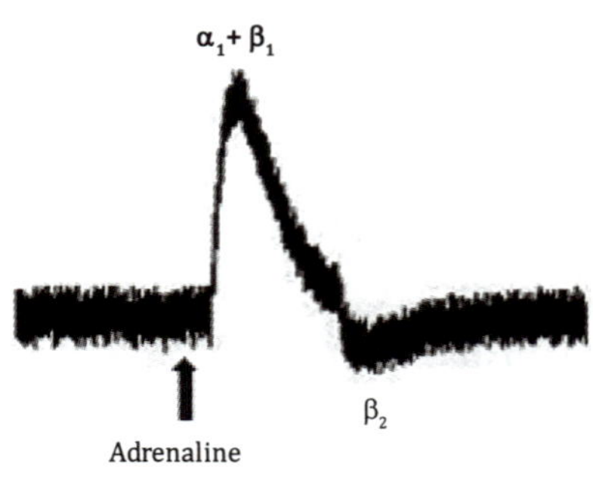


which is due to predominant $\beta_2$ stimulation at skeletal muscle blood vessels causing decrease in peripheral resistance. This is the reason why adrenaline is not used for treating hypovolumic shock as it causes rise in systolic blood pressure and fall in diastolic blood pressure, so it has minimal impact on mean arterial pressure.

- **Dale's vasomotor reversal :** Adrenaline causes rise in BP due to stimulation of $\alpha_1$ and $\beta_1$ receptors followed by a fall in BP due to $\beta_2$

action (biphasic response). Then an α-blocker like Tolazoline is administered followed by the same dose of adrenaline. This results in conversion of biphasic response to depressor response due to α-receptor blockade by Tolazoline and stimulation of peripheral $\beta_2$ receptors by adrenaline. Therefore, only fall in BP is seen.

**Dale's vasomotor reversal**

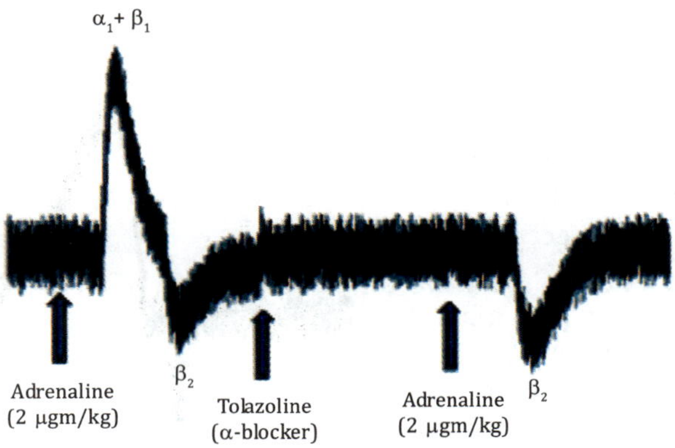


- ***Respiratory system :*** Powerful bronchodilator, relaxes bronchial smooth muscle ($\beta_2$ effect). Adrenaline is physiological antagonist to mediators of bronchoconstriction *e.g.* Histamine.
- ***GIT and Urinary tract smooth muscles :*** are relaxed but are clinically unimportant.
- ***Uterus :*** non-pregnant uterus contracts ($\alpha_1 > \beta_2$) and in the pregnant uterus there is inhibition of tone and contractions ($\beta_2 > \alpha_1$).
- ***Metabolic effects :*** Hyperglycemia due to glycogenolysis, increased free fatty acids due to lipolysis, Inhibition of insulin secretion, calorigenesis.
- ***Other effects :*** Mydriasis due to contraction of radial muscle of iris ($\alpha_1$), piloerection, sweating of palms and soles, inhibition of histamine release from mast cells, anxiety and tremors (CNS effect).

**Uses :**

- Injectable preparations are available in dilutions 1:1000, 1:10000 and 1:100000.
- Usual dose is 0.3-0.5 mg SC of 1:10000 solution.
- Used in :
  - Anaphylactic shock.
  - Prolong action of local anesthetics.
  - Cardiac arrest.

- Topically, to stop bleeding (*E.g.* epistaxis).
- Bronchial asthma.

### Adverse effects :

- Restlessness, throbbing headache, tremors, palpitations, increased BP, cerebral hemorrhage, cardiac arrhythmias.

## NORADRENALINE :

- It is released from postganglionic adrenergic nerve endings and is the main neurotransmitter secreted from adrenal tumor like pheochromocytoma (97%).
- Has $\alpha_1$, $\alpha_2$, $\beta_1$, $\beta_3$ effect and no $\beta_2$ action.
- Increases systolic and diastolic BP, mean pressure, pulse pressure and stroke volume. Hence, total peripheral resistance increases.

Effect of nor-adrenaline on BP

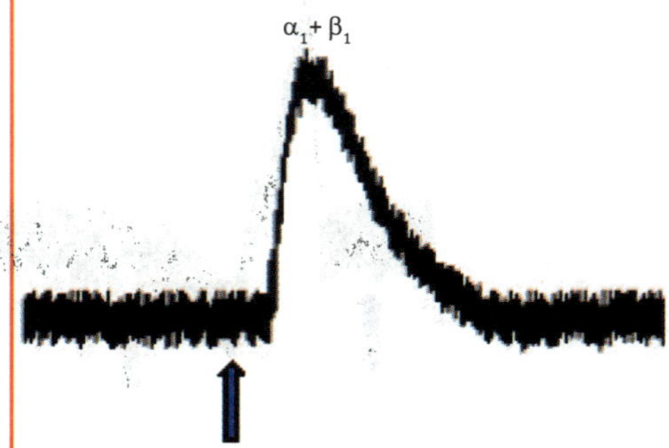


### Uses :

- Treatment of hypovolemic shock and other hypotensive states in order to raise BP.

### Adverse effects :

- Anxiety, palpitation, respiratory difficulty, rise in BP, headache, extravasations causes necrosis, gangrene, severe hypertension, violent headache, photophobia, anginal pain.

## DOPAMINE :

- Has $D_1$, $D_2$, $\beta_1$ effects. $\alpha_1$ effect in high doses (no $\beta_2$ or $\beta_3$ action).
- Immediate metabolic precursor of Noradrenaline.
- High concentration in basal ganglia, limbic system and hypothalamus.
- Central neurotransmitter regulates body movements.
- Ineffective orally, IV use only.
- Short $T_{1/2}$ (3-5 minutes).

### Actions :

- ***Low dose (2-5 μg/kg/min) :*** *$D_1$ effects.* It stimulates $D_1$ receptor and causes dilatation of renal vessels, increasing renal blood flow and GFR.
- ***Therapeutic dose (5-10 μg/kg/min) :*** *$D_1$ and $\beta_1$ effects.* It stimulates cardiac $\beta_1$ receptors resulting in increased cardiac output but the BP is not elevated because there is simultaneous dilatation of renal and splanchnic blood vessels due to stimulation of $D_1$ receptors.

- ***High dose (>10 µg/kg/min) :*** *$\alpha_1$ effect.* It stimulates $\alpha_1$ receptors on blood vessels in higher doses causing vasoconstriction and decreased renal blood flow thereby nullifying the beneficial effect of lower dose of DA.

**Uses :**

- Congestive cardiac failure with compromised renal functions.
- Cardiogenic shock after myocardial infarction, trauma or surgery.

**Note :** Before giving DA in patients of shock, hypovolemia must be corrected first. It is usually as an infusion. BP, HR and urine output should be monitored.

**Adverse effects :**

- Nausea, vomiting, tachycardia, elevated BP, cardiac arrhythmias.

## ISOPRENALINE :

- Has $\beta_1$, $\beta_2$, $\beta_3$ and no $\alpha$ action.
- ***Main Actions :*** It causes rise in systolic but marked fall in diastolic pressure, fall in mean BP. It also causes bronchodilatation and relaxation of Gut.

**Action of Isoprenaline on BP**

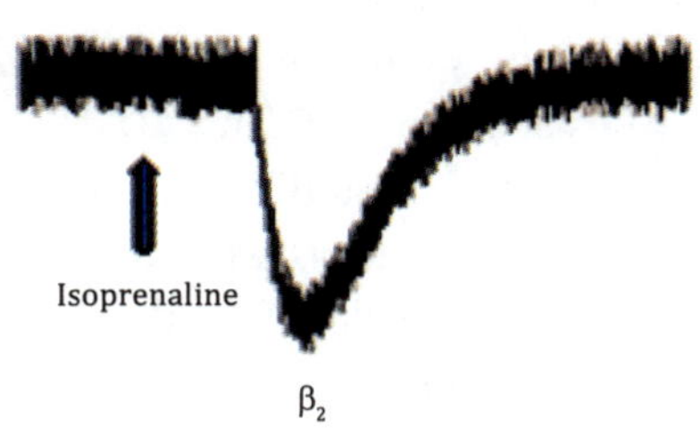


**Use :**

- Used as Bronchodilator and for treatment of AV block, etc. – but not preferred anymore.

## DIPIVEFRINE :

- It is a prodrug of adrenaline.
- It has enhanced corneal permeability.

**Use :**

- Glaucoma.

**Adverse effects :**

- Photosensitivity, conjunctival hyperemia.

## DOBUTAMINE :

- Has predominant $\beta_1$ action (selective $\beta_1$ agonist).
- Increase in force of contraction and cardiac output but no change in heart rate.

**Uses :**

- Clinically given in dose of 2-8 mcg/kg/min IV infusion for :
  - Heart failure in cardiac surgery.
  - Septic and cardiogenic shock.
  - Congestive cardiac failure.

### Adverse effects :

- Tachycardia, hypertension, angina and cardiac arrhythmia.

### FENOLDOPAM :

- It is a peripheral $D_1$ receptor agonist which reduces BP without causing tolerance, rebound HTN or deterioration of renal functions. It is used in hypertensive emergencies associated with impaired renal functions.

### NASAL / MUCOSAL DECONGESTANTS (Selective $\alpha_1$ agonists) :

- Nasal and bronchial decongestants are the drugs used in allergic rhinitis, colds, coughs and sinusitis as nasal drops. They are sympathomimetic vasoconstrictors with $\alpha$1 effects that reduce congestion and hyperemia in mucosa.

### Drugs :

Phenylephrine, Naphazoline, Xylometazoline, Oxymetazoline, Phenylpropalamine, Ephedrine, Pseudoephedrine.

### PHENYLEPHRINE :

- Actions similar to noradrenaline. Has long duration of action.
- Resistant to MAO and COMT.
- Does not cross BBB, so no CNS effects.
- Peripheral vasoconstriction leads to rise in BP but Reflex bradycardia occurs.
- Produces mydriasis and nasal decongestion.
- Administered parenterally & topically (eye, nose).

### Use :

- Sinusitis & Rhinitis as nasal decongestant (common in oral preparations), hypovolemic shock as pressor agent and as mydriatic in the form of eye drops for retinal examination.

### Adverse effects :

- Photosensitivity, conjunctival hyperemia and hypersensitivity.

### NAPHAZOLINE, OXYMETAZOLINE, XYLOMETAZOLINE :

- They are exclusively used as nasal decongestants.
- However, mucosal ischemic damage occurs if used excessively or for prolonged periods (> 3 weeks).
- Rebound congestion is a problem with their use.
- Used only for a few days since longer application reduces ciliary action.

### Use :

- Allergic rhinitis with rhinorrhea, epistaxis.

### PHENYLPROPALAMINE :

- It was earlier used as decongestant along with antihistaminics.
- It leads to hemorrhagic stroke, therefore withdrawn from the market.

## EPHEDRINE, PSEUDOEPHEDRINE :

- **Ephedrine :** Plant alkaloid obtained from *Ephedra vulgaris.*
- Has indirect action but also acts on $\alpha$ and $\beta$ receptors.
- **Central action :** Increased alertness, anxiety, insomnia, tremor and tachyphylaxis occur on repeated dosing.
- **Pseudoephedrine** is similar but less CNS and cardiac effects.
- **Use :** Used as bronchodilator, mydriatic, decongestant. Given in combination with antihistaminics, antitussives and NSAIDs in common cold and, allergic rhinitis, rhinorrhea etc.

## SELECTIVE $\alpha_2$ AGONISTS (Central sympatholytics) :

- They are agonist at pre-synaptic $\alpha_2$ receptors which reduces release of nor-adrenaline from sympathetic neurons and decreases central sympathetic outflow.

### Clonidine :

- It mainly stimulates $\alpha_2$ adrenoceptors in vasomotor center in brainstem. This reduces central sympathetic outflow. This decreases in BP and heart rate.
- It also activates peripheral presynaptic $\alpha_2$ adrenoceptors on adrenergic nerve ending and suppresses noradrenaline release.
- Overdose stimulates peripheral postsynaptic $\alpha_1$ adrenoceptors & cause hypertension by vasoconstriction.
- ***Uses :***
    - Moderate hypertension (100-300 μg BD orally).
    - Prophylaxis of migraine.
    - Nicotine, alcohol and opiate withdrawal.
    - Diabetic diarrhea.
    - Menopausal hot flushes.
    - ADHD (Attention deficit hyperactivity disorder), restless leg syndrome.
- ***Adverse effects :*** Sedation, abrupt withdrawal causes rebound hypertension, dry mouth, constipation etc.
- ***Moxonidine and Rilmenidine :*** They are newer congeners of clonidine having longer plasma half life and are selective for Imidazoline ($I_1$) receptors rather than $\alpha_2$ receptors. Incidence of rebound hypertension is significantly less with these drugs.
- ***Dexmedetomidine :*** It is a newly launched selective $\alpha_{2A}$ agonist. It is used for pre-anesthetic medication to provide sedation, analgesia and anti-anxiety effects and also reduces bronchial secretions. It is also used to provide conscious sedation in ICU patients who require ventilator or mechanical ventilation.

### α-Methyldopa :

- It is also a selective $\alpha_2$ adrenoceptor agonist, but the actions are mediated by its active metabolite.
- α-Methyldopa is metabolised to α-Methyldopamine in adrenergic neurons. It then enters into presynaptic storage vesicles in place of dopamine and gets converted to α-Methylnoradrenaline. It is then stored in the vesicles and released whenever there is an action potential. α-Methylnoradrenaline is a false neurotransmitter in place of nor-adrenaline and does not produce adrenergic effects.
- ***Use :*** Hypertension during pregnancy (safe to mother and baby).
- ***Adverse effects :*** sedation, dryness of mouth, gynecomastia in males and galactorrhea in females, reduced libido and Hepatotoxicity. *Due to these reasons, its use as an anti-hypertensive in pregnancy is reduced and now other drugs like β-blockers like labetalol and calcium channel blockers are being used.*

### Apraclonidine, Brimonidine :

- They have selective agonistic action on $\alpha_2$ present on ciliary body. This reduces aqueous humor production.
- They are potent ocular hypotensives which do not cross blood-brain-barrier and hence have negligible systemic side effects.
- ***Use :*** Glaucoma (used topically as eye drops).

### SELECTIVE $\beta_2$ AGONISTS :

- *Salbutamol, Terbutaline, Salmeterol, Formeterol, Isoxuprine, Ritodrine.*
- They are mainly used in bronchial asthma, COPD and as uterine relaxants (tocolytics).
- They are covered in detail in chapters on drugs for bronchial asthma and tocolytics.

### SELECTIVE $\beta_3$ AGONISTS :

- *Mirabegron.*
- It is agonist at $\beta_3$ receptors in detrusor muscle of urinary bladder. Stimulation of these $\beta_3$ receptors increases the bladder capacity to store more urine.
- It is sometimes used for urinary urge incontinence.

### INDIRECTLY ACTING SYMPATHOMIMETICS :

- They are taken up in the adrenergic neurons. They then enter the storage vesicles from where they displace the nor-adrenaline. This nor-adrenaline which is released now acts on the adrenoreceptors causing sympathetic symptoms. Repeated dosing can cause tachyphylaxis (Acute tolerance / decreased response).
- When indirectly acting sympathomimetic agents like Tyramine, Ephedrine, etc are administered in the same dose and at frequent intervals in quick succession, there is reduction in response. These drugs act by releasing catecholamines in the body, synthesis of which is unable to match the rate of

Tachyphylaxis

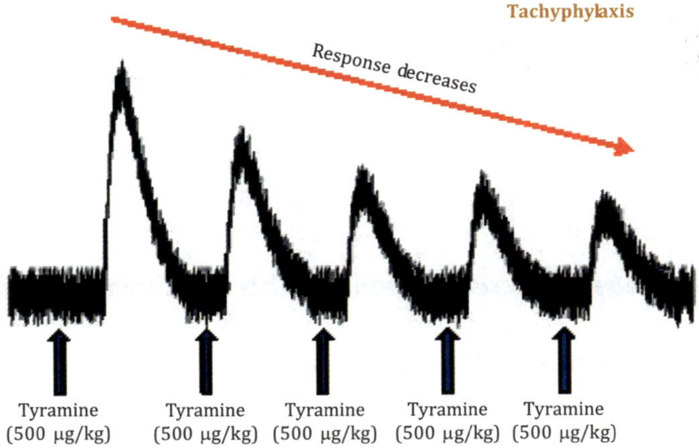


release. As such, stores get depleted. This results in reduction of response. This phenomenon is called tachyphylaxis or acute tolerance.

### Tyramine :

- It is indirectly acting sympathomimetic. It is not used clinically.
- Tyramine is found in cheese, wine, banana, yoghurt etc and can cause 'cheese reaction' if taken along with MAO inhibitors (for details refer chapter on antidepressant drugs).

### Amphetamines, Methamphetamine, Methylphenidate, Modafinil (CNS stimulants)

- They are potent CNS stimulants.
- ***Actions :*** Increased alertness, euphoria, talkativeness, increased performance (Banned drug and included in the list of drugs of "Dope Test), decreased fatigue (acts on DA and NA neurotransmitters in reward and re-enforcement pathway), BP is elevated and suppression of appetite.
- ***Uses :*** Narcolepsy, ADHD, weight reduction.
- ***Adverse effects :*** Restlessness, tremors, hyperactive reflexes, euphoria, hallucinations, psychosis in higher doses, palpitations, headache, arrhythmias, anorexia, dry mouth, dependence and tolerance.

## ANORECTICS :

Fenfluramine, dexfenfluramine and sibutramine :

- Drugs used for suppression of appetite are called anorectics.
- **Mechanism :** Inhibition of Noradrenaline/Dopamine/Serotonin uptake : enhancement of monoaminergic transmission.
- Noradrenergic agents affect the appetite centre and Serotonergics act on satiety centre.
- All these drugs are banned now due to occurrence of serious adverse effects like heart valve defects, pulmonary fibrosis and pulmonary hypertension etc.

# 15 DRUGS ACTING ON THE SYMPATHETIC NERVOUS SYSTEM : ADRENERGIC RECEPTOR ANTAGONISTS (Anti-adrenergic drugs)

These are the drugs which antagonise the actions of adrenaline and related drugs. They are either competitive antagonist of receptors $\alpha$ or $\beta$ or both.

## $\alpha$-BLOCKERS *($\alpha$-adrenergic receptor antagonists / $\alpha$-adrenergic blockers) :*

### Classification :

- ***Non selective $\alpha$-blockers (Blocks $\alpha_1$ and $\alpha_2$) :***
  - **Reversible :** Phentolamine, Tolazoline.
  - **Irreversible :** Phenoxybenzamine.
- ***Selective $\alpha_1$-blockers :*** Prazosin, Terazosin, Doxazosin, Alfuzosin, Tamsulosin, Silodosin.
- ***Selective $\alpha_2$-blockers :*** Yohimbine.
- ***Others :*** Ergot alkaloids.

### General pharmacological effects :

- ***CVS :*** $\alpha_1$-blockade reduces peripheral resistance; fall in BP, reflex tachycardia, postural hypotension (due to $\alpha_1$-blockade, there is peripheral vasodilatation leading to peripheral pooling of blood leading to cerebral hypoxia). $\alpha_2$-blockade in brain increases vasomotor tone. They also block pressor action of adrenaline *("vasomotor reversal of Dale")* - refer chapter on adrenergic drugs.
- ***Nose :*** nasal stuffiness (vasodilatation and congestion of nasal mucosa).
- ***Eye :*** miosis ($\alpha_1$-receptor blockade on radial muscles of iris).
- ***GIT :*** nausea, vomiting and diarrhea.
- ***Kidney :*** Hypotension which reduces GFR. This causes salt and water retention.
- ***Urinary bladder :*** $\alpha_{1A}$-blockade decreases the tone of smooth muscle in trigone, sphincter & prostate. This improves urine flow and thus $\alpha$-blockers are used in benign prostatic hyperplasia (BPH).
- ***Reproductive system :*** Contraction of vas deferens results in ejaculation. Blockade of these $\alpha$-receptors results in impotence and failure to ejaculate.

### Non-selective $\alpha$-blockers (Blocks $\alpha_1$ and $\alpha_2$) :

***Phenoxybenzamine :***

- It is an irreversible $\alpha$-blocker which binds covalently to $\alpha$-receptors (both $\alpha_1$ and $\alpha_2$) and produces irreversible competitive blockade of $\alpha$-receptors. Blockade is slow in onset and of longer duration (3-4 days). This blockade cannot be reversed by catecholamines (even in increasing amounts) as the receptor binding is covalent. This makes it the drug of choice for treating pheochromocytoma where there is excess production of catecholamines like nor-adrenaline.

- ***Uses :*** Pheochromocytoma, occasionally used in secondary shock, frostbite, peripheral vascular disease (PVD).
- ***Dose :*** 10-20 mg TDS orally or 1 mg/kg/1 hr slow IV infusion.
- ***Adverse effects :*** marked hypotension (with initial few doses), salt and water retention, failure of ejaculation, sedation etc.

***Tolazoline :***

- Block is modest & short lasting. It is a direct vasodilator and also stimulates the heart. It also has histamine like gastric secretagouge action.
- ***Use :*** PVD, pulmonary hypertension in newborn.
- ***Adverse effects :*** Nausea, Vomiting, cramps, diarrhea, nervousness, tachycardia, exacerbation of myocardial infarction, peptic ulcer.

***Phentolamine :***

- It is a more potent $\alpha$-blocker than tolazoline. Duration of action is shorter (min). Equally blocks $\alpha_1$ & $\alpha_2$ receptors.
- ***Uses :*** Diagnosis (Phentoalamine test) and intraoperative management of pheochromocytoma (5 mg is given as IV; If B.P falls by 25 mm of Hg diastolic or 35 mm Hg Systolic, it is diagnostic), hypertension due to clonidine withdrawal, cheese reaction, dermal necrosis due to extravasated IV noradrenaline (Given S.C. as local infiltration).

**Selective $\alpha_1$-blockers :**

***Prazosin :***

- It is a highly selective $\alpha_1$-blocker, $\alpha_1 : \alpha_2$ selectivity 1000:1. There is fall in BP with only mild tachycardia. It dilates arterioles more than veins. Postural hypotension occurs as *1st dose effect*, minimized by starting with low doses at bed time. It also inhibits PDE; Increases cAMP in the smooth muscle. It has also favorable effect on lipid profile; increases HDL and decreases LDL cholesterol and triglycerides. Being a selective $\alpha_1$-blocker, it relaxes the smooth musces in the bladder neck, prostatic urethra and improves urine flow in BPH.
- ***Uses :*** Hypertension, BPH, Raynaud's disease, LVF not controlled by diuretics & digitalis. Prazosin has also been used in scorpion bite cases to reduce the incidence of autonomic symptoms.
- ***Dose :*** 1-5 mg BD.
- ***Adverse effects :*** Postural hypotension (*1st dose effect),* impotence, GI upset etc.

***Terazosin, Doxazosin :***

- They are highly selective $\alpha_1$-blocker like prazosin. Have longer duration of action, hence given as OD.
- ***Use :*** Hypertension, BPH.

***Alfuzosin :***

- Similar to prazosin in pharmacological actions, use and adverse effects.
- The drawback is that it has to be given as TDS.

***Tamsulosin, Silodosin :***

- They are Uroselective $\alpha_{1A}$-blockers.
- $\alpha_{1A}$-receptors are located in the bladder neck, prostate and urethra and $\alpha_{1B}$-receptors are located in the blood vessels. $\alpha_{1A}$ selectivity does not cause significant changes in BP & HR (as $\alpha_{1B}$-receptors are located in the blood vessels are spared). Though plasma half life is only 6-9 hr, sustained release capsules can be given OD.
- ***Use :*** BPH, prostatic carcinoma.
- It is usually used in combination with *Finasteride and Dutasteride* (Competitive inhibitor of 5-$\alpha$-reductase enzymes) – refer chapter androgens and antiandrogens.
- ***Dose :*** Tamsulosin (0.2-0.4 mg) sustained release.
- ***Adverse effects :*** retrograde ejaculation, dizziness, floppy iris syndrome (blockade of $\alpha_{1A}$-receptors on iris).
- ***Silodosin*** is a weaker but longer acting analogue of Tamsulosin.

***Yohimbine :***

- It is a selective $\alpha_2$-blocker. It has no therapeutic use.

***Ergot alkaloids :***

- **Ergotamine & Dihydroergotamine.**
- Competitive $\alpha$-receptor blockers.
- ***Use :*** migraine.

**Uses of $\alpha$-blockers :**

- ***Pheochromocytoma :*** It is a tumor of adrenal medullary cells in which there is excess catecholamines (NE) synthesis and causes intermittent or persistent hypertension. Diagnosis is by increased 24 hour urinary VMA. Phentolamine test can also be performed. Treatment : Phenoxybenzamine (preoperatively and also during surgery), $\beta$-blockers are also used.
- ***Hypertension :*** Selective $\alpha_1$-blocker prazosin is preferred.
- ***Secondary shock :*** Fluid loss leads to vasoconstriction. Should not be given without fluid replacement.
- ***Peripheral vascular disease :*** Little benefit in Buerger's disease & intermittent claudication. More useful in Raynaud's disease where vasoconstriction is prominent. Prazosin or phenoxybenzamine are useful.

- ***CHF :*** Provides only short term benefit, leads to $Na^+$ & $H_2O$ retention.
- ***Migraine :*** Ergot alkaloids more effective.
- ***BPH :*** Tamsulosin or Silodosin are used. Usually used in combination with *Finasteride and Dutasteride* (Competitive inhibitor of 5-α-reductase enzymes).
- ***Scorpion bite :*** Prazosin is used to prevent autonomic symptoms. This use was proposed by **Dr. Himmatrao Bawaskar** from Mahad, Maharashtra.

**Adverse effects of α-blockers :**

- Palpitation.
- Postural hypotension.
- Dizziness.
- Nasal blockade
- Diarrhea.
- Fluid retention.
- Inhibition of ejaculation & impotence.
- Retrograde ejaculation (Tamsulosin).

## β-BLOCKERS (β-adrenergic receptor antagonists / β-adrenergic blocking drugs) :

**Classification :**

- ***Nonselective β-blockers (blocks both $\beta_1$ & $\beta_2$) :***
  - **Without intrinsic sympathomimetic activity :** Propranolol, Sotalol, Timolol, Nadolol.
  - **With intrinsic sympathomimetic activity :** Pindolol, Oxprenolol.
  - **With additional α-blockade activity (blocks α+β) :** Labetalol, Carvedilol.
- ***Cardioselective β-blockers (blocks only $\beta_1$) :***
  Metoprolol, Atenolol, Acebutolol, Esmolol, Celiprolol, Bisoprolol, Betaxolol, Nebivolol.

**How to remember ?**

- **Nonselective β-blockers :**
  - Without intrinsic sympathomimetic activity : PSTN
  - With intrinsic sympathomimetic activity : PO
  - With additional α-blockade activity : LC
- **Cardioselective β-blockers :** MAAEC-BBN

### Non-selective β-blockers :

***Propranolol (Prototype) :***

**Pharmacological actions :**

- *CVS :*
  - *Heart :* decreases heart rate, force of contraction and oxygen consumption.

- *Blood vessels :* fall in both diastolic and systolic BP. Other factors that also contribute in the anti-hypertensive action are :
  - ❑ Decrease in renin release ($\beta_1$ effect).
  - ❑ Decreased central sympathetic outflow.

- ***Respiratory system :*** Bronchoconstriction (Due to $\beta_2$-blockade. $\beta_2$-receptors cause bronchodilation. Blockade of $\beta_2$-receptors cause bronchoconstriction), especially seen with nonselective β-blockers.
- ***CNS :*** Decreases anxiety, performance anxiety, tremors and causes lethargy.
- ***Metabolic :*** Increases LDL, triglycerides, decreases HDL. Inhibition of glycogenolysis in heart, muscle and liver. Masks the symptoms of hypoglycemia like palpitations, tremors and sweating.
- ***Membrane stabilising effect :*** It has membrane stabilising effect like local anesthetics.
- ***Skeletal muscles :*** Propranolol inhibits adrenergically evoked tremors.
- ***Eye :*** Decreases synthesis and release of aqueous humor and reduces IOP. This property is used in treating glaucoma (Timolol and betaxolol are used).
- ***Other actions :***
  - It prevents platelet aggregation.
  - It increases synthesis of prostaglandins in vascular bed (NSAIDs can counteract anti-hypertensive effect of β-blockers).
  - It reduces portal venous pressure.

***Sotalol :***

- It has low lipid solubility, therefore lesser CNS side effects.
- It has additional $K^+$ channel blocking property (class III anti-arrhythmic).
- Other actions, uses and side effects are similar to propranolol.

***Timolol :***

- Used in glaucoma as eye drops (0.25-0.5%). It may be absorbed from eye to cause systemic side effects.

***Nadolol :***

- It has longer half life, therefore given OD. Other actions, uses and side effects are similar to propranolol.

***Pindolol, Oxprenolol :***

- They are non-selective β-blockers like propranolol but, have *additional intrinsic sympathomimetic activity* (they themselves stimulate $\beta_1$ and $\beta_2$-receptors submaximally).

- **Benefits of intrinsic sympathomimetic activity :**
  - Lesser incidence of bradycardia (useful in patients with low cardiac reserve like CHF or patients who are prone to bradycardia).
  - Rebound hypertension after withdrawal is less.
  - Lipid profile is less worsened.
  - Better option in asthmatic patients due to stimulation of $\beta_2$-receptors.

### *Labetalol ($\alpha$ +$\beta$-blocker) :*

- $\beta_1$ + $\beta_2$+ $\alpha_1$ blocker along with $\beta_2$ agonism. It is more potent $\beta$-blocker than $\alpha$.
- Effects at low dose resemble propranolol while at high dose propranolol + prazosin ($\alpha$-blocker). Fall in BP is due to decrease in cardiac output and peripheral resistance.
- ***Use :*** Used especially in pheochromocytoma, rebound hypertension after clonidine withdrawal, hypertension in elderly patients.
- ***Dose :*** 100-200 mg BD.
- ***Adverse effects :*** Postural hypotension and Hepatotoxicity.

### *Carvedilol ($\alpha$+$\beta$-blocker) :*

- $\beta_1$ + $\beta_2$+ $\alpha_1$ blocker. It is more potent $\beta$-blocker than $\alpha$.
- It has also got antioxidant property.
- ***Use :*** It is used as anti-hypertensive, due to its cytoprotective and antioxidant property it is used in CHF.
- ***Dose :*** 6.25-12.5 mg BD orally.

## Cardioselective $\beta$-blockers (blocks only $\beta_1$) :

- They selectively block $\beta_1$-receptor without blocking $\beta_2$-receptors.
- ***Advantages :***
  - Lower chances of bronchoconstriction (as no $\beta_2$-blockade); safer in patients of bronchial asthma and COPD.
  - Lesser interference with carbohydrate metabolism and does not mask symptoms of hypoglycemia; safer in diabetics.
  - Lower incidence of cold hand and feet.
  - Lesser impairment of exercise capacity.
- ***Disadvantages :***
  - They are ineffective in essential tremors and migraine (as no $\beta_2$-blockade).

### *Metoprolol :*

- Prototype of cardioselective blockers.
- Safer in patients with asthma, COPD and diabetes.
- Less first pass metabolism. Though it has short plasma half life (4 hours), sustained release preparations are used as OD.

- Available as sustained or extended release 25/50/100 mg tablets and IV injection.
- Uses are similar to propranolol.

***Atenolol :***

- Selective $\beta_1$-blocker with low lipid solubility and longer duration of action; once daily dosing. Uses are similar to metoprolol.

***Esmolol :***

- Ultra short acting cardioselective β-blocker. Duration of action is only 15-20 minutes after IV infusion. Rapid onset short lasting fall in BP.
- ***Uses :*** To terminate supraventricular tachycardia, atrial fibrillation or flutter, during cardiac surgery to decrease heart rate and BP.

***Celiprolol :***

- Selective $\beta_1$-blocker with additional $\beta_2$-agonistic activity (Preferred anti-hypertensive in asthmatics). Causes vasodilatation by NO production which confers additional benefit as antihypertensive.
- ***Dose :*** 200-400 mg OD orally.

***Nebivolol :***

- Selective $\beta_1$-blocker with NO producing property.
- Acts as NO donor, improves endothelial function and delays atherosclerosis.
- No deleterious effects on carbohydrate and lipid metabolism.
- ***Uses :*** CHF and hypertension.
- ***Dose :*** 5-10 mg OD orally.

## β-blockers with additional properties :

| β blocker | Additional properties |
|---|---|
| Sotalol | $K^+$ channel blocking property |
| Pindolol, Oxprenolol | Intrinsic sympathomimetic activity |
| Labetalol | $\alpha_1$-blocking property |
| Carvedilol | $\alpha_1$-blocking property, antioxidant property |
| Celiprolol | $\beta_2$-agonistic, NO production |
| Nebivolol | NO production |

## Uses of β-blockers :

- ***Hypertension :*** β-blockers are used alone or in combination with a diuretic or calcium channel blocker. Propranolol in the dose of 20-40 mg TDS or 80 mg sustained release OD orally is used. Nowadays, cardioselective β-blockers are increasingly used due to $\beta_1$ selectivity.
- ***Angina pectoris :*** decreases cardiac workload and oxygen demand.
- ***Cardiac arrhythmias :*** arrhythmias in digitalis toxicity, arrhythmias of phaochromocytoma, thyrotoxicosis, supraventricular tachycardias.

- ***Acute myocardial infarction :*** They significantly reduce the mortality in AMI patients. It also has benefit by inhibiting platelet aggregation.
- ***CHF :*** Theoretically, β-blockers should not be given in cardiac failure because it decreases heart rate and force of contraction but, they are used in CHF because of following reasons :
  - Reduces cardiac load and oxygen consumption.
  - Prevents fatal arrhythmias.
  - Some also have antioxidant property (carvedilol) which protects the heart.
- ***Pheochromocytoma :*** they are used in combination with a α-blocker prior to and during removal of adrenal tumor.
- ***Thyrotoxicosis :*** they reduce the sympathetic symptoms like palpitations, tachycardia, tremors, arrhythmias. A non-selective β-blocker like propranolol is preferred (20-40 mg TDS).
- ***Migraine prophylaxis :*** Propranolol 20-40 mg TDS is used for prophylaxis.
- ***Anxiety/social anxiety/stage anxiety/performance anxiety :*** They prevent anxiety states like an interview, examinations. They also control peripheral manifestations of anxiety like sweating, tremors and palpitations. Propranolol 10-20 mg TDS is used.
- ***Essential tremors :*** A non-selective β-blocker like propranolol in the dose of 10-20 mg TDS is used. This action is due to $\beta_2$-blockade in skeletal muscles. However, they are not effective in parkinsonian tremors.
- ***Alcohol withdrawal symptoms :*** Propranolol 10-20 mg TDS is used.
- ***Glaucoma :*** Timolol and betaxolol as eye drops are used.
- ***Esophageal varices, portal hypertension :*** propranolol reduces portal venous pressure.

### Adverse effects :

- Bradycardia, reduced cardiac output, heart failure, AV block.
- Bronchoconstriction (especially seen with nonselective β-blockers).
- Tiredness, fatigue, reduced exercise capacity.
- Rebound hypertension on abrupt withdrawal.
- Cold hands and feets.
- Adverse lipid profile.
- Masks the symptoms of hypoglycemia (nonselective β-blockers).
- *Others :* lack of drive, lightheadedness, forgetfulness, rarely hallucinations.

### Contraindications :

- Bradycardia.
- Bronchial asthma, COPD (nonselective β-blockers avoided).
- Diabetes mellitus (nonselective β-blockers avoided).
- Hypertriglyceridemia (nonselective β-blockers avoided).
- Partial or complete heart block.

# 16 DRUGS ACTING ON AUTONOMIC GANGLIA

Drugs can act on sympathetic and parasympathetic ganglia producing either stimulation or blockade.

## GANGLIONIC STIMULANTS :

### Classification :

- ***Selective agonists :*** Nicotine (small doses), Lobelline, DMPP (Dimethyl phenyl piperazenium), TMA (Tetramethylammonium) and Varenicline.
- ***Non-selective agonists :*** Acetylcholine, Pilocarpine, Carbachol and Anticholinesterase.

### Use :

- These drugs have little or no therapeutic use.
- Nicotine has been used in tobacco cessation programmes.
- Recently, Varenicline is also being used in tobacco cessation programmes.

### Tobacco (nicotine) withdrawal / cessation treatment :

- Counselling and motivation.
- Health education.
- Nicotine chewing gum and transdermal patches.
- Varenicline.
- Bupropion (atypical antidepressant).
- Nortriptyline (Tricyclic antidepressant).
- Clonidine ($\alpha$-2 adrenergic agonist)

## GANGLIONIC BLOCKERS :

### Classification :

- ***Competitive blockers :*** Hexamethonium, Pentolinium, Mecamylamine, Pempidine and Trimethaphan camphorsulphonate.
- ***Persistent depolarising blockers :*** Nicotine (large doses), Anticholinesterases (large dose).

### Uses :

- The competitive ganglion blockers were previously used for hypertension and peptic ulcer, but have been totally replaced now because they produce a number of intolerable side effects.
- ***Trimethaphan :*** is an ultrashort acting ganglion blocker and has been occasionally infused intravenously to produce controlled hypotension and in hypertensive emergency due to aortic dissection.

❑❑❑❑❑

# DRUGS ACTING ON PERIPHERAL NERVOUS SYSTEM (PNS)

# 17 LOCAL ANESTHETICS

Local anesthetics (LAs) are drugs which upon topical application or local injection cause reversible loss of sensory perception, especially of pain in a localised area of the body. Blocks generation and conduction of nerve impulses at a localised site of contact without structural damage to neurons.

## CLASSIFICATION :

### Amide type :

- ***Long acting :*** Bupivacaine, Levo-bupivacaine, Ropivacaine.
- ***Intermediate acting :*** Lignocaine (Lidocaine), Mepivacaine, Prilocaine.

### Ester type :

- ***Long acting :*** Tetracaine.
- ***Intermediate acting :*** Cocaine.
- ***Short acting :*** Procaine, Chlorprocaine, Benzocaine.

### Miscellaneous :

- Pramocaine, Oxethazaine (Oxetacaine).

### Advantages of Amide type LAs :

1. More intense and longer lasting anesthesia.
2. Not hydrolysed by plasma esterase.
3. Less chances of hypersensitivity reactions.

### Pharmacokinetics :

- **Absorption :** LA generally have good absorption from mucous membranes and abraded skin (From intact skin – poor). Systemic absorption terminates local action. Factors influencing peak plasma concentration are site of injection, total dose, blood supply to the part and presence of vasoconstrictor (*e.g.* Adrenaline).

- **Effect of adding Vasoconstrictor :** (Inj. Lignocaine 1% + Adrenaline 1:100000) :
  - Decrease rate of systemic absorption.
  - Increase local duration of action.
  - Decrease systemic toxicity.
  - Decreased blood loss.

- **Potential adverse effects of vasoconstrictors :**
  - Don't use in areas of toes, fingers, ear lobes, penis as these areas are having end arteries and due to vasoconstriction caused by adrenaline, it can cause ischemia and gangrene of the part.
  - May produce tissue necrosis.
  - May produce cardiovascular toxicity.
- **Distribution :** Widely distributed to all parts of the body including CNS.
- **Metabolism :** Ester type LA : Hydrolysis by plasma cholinesterase. Amide type LA : Hydrolysed by liver microsomal enzymes (P450).
- **Excretion :** Urine.

### Mechanism of action :

- LA blocks the voltage gated $Na^+$ channels and consequently blocks the nerve conduction by reducing the permeability of $Na^+$ ions during depolarisation.
- This is also called as membrane stabilising effect.

### Order of Loss of sensations :

- Autonomic sensation → pain → touch → vibration → deep pressure → motor sensations. *(Recovery in reverse order).*

### Uses :

- **Surface anesthesia :** Eye, ear, larynx – drops & spray. Lidocaine, Tetracaine are used.
- **Infiltration anesthesia :** Infiltrated s/c & nerve is anesthetised directly. Lidocaines, Tetracaine are used.
- **Nerve block or conduction block :** Drug is injected very close to nerve *e.g.* brachial plexus. Bupivacaine is used.
- **Spinal / epidural anesthesia :** Drug is injected into the sub-arachnoid / epidural space. Lidocaine (3-5%), Bupivacaine (0.5-0.7%) are used.
- **Epidural anesthesia for pain less child birth :** Lidocaine, Bupivacaine used.
- **Intravenous Regional Anesthesia :** Lidocaine, Prilocaine used.
- **Systemic uses :** Treatment of cardiac arrhythmias, I/V analgesia in pain due to malignancy. Lignocaine is used.
- **Other uses :** Scorpion bite, Neuropathic pain (lignocaine 5% patch), along with antacids (Oxethazaine).

### Adverse effects :

- **CNS :** Sleepiness, light-headedness, visual & auditory disturbances, restlessness, tongue numbness, convulsions and death. (Cocaine – drug of abuse).
- **CVS :** Bupivacaine is more cardiotoxic than other LA. Severe hypotension & cardiac arrhythmias.
- **Allergic reactions :** Common with ester LA.

# 18 SKELETAL MUSCLE RELAXANTS

A muscle relaxant is a drug that can decrease the muscle tone and relaxes skeletal muscles. It may be used to improve symptoms such as muscle spasms, pain, for endotracheal intubation, and in relaxation of muscle during surgery.

## CLASSIFICATION :

### Peripherally acting muscle relaxants (Neuromuscular blocking agents) :

- ***Nondepolarising (Competitive) blockers :***
  - **Long acting :** d-Tubocurarine, Pancuronium, Pipecuronium.
  - **Intermediate acting :** Vecuronium, Atracurium, Cisatracurium, Rocuronium.
  - **Short acting :** Mivacurium.
- ***Depolarising blockers :***
  - Succinylcholine (Sch), Decamethonium.

### Centrally acting muscle relaxants :

- ***Mephenesin congeners :*** Mephenesin Carisoprodol Chlorzoxazone.
- ***Benzodiazepines :*** Diazepam and others.
- ***GABA mimetic :*** Baclofen Thiocolchicoside.
- ***Central $\alpha_2$ agonist :*** Tizanidine.

### Directly acting muscle relaxants :

- ***Dantrolene sodium.***

## PERIPHERALLY ACTING SKELETAL MUSCLE RELAXANTS :

### Non-depolarising (competitive) blockers :

***Mechanism of action :***

- They prevent binding of Ach to the $N_M$ receptor.
- Binding of Ach is needed for $Na^+$ channel opening and thus prevents $Na^+$ channel opening and depolarisation and thus the action potential is not generated and muscle doesn't contract

***Pharmacological actions :***

- **Skeletal muscles :** Causes Progressive flaccid paralysis. It starts with the smaller muscles (eyes, jaws and face) and then moves to the larger muscle (limbs and trunk), and finally to the respiratory muscles (intercostal and

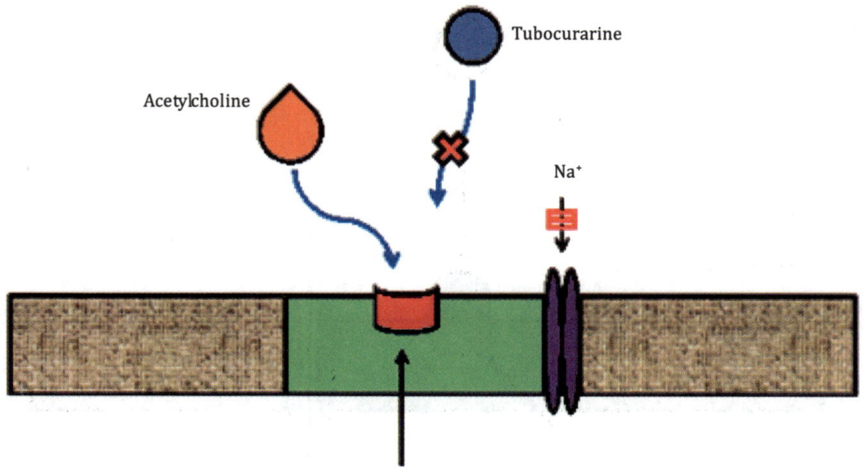

Nicotinic receptor at neuromuscular junction

diaphragm). Recovery from neuromuscular blocking drugs occurs in the reverse order.

- **Histamine release :** d-TC releases histamine from mast cells. Histamine release causes hypotension, flushing, bronchospasm and increased respiratory secretions.
- **CVS :** fall in BP. This is due to ganglionic blockade and histamine release.
- **GIT :** constipation.
- **CNS :** All are quaternary compounds and hence, do not cross blood-brain barrier.

### *Reversal of blockade :*

- **Neostigmine** is used.
- Inhibits Acetylcholine esterase in synaptic cleft and increases availability of Acetylcholine and thus reverses the effect.

## Depolarising muscle relaxants (persistent depolarisers) :

### *Succinylcholine :*

- SCh is the most commonly used muscle relaxant for passing endotracheal tube.
- It induces rapid, complete paralysis with spontaneous recovery in 5 min.

### *Mechanism of action :*

- Succinylcholine is Ach analogue (At NMJ it acts like Ach).
- Binds to $N_M$ receptor, opens $Na^+$ channel, and causes depolarisation.
- Now, the Ach released during action potential also binds to $N_M$ receptor causing persistent depolarisation.
- A flaccid paralysis thus ensures.

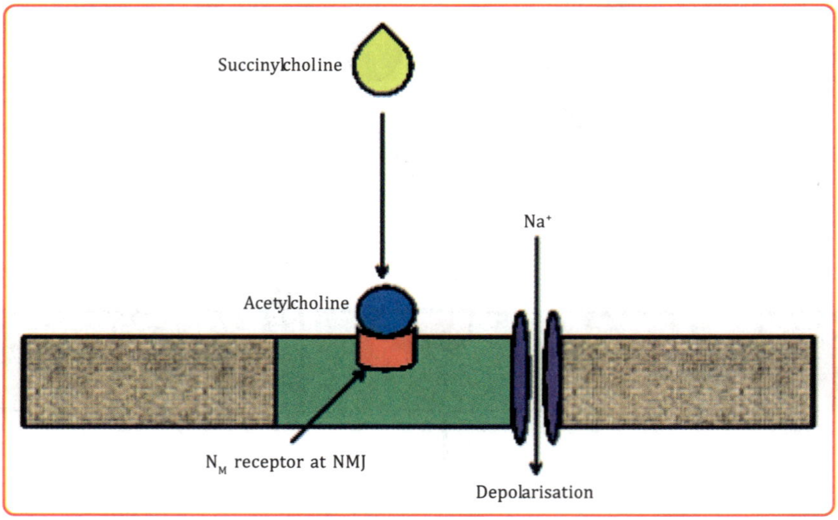


### *Adverse effects :*

- Prolonged apnea in patients with atypical pseudocholinesterase.
- Hyperkalemia and cardiac arrhythmia.
- Malignant hyperthermia (genetically mediated, ↑ $Ca^{+2}$ release from SR, ↑ muscle contraction, ↑ heat release).
- Muscle soreness (due to fasciculations).

### Uses of peripherally acting muscle relaxants :

- As an adjuvant in GA (intubation, scopies, Surgeries), ECT (Electroconvulsive therapy), Status epilepticus and assisted ventilation.

## CENTRALLY ACTING SKELETAL MUSCLE RELAXANTS :

### Mephenesin Congeners :

- ***Mechanism :*** Inhibits polysynaptic reflexes.
- Carisoprodol also has analgesic, antipyretic and antimuscaranic action.
- Chlorzoxazone has longer duration of action.

### Benzodiazepines :

- Discussed in detail in sedatives and hypnotics chapter.

### Baclofen :

- This analogue of the inhibitory transmitter GABA acts as a selective $GABA_B$ receptor agonist. As such, it does produce muscle weakness, but is less sedative than diazepam.

### Tizanidine :

- This clonidine congener is a **central $\alpha_2$ adrenergic agonist** which inhibits release of excitatory amino acids in the spinal interneurones.

- ***Adverse effects*** are dry mouth, drowsiness, dizziness, night-time insomnia and hallucinations. Dose-dependent elevation of liver enzymes also occurs.

**Uses of centrally acting muscle relaxants :**

- Acute muscle spasms, torticollis, lumbago, backache, neuralgias, spastic neurological diseases like cerebral palsy, tetanus, electroconvulsive therapy and orthopedic manipulations during fracture reduction.

## DIRECTLY ACTING MUSCLE RELAXANTS (DANTROLENE) :

- Acts directly at the contractile mechanism of muscles.
- Inhibits release of calcium from the calcium channels in the sarcoplasmic reticulum of skeletal muscles.
- It is the drug of choice for malignant hyperthermia.

# AUTOCOIDS AND RELATED DRUGS

# 19 AUTOCOIDS

- It is a term derived from Greek words : *autos* meaning self and *akos* which means healing substance or remedy.
- These are different substances, produced by a wide variety of cells and act locally.
- They mediate various physiological and pathological processes and also are transmitters in CNS.
- They are *Histamine, 5-HT, Bradykinin, Prostaglandins, Leukotrienes and Platelet activating factor*.

❑❑❑❑❑

# 20 ANTIHISTAMINICS

## HISTAMINE :

It is an important mediator of hypersensitivity and potential tissue injury. The primary sites for histamine synthesis and storage are the mast cells which are found in skin, intestinal and gastric mucosa, lungs, liver and placenta.

## MECHANISM OF ACTION AND RECEPTORS OF HISTAMINE :

| Receptor | Mechanism | Actions |
|---|---|---|
| $H_1$ Receptors | ↑ $Ca^{+2}$ | • Smooth muscle contraction (Bronchi, uterus, intestine).<br>• Increased capillary permeability<br>• Vasodilatation.<br>• Sensory nerve endings : itching and pain. |
| $H_2$ Receptors | ↑ cAMP | • Gastric acid secretion.<br>• Increased capillary permeability.<br>• Vasodilatation.<br>• ↑ Heart rate, force of contraction.<br>• Neurotransmitter. |
| $H_3$ Receptors (presynaptic release auto receptors) | ↓ cAMP | • ↓ Histamine, NE and Ach.<br>• ↓ Secretions.<br>• Vasodilatation. |

## PHARMACOLOGICAL ACTIONS OF HISTAMINE :

- **$H_1$ Receptors mediated :** Itching, pain, bronchoconstriction, contraction of intestine and uterus, fall in BP, increased capillary permeability, triple response on intradermal injection (flush-wheal-flare).
- **$H_2$ Receptors mediated :** Increased gastric acid secretion (Therefore, $H_2$ receptor antagonists are used in the treatment of gastritis, hyperacidity and peptic ulcer).

## $H_1$ RECEPTOR AGONISTS :

### Betahistine :

- It causes vasodilatation and improves blood flow to labyrinth and brain stem.
- ***Dose :*** 8-16 mg BD.
- ***Use :*** used in vertigo, Meniere's disease.

- ***Adverse effects :*** being an $H_1$ receptor agonist, it can aggravate peptic ulcer and bronchial asthma.

## ANTIHISTAMINICS ($H_1$ RECEPTOR ANTAGONISTS) :

### Classification :

- ***1st Generation Antihistaminics :***
  - **Highly sedative** : Promethazine, Hydroxyzine, Doxylamine, Pheniramine, Diphenhydramine, Cyproheptadine.
  - **Less sedative** : Meclizine, Buclizine, Chlorpheniramine, Tripolidine, Cinnarizine.

- ***2nd Generation Antihistaminics :***

  Cetirizine, Loratidine, Rupatidine, Olapatadine, Azelastine, Ebastine, Astemizole, Terfenadine.

- ***3rd Generation Antihistaminics :***

  Levocetirizine, Desloratidine, Fexofenadine.

### 1st generation antihistaminics :

***Disadvantages :***

- Sedation.
- Anticholinergic side effects like dry mouth, constipation, blurring of vision, urinary retention.

### 2nd and 3rd generation antihistaminics :

***Advantages :***

- Non-sedating.
- No anticholinergic side effects.
- No psychomotor impairment : driving, working on a machinery can be performed.
- No sleep induction.
- Do not potentiate Benzodiazepine and alcohol.

***Uses :***

- Allergic rhinitis, Common cold.
- Allergic dermatitis, Itching, Urticaria.
- *Bee sting :* Pain and itching decreases.
- Anaphylactic shock (Adrenaline is the drug of choice).
- Mild blood transfusion reactions.
- Allergic conjunctivitis.
- *Motion sickness :* Diphenhydramine, Promethazine.
- *Sea sickness :* Meclizine.
- Morning sickness in pregnancy : Doxylamine.
- *Vertigo :* Cinnarizine.

- *Appetite stimulant :* Cyprohepatidine, Buclizine.
- Drug induced parkinsonism : Diphenhydramine.

**Adverse effects :**

- Sedation (1st generation).
- Anticholinergic effects (1st generation).
- Dermatitis on local use.
- Cyclizine, Meclizine : teratogenicity.
- *Terfenadine :* ventricular tachycardia, torsades de pontes.

**$H_2$ RECEPTOR ANTAGONISTS :**

- **Cimetidine, Ranitidine, Famotidine and Roxatidine.**
- Discussed in detail in drugs acting on gastritis and peptic ulcer.

# 21 DRUG THERAPY OF MIGRAINE

## MIGRAINE :

It is a disorder characterised by recurrent attacks of headaches variable in intensity, frequency and duration. Attacks are unilateral and are usually associated with anorexia, nausea, vomiting, sensitivity to light (photophobia) and sensitivity to sound (phonophobia).

### Phases of migraine :

- ***Prodrome :*** Occurs hours to days before migraine without headache. It is characterised by difficulty concentrating, yawning, fatigue and/or sensitivity to light and noise.
- ***Aura :*** Stage of migraine that is characterised by visual illusions of sparks and lights, often followed by blind or dark spots in the same place as the bright hallucinations.
- ***Pain phase :*** Headache on one side of head with nausea, photophobia and other classic migraine symptoms.
- ***Postdrome :*** Characterised by exhaustion, lethargy, irritability, depression.

### Types of migraine :

- ***Classic migraine (migraine with aura) :*** In this type, the pulsatile throbbing headache is preceded by aura.
- ***Common migraine (migraine without aura) :*** In this type, there is severe, unilateral, pulsating headache. These headaches are often aggravated by physical work and are accompanied by nausea, vomiting and intolerance to sound and light

### Common triggers :

Hormonal like estrogen and progesterone, foods like alcohol, chocolate, etc, stress, physical activity, lack of sleep, travel, environmental stimulus like sight, smells, medications *e.g.* OC pills.

### Pathophysiology of migraine :

Exact mechanism still not known. However, there are many theories postulated in etiopathogenesis of migraine. Few of them are :-

- Intracranial / Extracranial blood vessel vasodilation.
- Activation of trigeminal nerve terminals.
- Neurogenic inflammation.

- Increased excitability of CNS.
- Cortical spreading depression.
- Decreased serotonin (5-HT) levels linked to migraine.

**Treatment :**

***Non-pharmacological treatment :***

- Avoid triggers, massage, ice application.

## DRUGS FOR MIGRAINE :

**For acute attack :**

- ***Triptans :*** Sumatriptan, Naratriptan, Almotriptan, Rizatriptan.
- ***Ergots :*** Ergotamine, Dihydroergotamine.
- ***NSAIDs :*** Aspirin, Paracetamol, Ibuprofen, Diclofenac.
- ***Anti-emetics :*** Metoclopramide.

**For prophylaxis :**

- ***$\beta$ Blockers :*** Propranolol.
- ***Tricyclic Antidepressants :*** Amitriptyline, Nortriptyline.
- ***Calcium channel blocker :*** Flunarizine.
- ***5HT antagonists :*** Methysergide, Cyproheptadine.
- ***$\alpha_2$ receptor agonist :*** Clonidine.
- ***Anticonvulsants :*** Valproic acid, Gabapentin, Topiramate.

## TRIPTANS (SELECTIVE $5HT_{1B/1D}$ RECEPTOR AGONISTS) :

- *Sumatriptan, Naratriptan, Almotriptan, Rizatriptan.*
- **Mechanism of action :** They bind to the serotonin $5\text{-}HT_{1B}$ receptors in the walls of blood vessels and leads to constriction of arteries, particularly at cerebral and dura arteries. Triptans also inhibit inflammation of vessels of the dura matter that are stimulated by the trigeminal ganglion by acting as a $5\text{-}HT_{1D}$ receptor agonist.
- Sumatriptan has poor oral bioavailability, therefore given as SC injection or as nasal spray. Other triptans can be given orally also.
- **Use :** Acute attack of migraine.
- **Adverse effects :** Sumatriptan can cause coronary vasospasm (risk of angina and myocardial infarction), paraesthesia and muscle weakness. These adverse effects are less with other triptans.

## ERGOTS :

- *Ergotamine, Dihydroergotamine.*
- **Mechanism of action :** They are partial agonist $5HT_{1B/1D}$ receptors. This leads to constriction of dilated cranial vessels, blocks trigeminal nerve transmission and suppresses neurogenic inflammation.
- It has got poor oral bioavailability. Caffeine 100 mg enhances its absorption.

Sublingual route is also preferred. 1 mg is given at half hours intervals till relief is obtained. Dihydroergotamine can be used as parenteral preparation.

- **Use :** Acute attack of migraine.
- **Adverse effects :** Nausea, vomiting, uterine contractions, coronary vasoconstriction, muscle cramps.
- **Contraindications :** Pregnancy, IHD.

## NSAIDs AND ANTIEMETICS :

- **Mechanism of action :** They inhibit prostaglandin synthesis and kinin release due to neurogenic inflammation.
- **Use :** Acute attack of migraine.
- **Adverse effects :** Nausea, vomiting, gastritis, peptic ulcer, allergic rash etc.
- **Role of antiemetic (metoclopramide) :** Besides reducing nausea and vomiting in acute attack, it also enhances absorption of NSAIDs.

## β BLOCKERS :

- *Propranolol, Nadolol etc.*
- **Mechanism of action :** Mechanism of action is uncertain.
- **Dose :** Start with 40 mg BD increased upto 160 mg BD.
- **Use :** Prophylaxis of migraine.
- **Adverse effects :** Mainly bronchoconstriction (should be avoided in asthma).

## TRICYCLIC ANTIDEPRESSANTS :

- *Amitriptyline, Nortriptyline.*
- **Mechanism of action :** Blocks the reuptake of 5-HT.
- **Use :** Prophylaxis of migraine.
- **Adverse effects :** Dry mouth, blurred vision, constipation, weight gain etc.

## CALCIUM CHANNEL BLOCKER :

- *Flunarizine.*
- **Mechanism of action :** It is weak but Cerebro-selective $Ca^{+2}$ channel blocker. It also inhibits $Na^{+}$ channels.
- **Dose :** 10-20 mg OD.
- **Use :** Prophylaxis of migraine.
- **Adverse effects :** Dry mouth, sedation, constipation etc.

## 5-HT ANTAGONISTS :

- *Methysergide, Cyproheptadine.*
- **Mechanism of action :** $5\text{-HT}_{2A/2C}$ receptor antagonist. Cyproheptadine also blocks histaminic $H_1$ receptor and muscaranic receptors.
- **Use :** Prophylaxis of migraine.
- **Adverse effects :** Sedation, weight gain. Continuous use of methysergide can cause retroperitoneal fibrosis.

- Due to lower efficacy and higher adverse effects, they are seldom used nowadays.

## $\alpha_2$ RECEPTOR AGONIST :

- *Clonidine.*
- **Mechanism of action :** $\alpha_2$ adrenergic receptor agonist action. The exact mechanism is unknown. Reduces cerebral blood flow.
- **Use :** Prophylaxis of migraine.
- **Adverse effects :** Dry mouth, sedation, constipation etc.

## ANTICONVULSANTS :

- *Valproic acid, Gabapentin, Topiramate.*
- They are recent additions to prophylactic management of migraine.
- Valproic acid (400-1200 mg/day), Gabapentin (300-1200 mg/day) are commonly used.
- Their detailed pharmacology is discussed in chapter on anti-epileptics.
- **Use :** Mostly used for recurrent and resistant cases of migraine.

❑❑❑❑❑

# 22 PROSTAGLANDINS AND LEUKOTRIENES (Eicosanoieds)

## BIOSYNTHESIS :

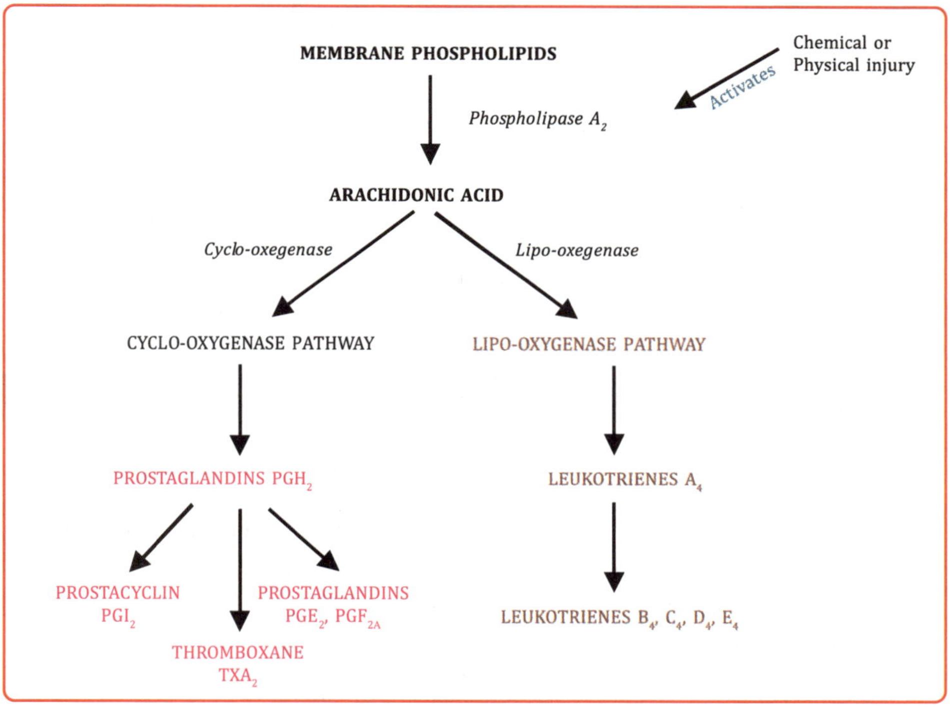


## PROSTAGLANDINS :

### Pharmacological actions :

| Target | $PGE_2$ | $PGF_{2a}$ | $PGI_2$ | $TXA_2$ |
|---|---|---|---|---|
| Blood vessels | Vasodilation | Vasoconstriction | Vasodilation | Vasoconstriction |
| Platelet aggregation | Inconsistent | ———————— | Inhibit | Stimulate |
| Uterus | Contracts uterus, softens cervix | Contracts uterus, softens cervix | —————— | ————————— |
| Bronchial muscles | Relaxation | Constriction | Relaxation | Constriction |

| Target | $PGE_2$ | $PGF_{2a}$ | $PGI_2$ | $TXA_2$ |
|---|---|---|---|---|
| GIT | ↓ gastric acid secretion, ↑ mucus production, ↑ mucosal blood flow | ———— | ↓ gastric acid secretion, ↑ mucus production, ↑ mucosal blood flow | ———— |
| Kidneys | Natriuresis, renal vasodilation | ———— | Natriuresis, renal vasodilation | ———— |
| Male reproductive system | Smooth muscle relaxing effect, penile erection ($PGE_1$) | ———— | ———— | ———— |
| Eye | ↓ intraocular pressure | ↓ intraocular pressure | ———— | ———— |

## Uses of prostaglandin preparations :

| Indication (use) | Prostaglandin preparation |
|---|---|
| Abortion | • Dinoprostone ($PGE_2$) – vaginally<br>• Misoprostol ($PGE_1$) – used along with Mifepristone (antiprogetin)<br>• Carboprost ($PGF_{2á}$) – intra-amniotic injection |
| Facilitate labor, cervical priming and post partum hemorrhage | • Dinoprostone ($PGE_2$)<br>• Carboprost ($PGF_{2á}$) |
| Peptic ulcer, NSAIDs induced ulcers | • Misoprostol ($PGE_1$)<br>• Enprostil ($PGE_2$) |
| Glaucoma | • Latanoprost ($PGF_{2á}$)<br>• Also Bimatoprost, Travoprost |
| Male impotence | • Alprostadil ($PGE_1$) – intracavernal injection or urethral suppository |
| Pulmonary hypertension | • Epoprostenol ($PGI_2$) |
| Maintain patency of ductus arteriosus prior to surgery | • Epoprostenol ($PGI_2$)<br>• Alprostadil ($PGE_1$) |
| To prevent platelet aggregation | • Epoprostenol ($PGI_2$) |

## Adverse effects of prostaglandin preparations :

- Vomiting, diarrhea, fever, bronchoconstriction, fall in BP, syncopal attack, flushing, headache, dizziness, anaphylactic shock, allergic reactions.

## LEUKOTRIENES :

- They act on leukotriene receptors : **cys-LT receptor.**

### Pharmacological actions :

- Chemoattractant for neutrophils, eosinophils, bronchoconstriction, increased mucus secretions and increased permeability.

### Drugs acting on leukotrienes :

#### *Leukotriene synthesis inhibitor :*

- Inhibit enzyme 5-lipooxygenase (Lipooxygenase).
- **Drug :** Zileuton.

#### *Leukotriene receptor antagonist :*

- Antagonist of cys-LT receptor.
- **Drugs :** Montelukast, Zafirlukast, Iralukast, Pranlukast.

These drugs are discussed in details in the chapter of drugs for bronchial asthma.

❑❑❑❑❑

# 23 NSAIDs (Non-Steroidal Anti-Inflammatory Drugs)

**Inflammation :**

- It is the complex biological response of vascular tissues to harmful stimuli which is a protective attempt by the body to remove the injurious stimuli as well as initiate the healing process for the tissue.
- Inflammation can be classified as either *acute* or *chronic*.
- It is mediated by several autacoids like Histamine, 5-HT, Bradykinin and Prostaglandins.
- When a tissue is injured, from any cause, prostaglandin synthesis in that tissue increases.

**Causes of inflammation :**

- Burns, chemical irritants, frostbite, toxins, infection by pathogens, physical injury, immune reactions due to hypersensitivity, radiation and foreign bodies.

**NSAIDs :**

- NSAIDs are chemically diverse class of drugs that have anti-inflammatory, analgesic and antipyretic properties.

**Mechanism of action :**

- ***Antiinflammatory effect :*** NSAIDs inhibit the enzyme *cyclooxygenase (COX),* the primary enzyme responsible for synthesis of prostaglandins which are important mediators of inflammation.
  - Cyclooxygenases are present in two isoforms : COX-1 (constitutive) and COX-2 (inducible).
  - **COX-1** is constitutively or normally present in most of the cells including GIT and platelets. COX-1 has a protective function like secretion of mucus, protection of gastric mucosa, hemostasis, maintenance of renal functions and acts as a physiological housekeeper.
  - **COX-2** is not normally present always and is induced by oxidative stress, injury, ischemia, infections and various diseases. COX-2 is responsible for inflammatory and pathological changes occurring after an injury or insult to the tissue.
  - Recently **COX-3** has also been found in CNS.
- ***Analgesic effect :*** The analgesic effect of NSAIDs is thought to be related to : the peripheral inhibition of prostaglandin (PG) production and may also be

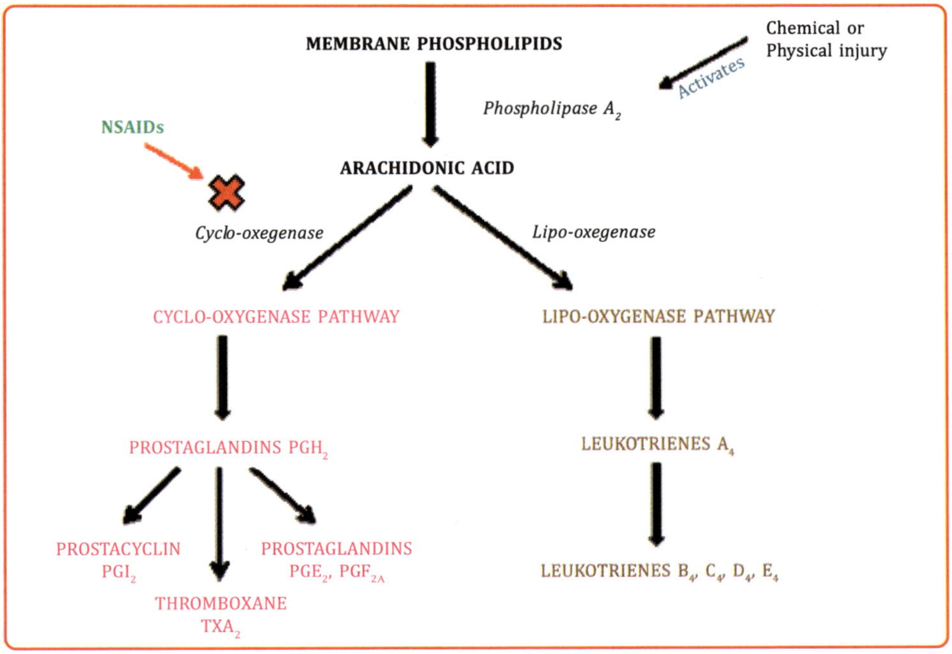


due to the inhibition of pain stimuli at a subcortical site. NSAIDs block the pain sensitising action of bradykinins on peripheral nerves.

- ***Antipyretic effect :*** The fever during infection is produced due to formation of interleukins, TNF-α and interferons which stimulate prostaglandin production in hypothalamus and raises its temperature set point. NSAIDs block the production of these pyrogens. They also cause the "resetting" of the thermoregulatory system in the hypothalamus, leading to vasodilatation and increased heat loss.

## CLASSIFICATION OF NSAIDS :

- **Nonselective COX inhibitors (Inhibit both COX-1 and COX-2) :**
  - ***Salicylates :*** Aspirin.
  - ***Pyrazolone derivatives :*** Phenylbutazone.
  - ***Indole derivatives :*** Indomethacin.
  - ***Propionic acid derivatives :*** Ibuprofen, Flurbiprofen, Ketoprofen, Naproxen.
  - ***Anthranilic acid derivatives :*** Mephenemic acid.
  - ***Aryl-acetic acid derivatives :*** Diclofenac, Aceclofenac.
  - ***Oxicam derivatives :*** Piroxicam, Tenoxicam.
  - ***Pyrrole derivatives :*** Ketorolac.

- **Preferential COX-2 inhibitor (Inhibit COX-2 > COX-1) :**
  Nimesulide, Meloxicam, Nabumetone.

- **Selective COX-2 inhibitors (Inhibit only COX-2) :**
  Celecoxib, Rofecoxib, Valdecoxib, Etoricoxib, Parecoxib.
- **Analgesics-Antipyretics with poor antiinflammatory action :**
  Paracetamol, Metamizol, Nefopam.

## NON-SELECTIVE COX INHIBITOR (INHIBIT BOTH COX-1 AND COX-2) :

### Aspirin :

Aspirin is Acetylsalicylic acid & converts to salicylic acid in the body (active form).

### *Pharmacological actions :*

- ***Analgesic, antipyretic, antiinflammatory actions :*** Aspirin is a weaker analgesic than opioids like morphine. It effectively relieves inflammation, tissue injury, connective tissue and integumental pain, but is relatively ineffective in severe visceral and ischemic pain.
- ***Antiplatelet action :*** Aspirin irreversibly inhibits $TXA_2$ synthesis by platelets. Thus, it interferes with platelet aggregation and bleeding time is prolonged.
- ***Respiration :*** Effects are dose dependent. At antiinflammatory doses, respiration is stimulated. Hyperventilation is prominent in salicylate poisoning. Further rise in salicylate level causes respiratory depression; death is due to respiratory failure.

**DOSES OF ASPIRIN**

| Action | Dose |
|---|---|
| Antiplatelet | 75-300 mg |
| Analgesic | 300-600 mg |
| Antiinflammatory | 3-6 g |
| Uricosuric | > 5 g |

- ***Acid-base balance :*** Higher doses initially cause respiratory stimulation and tend to wash out $CO_2$ leading to respiratory alkalosis, which is compensated by increased renal excretion of $HCO_3^-$. Still higher doses cause respiratory depression with $CO_2$ retention leading to respiratory acidosis.
- ***CVS :*** Larger doses increase cardiac output and causes direct vasodilatation. Toxic doses depress the vasomotor centre : BP may fall. Because of increased cardiac work as well as $Na^+$ and water retention, CHF may be precipitated.
- ***GIT :*** $PGE_2$ and $PGI_2$ inhibit gastric acid secretion and stimulate mucus and bicarbonate production and increase mucosal blood flow. Aspirin inhibits COX-1, therefore nullifies these protective effects & hence, can cause gastritis, vomiting, dyspepsia and peptic ulcer. Besides PG synthesis inhibition, there is local *ion trapping* of aspirin (Aspirin being acidic drug, remains unionised in gastric acid and can enter gastric mucosal cells. Once inside the mucosal cells, the alkaline pH makes it ionized and it gets trapped inside) which leads to even more gastritis.

- ***Uric acid excretion :*** Low doses decreases uric acid excretion and higher doses has uricosuric effect (increases uric acid excretion).
- ***Metabolic effects :*** Significant only at high doses. There is increased utilisation of glucose; blood sugar may decrease (especially in diabetics). Chronic use of large doses causes negative nitrogen balance.

*Uses :*

- As analgesic for various painful conditions like headache, backache, pulled muscle, toothache etc.
- As antipyretic for fever (Paracetamol is a better option).
- As Antiplatelet drug (low dose) especially after a vascular event like myocardial infarction, stroke, or any vascular procedures like angioplasty, bypass grafting etc.
- As antiinflammatory drug in rheumatoid arthritis, gout, osteoarthritis etc.
- Acute rheumatic fever.
- ***Patent ductus arteriosus :*** during fetal circulation, ductus arteriosus is kept patent by $PGE_2$ and $PGI_2$. This synthesis is switched off at birth of the baby. Low dose aspirin can bring about this closure by inhibiting synthesis of $PGE_2$ and $PGI_2$ if closure fails to occur at birth.
- ***Colonic and rectal cancer :*** studies have shown that it reduces the risk.
- ***Familial colonic polyposis :*** aspirin suppresses polyp formation.
- Pregnancy induced hypertension and pre-eclampsia.
- Dysmenorrhea.
- To prevent niacin induced flushing of face.

*Adverse effects :*

- ***GIT :*** Nausea, vomiting, diarrhea, dyspepsia, epigastric pain, gastritis, GI bleeding, peptic ulceration. This is due to inhibition of COX-1, therefore nullifies its gastroprotective effects.
- ***Hypersensitivity :*** Rash, rhinitis, edema or an anaphylactic reaction.
- ***Reye's syndrome :*** The use of aspirin for fever during viral infections in children is associated with Reye's syndrome, where there is vomiting, hepatic disturbances, and encephalopathy that has high mortality.
- ***Bleeding :*** By suppressing platelet adhesion and aggregation.
- ***Acute salicylate poisoning (Salicylism) :*** It is the overdose or toxicity of aspirin or salicylates. The features are vomiting, dehydration, electrolyte imbalance, acidotic breathing, petechiae, delirium, hyperpyrexia, convulsions, coma and death due to respiratory failure. Treatment is symptomatic and supportive along with stomach wash, forced alkaline diuresis and hemodialysis.
- ***CVS :*** Fluid retention, edema, hypertension.
- ***CNS :*** Dizziness, tinnitus.

- ***Hepatotoxicity***, especially in high doses.
- ***Nephrotoxicity*** and renal failure on prolonged use.
- ***Bronchospasm*** (especially in asthmatics).

***Contraindications :***
- Gastritis, Peptic ulcer and GI bleed.
- Elective surgery (1 week prior to surgery aspirin should be stopped).
- Liver and kidney diseases.
- Children in viral infections.
- Diabetics.

***Drug interactions :***
- Displacement reaction with sulfonylureas (antidiabetic drugs) may lead to hypoglycemia.
- Displacement reaction with warfarin (anticoagulant drugs) may lead to bleeding.
- It blunts diuretic action of diuretics.

**OTHER NON-SELECTIVE COX INHIBITORS :**

- **Indomethacin :** It is indole derivative with a feature that it inhibits phospholipase-$A_2$ also and has some immunosuppressive action also. It is effective in gout and ankylosing spondylitis. It causes severe GI upset and is contraindicated in psychiatric patients and epilepsy because it causes neuropsychiatric symptoms. It is also contraindicated in pregnancy. ***Dose :*** 25 mg TDS.
- **Ibuprofen :** Adverse effects are lesser than aspirin in ibuprofen. Used in musculoskeletal pain, dental pain etc. ***Dose :*** 200-400 mg TDS. It is also available as gel preparation for topical application. Ibuprofen is used as a simple analgesic and antipyretic in the same way as low dose of aspirin. It is particularly effective in dysmenorrhea. In which the action is clearly due to PG synthesis inhibition.
- **Ketoprofen :** Same as ibuprofen with additional lysosomal stabilising action.
- **Flurbiprofen :** It is similar to aspirin and ibuprofen. It is also available as eye drops for inflammatory eye conditions and as gel for topical application.
- **Naproxen :** It is also good analgesic antiinflammatory drug. It also inhibits leucocyte migration and causes moderate GIT adverse effects. ***Dose :*** 250 mg BD.
- **Mefenemic acid :** It is a very good drug especially in dysmenorrhea. Besides COX-1 inhibition, it also acts as PG receptor antagonist and inhibits leukotriene synthesis as well. ***Dose :*** 250-500 mg TDS.
- **Diclofenac :** It is a good analgesic with moderate GIT adverse effects. ***Dose :*** 50 mg TDS. It also reduces free radicals at the site of injury or inflammation.

Also used as cream or gel for topical application in various musculoskeletal conditions.

- **Aceclofenac :** It is similar to diclofenac but is long acting. ***Dose :*** 100 mg BD. Causes lesser GI effects than diclofenac.
- **Piroxicam :** It is a longer acting analgesic antiinflammatory drug. It is given once daily. ***Dose :*** 20 mg OD. It inhibits activation of neutrophils and decreases IgM rheumatoid factor. GI adverse effects and allergic rash is common.
- **Ketorolac :** It is primarily used as eye drops for seasonal allergic conjunctivitis. Orally it is given short term management of pain.

### PREFERENTIAL COX-2 INHIBITOR (INHIBIT COX-2 > COX-1) :

#### Nimesulide :

- Its antiinflammatory action apart from PG synthesis, is by other mechanisms as well like reduced generation of superoxide, reduced TNF-$\alpha$ release, free radical scavanging, inhibition of metalloproteinase activity in cartilage.
- The analgesic, antipyretic and antiinflammatory activity of nimesulide is good.
- It is used for various painful inflammatory conditions like musculoskeletal pain, dental pain, low backache, dysmenorrhea, postoperative pain, osteoarthritis, joint pain and for fever.
- Due to lesser inhibition of COX-1, it causes lesser GI adverse effects. But, still some GI adverse effects occur. It also causes rash, dizziness etc.
- It also causes fulminant hepatitis especially in children, therefore not used in pediatric population.

### SELECTIVE COX-2 INHIBITORS (INHIBIT ONLY COX-2) :

- *Celecoxib, Rofecoxib, Valdecoxib, Etoricoxib, Parecoxib.*
- They are selective inhibitor of inducible COX-2 without inhibiting the physiological housekeeper COX-1.

#### Advantages of Selective COX-2 inhibitors :

- Lesser chances of gastritis and peptic ulcers as seen in non-selective COX inhibitors like aspirin (They don't inhibit COX-1 which is gastroprotective).
- They do not inhibit platelet aggregation or prolong bleeding time as they do not inhibit $TXA_2$ production by platelets (COX-I dependent).

#### Uses :

- They are useful in all the painful conditions mentioned under Non-selective COX inhibitors especially in patients with peptic ulcers, gastritis and GI bleed.
- If used, they should be given in the lowest possible dose for the shortest period of time.

#### Adverse effects :

- Increased chances of thromboembolic phenomenon like stroke or myocardial infarction (should be avoided in patients with history or who are predisposed to cardiovascular and cerebrovascular events).

- Edema.
- Steven Johnson syndrome.
- Allergic rash.

***Celecoxib :***

- Celecoxib is metabolised primarily by CYP2C9. Therefore, caution must be taken while prescribing inhibitor of CYP2C9 like fluconazole, which can increase plasma levels of celecoxib.

***Rofecoxib and Valdecoxib :***

- They were withdrawn from market because of increased risks of heart attacks and strokes.

***Etoricoxib :***

- This COX-2 inhibitor has high COX-2 selectivity.
- It is suitable for once a day treatment of various painful and inflammatory conditions.
- The plasma half life is 24 hours.
- **Dose :** 60 mg, 90 mg, 120 mg OD.

***Parecoxib :***

- It is newer drug which is a prodrug of valdecoxib suitable for injection, and to be used in postoperative or similar short-term pain, with efficacy similar to ketorolac.

## ANALGESICS-ANTIPYRETICS WITH POOR ANTIINFLAMMATORY ACTION :

### Paracetamol (Acetaminophen) :

- It is one of the most commonly used analgesic and antipyretic drug.
- It has very poor antiinflammatory action.
- It poorly inhibits COX-1 in the periphery at the site of inflammation, but not in hypothalamus where the temperature regulating centre of the body lies.
- Recently, it has been suggested that paracetamol also inhibits COX-3 in the CNS. COX-3 is involved in pain perception and fever but not in inflammation.
- ***Advantages :*** It does not cause gastric mucosal damage and has no effect on platelet aggregation.
- ***Dose :*** 500 mg TDS.
- ***Uses :*** Mild to moderate pain such as headache, musculoskeletal pain, fever.
- ***Adverse effects :*** It is quite safe and well tolerated. In higher doses and in toxicities, it can cause hepatic damage (antidote used in treatment of paracetamol poisoning is N-acetyl cysteine).

# 24 DRUG THERAPY FOR GOUT AND RHEUMATOID ARTHRITIS

## DRUG THERAPY FOR GOUT :

### Gout :

- Gout is a metabolic disorder characterised by elevated uric acid levels along with recurrent episodes of acute and chronic arthritis due to deposition of monosodium urate crystals in joints and cartilages. There are also chances of formation of uric acid calculi in the kidneys.
- Gout usually affects the 1$^{st}$ metatarsophalangeal joint of the big toe, but can also affect other joints. After several years, the crystals can build up in the joints and surrounding tissues, forming large deposits, called tophi.
- Uric acid is a waste product produced during metabolism of purines (DNA and RNA). It is synthesised from xanthine by the enzyme xanthine oxidase. Uric acid is freely filtered by glomerulus of kidney and then reabsorbed from the tubules.

### Causes :

- Familial, genetic in origin, obesity, heavy alcohol use, high protein diet can increase risk of gout. Thiazide diuretics also increase uric acid levels.

### Normal uric acid levels :

- 2.4-6.0 mg/dL (females) and 3.4-7.0 mg/dL (males).

### Pathophysiology :

- Urate crystals are initially phagocytosed by synoviocytes, which then release prostaglandins, lysosomal enzymes and interleukin-1 which attract and activate polymorphonuclear leucocytes and mononuclear phagocytes (macrophages).
- In the later phases of the attack, increased numbers of mononuclear phagocytes (macrophages) appear and ingest the urate crystals, and release more inflammatory mediators.
- Another precipitating factor is the release of the lysosomal enzymes which cause more joint and cartilage destruction.

### Types of gout :

- ***Acute gout :*** It is a painful, arthritic, sudden attack, which usually occurs at night. The joint is painful, red, swollen and warm. There can be associated fever, chills and malaise.
- ***Chronic gout :*** Chronic hyperuricemia may lead the patients to develop tophi

deposition in joints, in the pinna of external ear, tip of the nose. There can be urate calculi, joint destruction.

**Treatment :**

***Non-pharmacological treatment :***

- Avoid high protein diet like red meat, seafood etc. drink plenty of water and fluids, lose weight and exercise regularly, avoid alcohol use, avoid thiazide diuretics.

## CLASSIFICATION OF DRUGS USED FOR GOUT :

**Drugs for acute gout :**

- **Colchicine.**
- ***NSAIDs :*** Ibuprofen, Diclofenac, Naproxen, Indomethacin etc.
- ***Corticosteroids :*** Prednisolone, Methylprednisolone etc.

**Drugs for chronic gout :**

- ***Uric acid Synthesis inhibitor :*** Allopurinol, Febuxostat.
- ***Uricosuric drugs :*** Probenecid, Sulfinpyrazone.
- **Uricase-mimetics :** Pegloticase, Rasburicase.
- ***URAT-1 inhibitor :*** Lesinurad.

### *Colchicine :*

- Is neither analgesic nor antiinflammatory, but it suppresses gouty inflammation.
- It does not inhibit the synthesis or promote the excretion of uric acid, and has no effect on blood uric acid levels.
- **Mechanism of action :** Colchicine acts by binding to the intracellular protein tubulin, thereby causing depolymerisation of microtubules in granulocytes (arresting neutrophil motility) and leading to the inhibition of leucocyte migration and phagocytosis.
- **Use :** Acute attack of gout.
- **Dose :** 1 mg orally followed by 0.5 mg every 3 hours until the pain is relieved or adverse effects of colchicines like nausea and diarrhea appear.
- **Adverse effects :** Diarrhea, nausea, vomiting, and abdominal pain. Rarely, hair loss and bone marrow depression as well as peripheral neuritis and myopathy.

### NSAIDs :

- **Mechanism of action :** Inhibit prostaglandin synthesis. In addition, some NSAIDs like Indomethacin also inhibit urate crystal phagocytosis.
- **Use :** Acute attack of gout.
- **Dose :** Ibuprofen 400 mg TDS orally, Diclofenac 50 mg TDS orally or IM, Indomethacin 25 mg TDS.
- **Adverse effects :** Nausea, vomiting, gastritis, GI bleed, abdominal pain etc.

## Corticosteroids :

- **Mechanism of action :** Inhibit prostaglandin synthesis as well as inhibit all processes of inflammation. Details are explained in the chapter on corticosteroids.
- They can be given orally, parenterally and as intra-articular injections.
- **Use :** Acute attack of gout.
- **Adverse effects :** Cushingoid features, hypertension, hyperglycemia, immuno-suppression etc.

## Uric acid synthesis inhibitors :

**Allopurinol :**

- ***Mechanism of action :*** It inhibits the rate limiting step in the synthesis of uric acid by inhibiting the enzyme *Xanthine oxidase*.

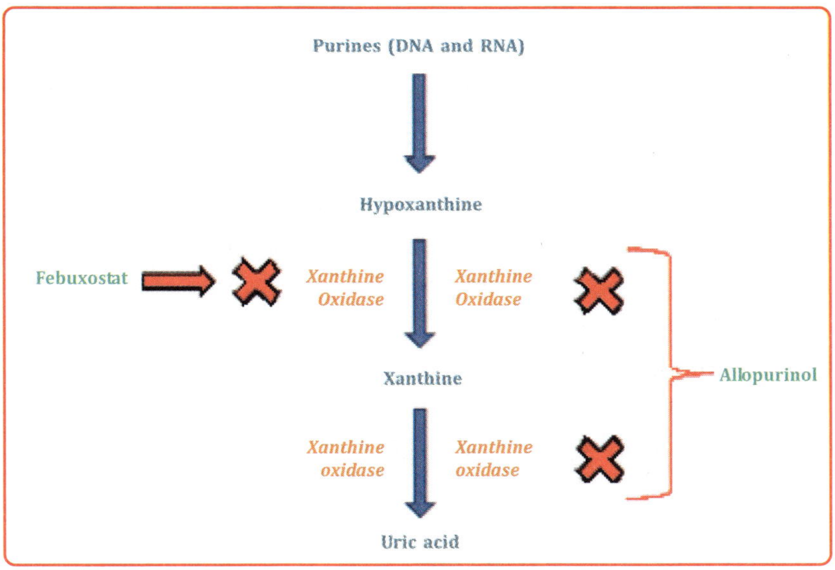


- Allopurinol inhibits xanthine oxidase and prevents conversion of hypoxanthine to xanthine and xanthine to uric acid.
- ***Use :*** prophylaxis of chronic gout and hyperuricemia, recurrent uric acid stones, secondary hyperuricemia due to cancer chemotherapy and thiazide diuretics. Allopurinol is also used with sodium stibogluconate in treatment of kala-azar.
- ***Dose :*** Allopurinol 100-300 mg / day orally.
- ***Adverse effects :*** Precipitation of acute attack, nausea, vomiting, diarrhea. Peripheral neuritis and necrotising vasculitis, depression of bone marrow, aplastic anemia may also occur. Allergic skin rash and exfoliative dermatitis is also reported.

**Febuxostat :**

- Febuxostat is a newer selective inhibitor of xanthine oxidase and thus prevents formation of uric acid.
- ***Uses :*** Prophylaxis of chronic gout and hyperuricemia, recurrent uric acid stones, secondary hyperuricemia due to cancer chemotherapy and thiazide diuretics.
- ***Dose :*** Febuxostat 80-120 mg OD.
- ***Adverse effects :*** Precipitation of acute attack, nausea, vomiting, diarrhoea and headache. Some cases of liver dysfunction are also reported.

### Uricosuric drugs :

- *Probenecid, Sulphinpyrazone.*
- ***Mechanism of action :*** They inhibit reabsorption of uric acid from renal tubules. This leads to more and more excretion of uric acid from the body.
- Plenty of fluid intakes should be there to prevent formation of renal urate calculi.
- ***Uses :*** Prophylaxis of chronic gout and hyperuricemia, secondary hyperuricemia due to cancer chemotherapy and thiazide diuretics. Probenecid is also used to prolong penicillins or cephalosporin levels in the blood. (probenecid inhibits tubular secretion of these drugs).
- ***Dose :*** Probenecid 250-500 mg BD.
- ***Adverse effects :*** Nausea, vomiting, allergic rash.

### Uricase-mimetics :

- *Pegloticase, Rasburicase.*
- In most mammals, uricase converts uric acid to the more soluble allantoin which is excreted by kidneys; this enzyme is absent in humans.
- Uricase mimetics are newer anti-gout drugs that mimic the action of uricase and metabolise uric acid to more soluble form.
- Worsening of gout symptoms can occur during its treatment and NSAIDs and corticosteroids can be needed.

### URAT-1 inhibitor : Lesinurad :

- This is a new entry to the list of anti-gout medications.
- Uric acid transporter (URAT-1) causes reabsorption of uric acid in the kidneys.
- By inhibiting URAT-1, this reabsorption is prevented and the levels of uric acid fall in the blood.

## DRUG THERAPY FOR RHEUMATOID ARTHRITIS :

### Rheumatoid arthritis :

- It is an Auto immune disease where there is joint inflammation, synovial proliferation and destruction of articular cartilage. It is a chronic progressive, crippling disorder with a waxing and waning course.

### Causes :

- Cause of rheumatoid arthritis remains unclear with hormonal, genetic and environmental factors playing a key role.

### Pathophysiology :

- Immune complexes composed of IgM activate complement and release cytokines which are chemotactic to neutrophils. IL-1, IL-6, TNF-α are important mediators of inflammation in RA.
- Inflammatory cells secrete lysosomal enzymes which damage cartilage and erode bone while prostaglandins cause vasodilatation and pain.
- The synovial membrane becomes highly vascularised and hypertrophied, creating a so called pannus formation. Ultimately, there is destruction of joints with progressive deformities.

### Clinical features :

- Morning stiffness, swelling in more than or equal to 3 joints, swelling in hand joints, symmetric joint involvement, erosions or decalcifications on X-ray of hand, rheumatoid nodules, deformities.
- Extra-articular features : Vasculitis, pulmonary complications, ocular manifestations, cardiac involvement, felty syndrome etc.

### Diagnosis :

- Clinical diagnosis, RA factor, anti-CCP antibody, anemia and elevated ESR, CRP, Radiological features.

### Treatment :

#### *Goals :*

- Symptomatic relief, slowing or prevention of joint damage, preserving and improving functional ability and achieving and maintaining disease remission.

#### *Non-pharmacological treatment :*

- Adequate rest, weight reduction, occupational therapy, physical therapy, use of assistive devices may improve symptoms and help maintain joint function, patients with severe disease may benefit from surgical procedures such as teno synovectomy, tendon repair and Joint replacements.

## DRUGS FOR RHEUMATOID ARTHRITIS :

### DMARDs (Disease modifying anti-rheumatoid drugs) :

#### *Non-biologics :*

- Immunosuppressants : Methotrexate, Azathioprine, Cyclosporin.
- Sulphasalazine.
- Chloroquine and Hydroxychloroquine.

- Leflunomide.
- D-Penicillamine.
- Gold compounds.

***Biologics :***

- TNF-α inhibitors : Etanercept, Infliximab, Adalimumab.
- IL-1 antagonist : Anakinra, Rilonacept.

***Others :***

- NSAIDs, Corticosteroids.

- **Methotrexate :**
  - DMARD of first choice in RA. The doses needed in RA are much lower than those needed in cancer chemotherapy.
  - ***Mechanism of action :*** It is a dihydrofolate reductase inhibitor. It causes selective inhibition of DNA synthesis and inhibits replication and function of T-cells. It also inhibits cytokine production.
  - ***Dose :*** 7.5-15 mg weekly (along with folic acid).
  - ***Uses :*** Rheumatoid arthritis, psoriasis, psoriatic arthritis, juvenile chronic arthritis, SLE.
  - ***Adverse effects :*** Mucosal ulcers, Hepatotoxicity.

- **Azathioprine :**
  - ***Mechanism of action :*** It is converted in the body to 6-thio GTP which gets falsely incorporated into DNA of lymphocyte, making it non-functional. Hence, T-cell activation and proliferation is prevented.
  - ***Dose :*** 50-150 mg/day.
  - ***Uses :*** Rheumatoid arthritis, organ transplant and inflammatory bowel disease.
  - ***Adverse effects :*** Bone marrow depression, alopecia, hepatotoxicity, increase in infection risk, GI disturbances.

- **Cyclosporin :**
  - ***Mechanism of action :*** It inhibits IL-1 and IL-2 receptor production. It also inhibits macrophages-T cell interaction.
  - ***Dose :*** 3-5 mg/kg/day.
  - ***Adverse effects :*** Nephrotoxicity, hepatotoxicity, gingival hyperplasia.

- **Sulphasalazine :**
  - ***Mechanism of action :*** Sulphasalazine is poorly absorbed from the intestine and gets converted in the GIT to 5-aminosalicylic acid (5-ASA) and sulphapyridine. This 5-ASA exerts local anti-inflammatory response in the GIT. Sulphapyridine is absorbed systemically and exerts its effects which are used in the treatment of rheumatoid arthritis. It inhibits

production of cytokines, PAF, TNF-α, prostaglandins and leukotrienes. Migration of inflammatory cells is interfered.

- ***Dose :*** 500-1500 mg BD.
- ***Uses :*** Rheumatoid arthritis, ulcerative colitis, Crohn's disease.
- ***Adverse effects :*** Neutropenia, thrombocytopenia and hepatitis.

- **Choloroquine and hydroxychloroquine :**
  - It is basically an antimalarial drug which is used in mild RA.
  - Onset delayed for up to 6 weeks. Hydroxychloroquine is preferred.
  - ***Mechanism of action :*** It traps free radicals, suppresses T-cell responses, stabilises lysosomal enzymes and decreases leucocyte migration.
  - ***Dose :*** HCQS (Hydroxychloroquine sulphate) 200 mg BD orally.
  - ***Uses :*** Rheumatoid arthritis (milder, non-erosive form).
  - ***Adverse effects :*** Corneal deposits and opacities, rashes, graying of hairs, neuropathy and myopathy.

- **Leflunomide :**
  - It is an immunomodulator.
  - ***Mechanism of action :*** It is rapidly converted to active metabolite which inhibits dihydroorotate dehydrogenase & pyrimidine synthesis in actively dividing cells. It inhibits proliferation of stimulated lymphocytes.
  - Arthritic symptoms are suppressed and radiological disease progression is retarded. Efficacy is comparable to methotrexate.
  - Onset of action is 4 weeks.
  - ***Dose :*** Loading dose 100 mg daily for 3 days followed by 20 mg OD.
  - ***Adverse effects :*** Diarrhea, nausea, thrombocytopenia, leucopenia, increased chances of infections.

- **D-Penicillamine :**
  - It is primarily a chelating agent which was previously used, but not used nowadays due to its toxicity and availability of better drugs.

- **Gold compounds :**
  - It reduces chemotaxis, phagocytosis and lysosomal activity.
  - Parenteral : Gold sodium thiomalate, Oral : Auranofin.
  - Gold compounds are not used nowadays due to its toxicity and availability of better drugs.
  - ***Adverse effects :*** **Oral :** diarrhea and abdominal cramps. **Parenteral :** hypoten-sion, dermatitis, rash, stomatitis, albuminuria, hepatitis, peripheral neuritis etc.

- **TNF-α inhibitors :**
  - TNF-α is a potent inflammatory cytokine produced mainly by macrophages and monocytes. It plays an important role in joint

destruction. It causes vasodilation, increases vascular permeability, platelet activation and adhesion. Blockade of TNF results in a reduction in a number of other pro-inflammatory cytokines (IL-1, IL-6 & IL-8).

- **Etanercept :**
  - It is a recombinant fusion protein of TNF receptor and Fc portion of human IgG. Slows erosive disease progression more than oral methotrexate. Used mainly in patients with inadequate response to methotrexate monotherapy.
  - ***Dose :*** 50 mg subcutaneous injection weekly.
  - ***Uses :*** Rheumatoid arthritis, chronic juvenile arthritis, psoriatic arthritis, scleroderma, sarcoidosis.
  - ***Adverse effects :*** Increased chances of infections, drug induced lupus.

- **Infliximab :**
  - It is a chimeric (25% mouse and 75% human) anti- TNF-α antibody. Combination of infliximab and Methotrexate is used. Halts progression of joint damage. Superior to Methotrexate monotherapy.
  - ***Dose :*** 3-5 mg/kg IV every 4-8 weeks.
  - ***Uses :*** Rheumatoid arthritis, chronic juvenile arthritis, psoriatic arthritis, scleroderma, sarcoidosis.
  - ***Adverse effects :*** Acute infusion reaction, increased chances of infections auto-antibodies and lupus-like syndrome has also been reported.

- **Adalimumab :**
  - It is a recombinant anti TNF-α monoclonal antibody. It is less immunogenic than Infliximab. Combination with Methotrexate improves response and decreases antibody formation.
  - ***Dose :*** 40 mg SC every 2 weekly.
  - ***Adverse effects :*** It is having same adverse effect profile as that of Infliximab.

- **IL-1 antagonist :**

  ***Anakinra :***
  - Clinically less effective than TNF-α inhibitors.
  - ***Use :*** Used in cases of failure of one or more DMARDs.
  - ***Dose :*** 100 mg subcutaneously.
  - ***Adverse effects :*** Local reaction to injection, chest infections.

- **NSAIDs :**
  - Ibuprofen 400 mg TDS orally, Diclofenac 50 mg TDS orally or IM, Indomethacin 25 mg TDS used.
  - Mechanism of action and adverse effects are explained in their respective chapter.

- **Corticosteroids :**
  - They can be given orally, parenterally and as intra-articular injections.
  - Mechanism and adverse effects are explained in their respective chapter.
- **NSAIDs and corticosteroids :**
  - Afford symptomatic relief
  - Reduce inflammation, pain, swelling and morning stiffness and improve joint function.
  - They do not halt the disease progression.

# DRUGS ACTING ON RESPIRATORY SYSTEM (RS)

# 25 DRUGS FOR BRONCHIAL ASTHMA

Asthma is a chronic inflammatory disease characterised by : A-B-C

**A** Airway Hyper responsiveness

**B** Bronchoconstriction (reversible)

**C** Chronic inflammation

There is also excessive secretion of mucus that may block the airway and worsen the condition.

### Clinical features :

- Breathlessness, cough, wheezing, chest tightness, in acute attack : tachypnea, tachycardia.

### Pathogenesis :

Antigens like pollen grains, dust mites, animal dander or any other allergen sensitise the individual and causes production of IgE antidody which remain in circulation or get attached to mast cells or basophils. On re-exposure to the same antigen, antigen-antibody reaction occurs and causes degranulation of mast cells releasing histamine, serotonin and leukotrienes which causes bronchoconstriction.

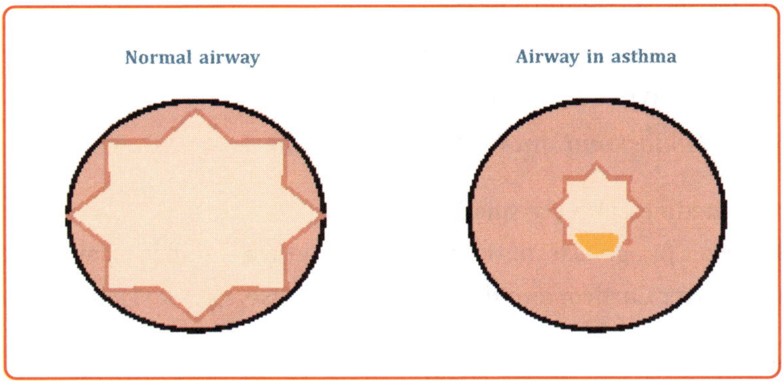

### Receptors on bronchial smooth muscles :

The main receptors that are present on the bronchial smooth muscles in the respiratory tract are :

| Receptor | Action |
|---|---|
| $\beta_2$ adrenergic | Bronchodilation |
| $M_3$ cholinergic receptors | Bronchoconstriction |

## CLASSIFICATION OF DRUGS FOR ASTHMA :

### Bronchodilators :

- ***$\beta_2$ agonists :***
  - **Short acting :** Salbutamol, Terbutaline.
  - **Long acting :** Salmeterol, Formeterol, Bambuterol.
  - **Ultralong acting :** Indicaterol.
- ***Methylxanthines :*** Theophylline, Aminophylline, Doxophylline.
- ***Anticholinergics :*** Ipratropium, Tiotropium.
- ***Sympathomimetics :*** Adrenaline, Ephedrine.

### Anti-inflammatory agents :

- ***Corticosteroids :***
  - **Oral :** Prednisolone, Methylprednisolone, betamethasone.
  - **Parenteral :** Hydrocortisone, Dexamethasone.
  - **Inhalational :** Beclomethasone, Budesonide, Ciclesonide, Fluticasone.
- ***Mast Cell Stabilisers :*** Sodium cromoglycate, Nedocromil, Ketotifen.
- ***Leukotriene Modulators :***
  - **Leukotriene receptor antagonist :** Montelukast, Zafirlukast, Pranlukast.
  - **5-Lipooxygenase inhibitor :** Zileuton.
- ***Anti-IgE Monoclonal Antibody :*** Omalizumab.

They are sometimes also classified as :

- **Relievers :** $\beta_2$ agonists, anticholinergics, methylxanthines, sympathomimetics.
- **Controllers :** Corticosteroids, mast cell stabilisers, leukotriene modulators.

### $\beta_2$ agonists :

- These are one of the most widely used drugs for bronchial asthma. Short acting are usually used in acute attack and long acting are used in prophylaxis.

☞ **Mechanism of action :**

**$\beta_2$ Agonists**

⇩

**Stimulation $\beta_2$ receptors**

⇩

**↑ cAMP**

⇩

**Bronchial smooth muscle relaxation**
**(Bronchodilation)**

☞ **Routes and modes of administration :**

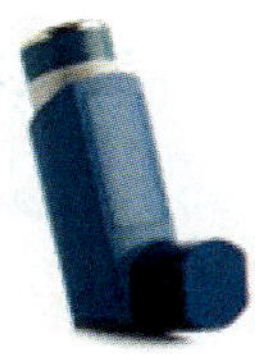

Metered dose inhaler (MDI)

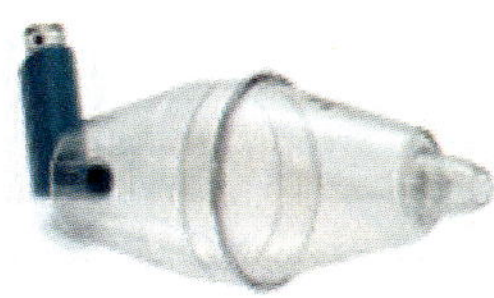

Inhaler with spacer

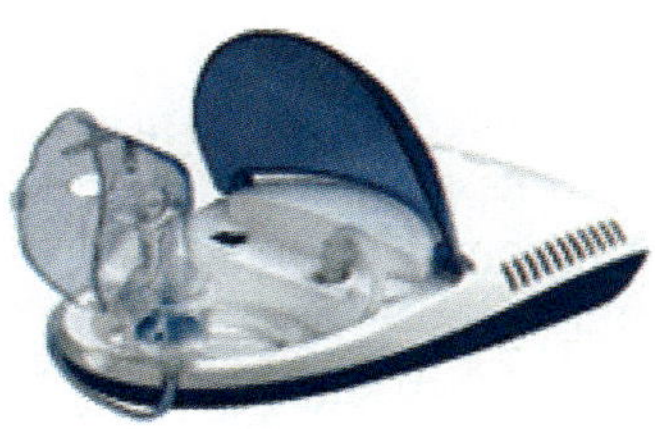

Nebuliser

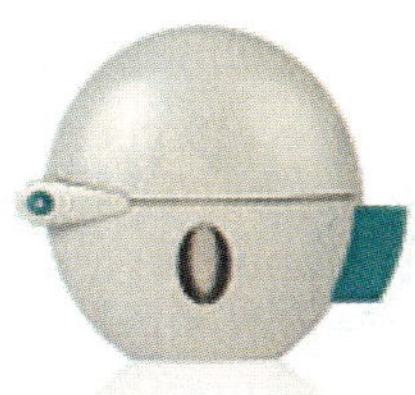

Dry power inhaler

$\beta_2$ agonists are usually delivered via a metered dose inhaler (MDI). The IV route is used for acute attack. Terbutaline is also given by SC route. Other inhalational mode of giving these is by nebulisation. Dry powdered forms can be given by dry powder inhalers. For better compliance especially in children and elderly, an inhaler with spacer is used. Inhalational route is most preferred. Advantage of inhalational route is the drug act directly on bronchial smooth muscle without causing systemic effects.

☞ Most short acting drugs act rapidly with onset of action of 5-15 minutes and duration of action of 4-6 hours and long acting drugs have delayed onset of action *i.e.* 30-60 minutes and duration of action of 12-24 hours. Therefore, short acting are usually used in acute attack and long acting are used in prophylaxis (chronic asthma).

- **Uses :** Acute attack of asthma, status asthmaticus, chronic asthma, COPD.
- **Adverse effects :** Skeletal muscle tremors, tachycardia (at high dose has $\beta_1$ effects), tolerance to $\beta$ agonist action (down-regulation of $\beta_2$ receptors), palpitations, restlessness, ankle edema.
- **Levosalbutamol :** This drug is an R enantiomer of salbutamol.

## Methylxanthines : *Theophylline, Aminophylline, Doxophylline :*

- **Mechanism of action :** They inhibit the enzyme phosphodiesterase-3 (PDE) in bronchial smooth muscles which metabolises cAMP to AMP. The cAMP levels therefore, get elevated leading to bronchodilatation.

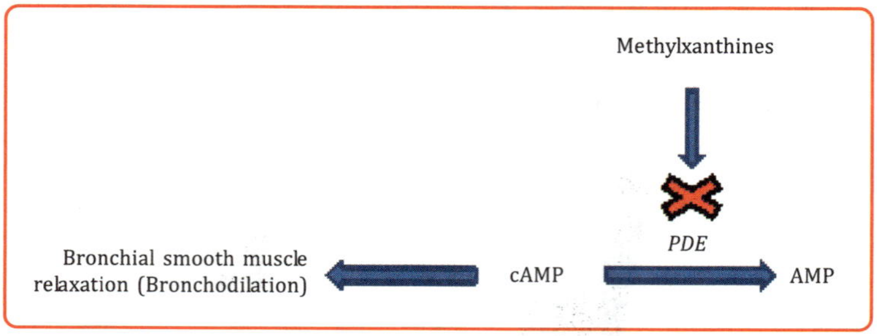


- **Uses :** Acute attack of bronchial asthma, status asthmaticus, chronic asthma, dyspnea of cardiac failure due to pulmonary edema (Theophylline), COPD.
- **Adverse effects :** They have a narrow therapeutic index. Its therapeutic and toxic effects are related to its plasma concentration. Adverse effects commonly seen are nausea, vomiting, headache, anxiety, abdominal discomfort. Cardiac arrhythmia are seen with parenteral use especially with Aminophylline (Therefore, Aminophylline is given as slow IV infusion of 500 mg of Aminophylline in 100 ml of 5% dextrose slowly over 30 min).
- **Drug interactions :** Smoking induces metabolism of theophylline, thus reduces its plasma levels. Antibiotics like erythromycin and ciprofloxacin decreases metabolism of theophylline, thus increase its plasma levels.

## Anticholinergics : *Ipratropium, Tiotropium :*

- **Mechanism of action :** They act by competitive blocking of muscarinic cholinergic $M_3$ receptors in bronchioles. They also decrease mucus gland secretion. They also reverse acute and vagally mediated bronchospasm.
- They cause less effective bronchodilation than $\beta_2$ agonists. They are usually given by inhalational route. This avoids systemic anticholinergic side effects. They are commonly used in combination of $\beta_2$ agonists like salbutamol. They are used when $\beta_2$ agonists are not tolerated or are contraindicated. Tiotropium is a longer acting congener of ipratropium.

- **Uses :** COPD, bronchial asthma.
- **Adverse effects :** Dryness of mouth, bad taste, cough.

## Sympathomimetics : *Adrenaline :*

- Unlike $\beta_2$ agonists they are non-selective agonist of $\alpha$ and $\beta$ receptors. They are less commonly used.
- **Use :** SC injection of 0.5 ml of 1:1000 adrenaline / nebulisation is used in non-responding acute attack of bronchial asthma and status asthmaticus.
- **Adverse effect :** Tachycardia, hypertension, worsening of angina and even arrhythmias.

## Corticosteroids :

- **Mechanism of action :** They are anti-inflammatory agents that depress the inflammatory response in bronchial mucosa thus, diminish bronchial hyper responsiveness. This is done by inhibiting phospholipase $A_2$ enzyme, a key enzyme in the inflammatory process. They also inhibit the

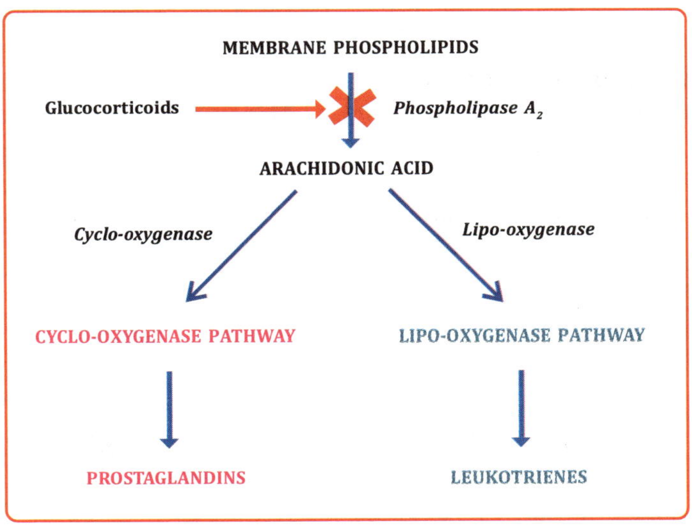


formation of leukotrienes which are potent bronchoconstrictors, thus causing bronchodilatation. They also decrease secretions and mucus formation in the bronchial tree. The//.y inhibit the release of histamine and other cytokines from the mast cells.

- **Routes and modes of administration :** *Inhalational* : Metered dose inhaler or nebulisation - Budesonide 200 to 400 µg BD or QID or Beclomethasone 50 µg or 100 µg per metered dose. *Intravenous* : used for severe asthma, status asthmaticus - Hydrocortisone hemisuccinate 100-200 mg every 8 hourly. *Oral* : Used for prophylaxis and chronic asthma - prednisolone 10 mg BD.

- **Uses :** Acute attack of asthma, status asthmaticus, chronic asthma, COPD.
- **Adverse effects :** *Local (with inhalational preparations)* : Cough, bad taste, oral candidiasis. *Systemic (with injectable and oral preparations)* : Adrenal suppression, hypertension, hyperglycemia, osteoporosis etc.

## Mast cell stabilisers : *Sodium cromoglycate, Nedocromil, Ketotifen :*

- **Mechanism of action :** They prevent antigen-IgE mediated transmembrane influx of $Ca^{+2}$ ions on mast cell. This prevents degranulation of mast cells and subsequent release of chemical mediators. They also decrease eosinophil recruitment. They are specific for lung mast cells and not the mast cells in the skin. Ketotifen has got additional antihistaminic property.
- **Dose and route :** Sodium cromoglycate 800 mcg per puff (2-4 puffs 4 times a day), Ketotifen (orally 1 to 2 mg BD).
- **Use :** These are reserved for prophylaxis of chronic and seasonal asthma but, are ineffective in acute attacks. They help in reducing the dose and frequency of corticosteroids and $\beta_2$ agonists.
- **Adverse effects :** Throat irritation, dryness of mouth, headache.

## Leukotriene modulators :

**Leukotriene receptor antagonist : *Montelukast, Zafirlukast, Pranlukast :***

- ***Mechanism of action :*** Leukotrienes are powerful bronchoconstrictor and act by activating cysteinyl leukotriene rerecptors (cys-LT receptor).

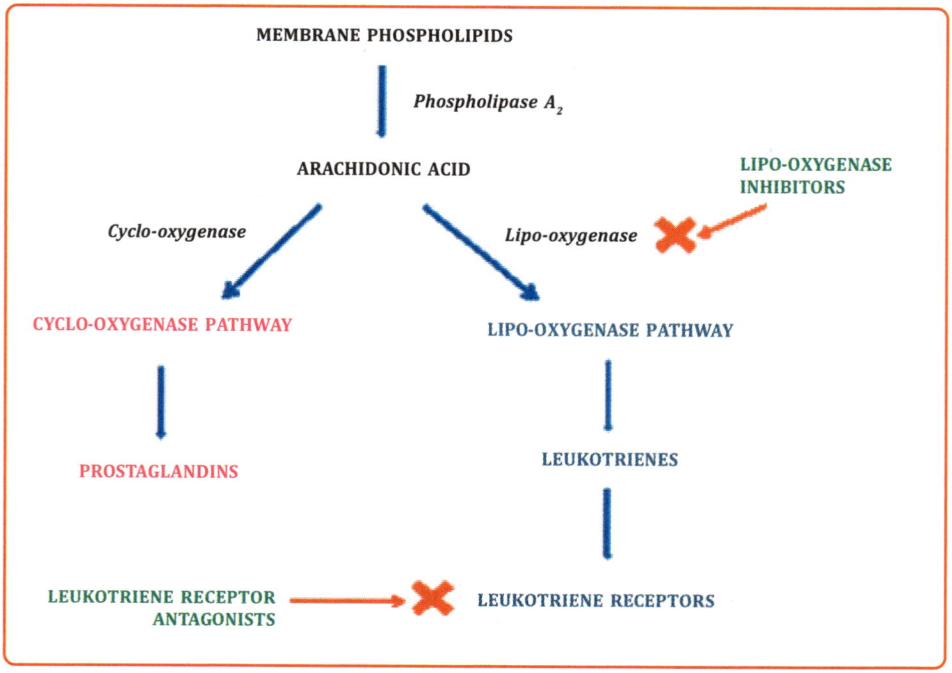

These drugs inhibit these leukotriene receptors and thus the action of Leukotrienes is not mediated and this results in bronchodilation.

- ***Zafirlukast :*** bioavailability is decreased after food, therefore taken 2 hrs before meal and 12 hrly. But, montelukast (10 mg) is taken just once daily and its bioavailability is not affected by food.
- ***Uses :*** As alternative to low dose steroids in mild persistent asthma for prophylaxis and allergic rhinitis (montelukast + levocetirizine).
- ***Adverse effects :*** Rarely, Churg-Strauss syndrome (vasculitis, eosinophilia and worsening of asthma). Some cases of neuropsychiatric symptoms were reported recently.

**5-Lipooxygenase inhibitor : *Zileuton :***

- ***Mechanism of action :*** It inhibits leukotriene production by blocking lipo-oxygenase enzyme.
- ***Use :*** As an alternatives to low dose steroids in mild persistent asthma.
- ***Adverse effects :*** Hepatotoxicity (hence, withdrawn from many countries).

### Anti-IgE Monoclonal Antibody Omalizumab :

- ***Mechanism of action :*** It prevents the binding of IgE to mast cell & thus prevents mast cell degranulation.
- ***Route of administration :*** IV or SC injection.
- ***Adverse effects :*** Redness, stinging, itching, induration.

## STATUS ASTHMATICUS :

It is a severe attack of acute asthma which is potentially life-threatening. The clinical features seen in these patients are severe breathlessness, cyanosis, exhaustion, bradycardia, hypotension, dehydration and metabolic acidosis. It is a medical emergency and has to be treated aggressively to prevent mortality and morbidity.

### Treatment :

- Inj. Hydrocortisone hemisuccinate 200 mg I.V stat followed by 100-200 mg 4-8 hourly.
- Nebulised salbutamol (2.5-5 mg) + ipratropium bromide (0.5 mg) intermittent inhalations driven by $O_2$.
- Inj. Aminophylline 500 mg in 100 ml of 5% dextrose slowly over 30 min in non-responding cases.
- Adrenaline SC injection of 0.5 ml of 1:1000 adrenaline / nebulisation is used if not responding to above drugs.
- High flow humidified oxygen inhalation 6-8 lit/min.
- Intubation & mechanical ventilation, if needed.

# 26 DRUGS FOR COUGH

Cough is a protective reflex for expulsion of respiratory secretions and foreign bodies from air passages.

## TYPES OF COUGH :

- Dry cough / non-productive cough.
- Cough with expectoration / productive cough.

### Causes of cough :

- Upper and lower respiratory tract infection, postnasal drip due to sinusitis, rhinitis, smoking and chronic bronchitis, pulmonary tuberculosis, asthmatic cough, gastrointestinal reflux, foreign body, drugs like ACE inhibitors.

### Treatment :

Let's make one thing very clear about treatment of different types of cough :

- **For dry cough – Antitussives / cough suppressants.**
- **For cough with expectoration – Expectorants and Mucolytics.**

**Note :** Cough with expectoration (productive cough) is associated with secretions, mucus and phlegm in the respiratory tract. We should never use Antitussives (cough suppressants) for cough with expectoration because, cough is a protective reflex in which attempts are made by the body to remove secretions from the respiratory tract and antitussives suppresses this protective reflex. This leads to accumulation of secretions inside the respiratory tract and this can worsen the condition and can also give rise to infections in the respiratory tract

### Some common terms :

- ***Antitussives :*** Drugs that suppress the cough.
- ***Expectorants :*** Drugs that increase volume of mucus secretion.
- ***Mucolytics :*** Drugs that reduce viscosity of mucus.
- ***Mucokinetics :*** Drugs that increase movement of secretions.

## CLASSIFICATION OF DRUGS FOR COUGH :

- **Antitussives (Cough suppressants) :**
  - ***Centrally acting :***
    - **Opioids :** Codeine, Pholcodeine.
    - **Non-opioids :** Noscapine, Dextromethorphan.

- ***Peripherally acting :*** Pharyngeal demulcents : Honey, lozenges, Liquorice.

- **Expectorants (Mucokinetics) :**

  Guaifenesin, Guaiacol, Sodium citrate, Ammonium chloride.

- **Mucolytic :**

  Bromhexine, Ambroxol, Acetylcysteine, Carbocysteine, Dornase alpha.

- **Others :**

  Antihistaminics, Bronchodilators, Local anesthetic.

## ANTITUSSIVES :

- ***Mechanism of action :*** They raise the threshold of cough centre in medulla. In respiratory tract reduce cough impulse.
- ***Use :*** All kinds of dry coughs (non-productive cough).
- ***Contraindication :*** Cough with expectoration.

### Codeine :

- It is a semi synthetic opioid analgesic but, less potent than morphine. It is more selective for cough centre. It shows potent cough suppressant action at low dose. Its antitussive action is blocked by opioid antagonists like Naloxone.
- ***Advantage :*** It has less addiction liability as compared to morphine.
- ***Adverse effects :*** Constipation, sedation, respiratory depression in large doses.
- ***Dose :*** 10 mg BD.

### Pholcodeine :

- It is structurally related to codeine and has antitussive efficacy similar to codeine. No analgesic or addictive effect. Causes lesser drowsiness and constipation as compared to codeine.
- ***Dose :*** 10-15 mg 3-4 times a day.

### Noscapine :

- It is an opium alkaloid and has no addictive, analgesic or constipating properties.
- ***Adverse effects :*** It can release histamine and can cause broncho-constriction, especially in asthmatics, nausea, headache, tremors.
- ***Dose :*** 15 mg.

### Dextromethorphan :

- It is one of the most commonly used antitussives. It raises threshold for cough centre. Its antitussive action is not blocked by Naloxone. Amongst the antitussives, it has got least addiction and constipation property. It has no analgesic action and no affect on mucociliary action.

- ***Adverse effects :*** Nausea, vomiting, ataxia, minimal drowsiness.
- ***Dose :*** 10 mg TDS.

**Pharyngeal demulcents :**

- They sooth the throat. They reduce afferent impulse from inflamed pharyngeal mucosa and offer symptomatic relief in dry cough arising due to throat irritation.

## EXPECTORANTS (Mucokinetics) :

**Guaifenesin, Guaiacol, Sodium citrate, Ammonium chloride :**

- ***Mechanism of action :*** These drugs stimulate the flow of respiratory secretions in productive cough patients by stimulating bronchial secretory cells which increases the volume of the secretions and also increases the mucociliary movements in the respiratory tract (mucokinetic action) to facilitate their removal.
- Guaifenesin and Guaiacol are obtained from creosote wood but now are made synthetically. Guaifenesin is less irritating than Guaiacol. The citrate from Sodium citrate after absorption gets converted into bicarbonate and mucus becomes less viscous in alkaline pH. Ammonium chloride is a gastric irritant. In larger doses, it causes metabolic acidosis.
- ***Use :*** Cough with expectoration (Productive cough).

## MUCOLYTICS :

- ***Mechanism of action :*** They decrease the viscosity of mucus in the respiratory tract and facilitate its removal.
- ***Use :*** Cough with expectoration (Productive cough).

**Bromhexine :**

- It is a synthetic derivative of *Vasaka plant.*
- ***Mechanism of action :*** It depolymerises mucopolysaccharides of the mucus secretion directly as well as by increasing lysosomal activity.
- ***Adverse effects :*** Nausea, vomiting, rhinorrhea, lacrimation.
- ***Dose :*** 8-16 mg TDS.

**Ambroxol :**

- It is a metabolite of bromhexine. It is having similar properties like that of bromhexine. It is especially helpful if mucus plugs are present like in asthma, emphysema and post-tracheostomy.
- ***Dose :*** 15-30 mg TDS.

**Acetylcysteine :**

- ***Mechanism of action :*** Reduce viscosity of sputum by breaking disulphide bond of mucoproteins and makes the mucus less viscid. It is directly administered in the respiratory tract by nebulisation.

- ***Adverse effects :*** Nausea, vomiting, stomatitis, bronchospasm, rhinorrhea.
- ***Dose :*** 200 mg / ml.

**Carbocysteine :**

- It is having similar pharmacological properties like acetylcysteine. It is administered orally. It is available in combination of antibiotics like amoxycillin for management of chronic bronchitis, sinusitis and bronchiectasis.

**Dornase alpha :**

- It is a recombinant human deoxyribonuclease (DNAse). This DNAse selectively cleaves DNA.
- ***Use :*** This property is useful in cystic fibrosis where there are purulent respiratory secretions which contain high amount of extracellular DNA which are released by degeneration of neutrophils in response to infections. It is given by inhalation.
- ***Dose :*** 2.5 mg OD.

## OTHERS :

**Antihistaminics : Chlorpheniramine, Levocetirizine etc.**

- They are usually added to antitussives / expectorant formulations and provide relief in cough due to sedative & anticholinergic actions (Decreases secretions).
- They lack selectivity for cough centre and have no expectorant action.
- They are suitable for allergic cough.
- ***Adverse effects :*** Sedation, anticholinergic effects etc.

**Bronchodilators : Salbutamol, Terbutaline etc.**

- Cough is aggravated if it is accompanied by bronchospasm. Hence, sometimes a bronchodilator is added to cough treatment especially in cases of bronchial asthma where, there is bronchospasm.

**Local anesthetics : Lignocaine.**

- They are used topically on pharyngeal and laryngeal mucosa in spray forms.
- They reduce the sensitivity of sensory receptors in these areas.
- ***Use :*** cough associated with endoscopy, bronchoscopy.

# HORMONES
# &
# RELATED DRUGS

# 27 ANTERIOR PITUITARY HORMONES

## GROWTH HORMONE, PROLACTIN, GONADOTROPINS (FSH & LH), TSH AND ACTH :

### GROWTH HORMONE :

- ***Physiological role :*** Promotes growth of all organs by inducing hyperplasia; proportionate increase in the size and mass of all parts except brain and eye, has positive nitrogen balance, indirect action is exerted mainly through Somatomedins or Insulin like growth factors (IGF-1 and IGF-2); promotes growth, retains nitrogen and promotes bone growth.
- ***Regulation :*** Hypothalamus secretes stimulatory GHRH (growth hormone releasing hormone) and also inhibitory GHRIH (growth hormone releasing inhibitory hormone / Somatostatin) which control GH secretion.
- ***GH related conditions :*** Deficiency produces : Dwarfism, Excess GH before epiphysis closes : Gigantism, Excess GH after 18 years : Acromegaly.
- ***Preparations :*** Natural GH not used. ***Somatropin*** and ***Somatrem*** are used which are synthetic GH analogues made by recombinant DNA technology.
- ***Uses :*** Replacement therapy in GH deficiency in hypothalamic or pituitary diseases, Turner's syndrome, AIDS associated wasting, Catabolic states like burns, renal failure, bed ridden patients and osteoporosis. It is also abused by athletes for increasing performance and also used off label as anti-ageing drug.
- ***Adverse effects :*** Type 2 diabetes, insulin resistance, arthralgia, pain at injection site, lipodystrophy. Leukemia, carpal tunnel syndrome, fluid retention.

#### Somatostatin (GHRIH) :

- Produce mainly by hypothalamus and also in GIT. Inhibits secretion of GH, TSH and prolactin by pituitary and insulin and glucagon by pancreas and all GIT secretions (Gastrin, HCl).
- ***Uses :*** Limited use due to short half-life (2-3 min) and non-specificity towards GH. Mostly synthetic analogues are used nowadays which are mentioned below.

### Octreotide :

- It is a long acting analogue of somatostatin. It inhibits GH release, but less potent in decreasing insulin secretion, therefore less chances of hyperglycemia.
- ***Uses :*** GH secreting pituitary tumors along with acromegaly, carcinoid syndrome, VIP secreting tumors, Gastrinoma, secretory diarrhea of diabetes, bleeding esophageal varices, insulinoma.
- ***Sandostatin :*** It is a slow release formulation of octreotide.
- ***Lanreotide :*** It is similar to octreotide but is used to treat thyroid tumors.

### Pegvisomant :

- It is a GH receptor antagonist. It prevents peripheral GH binding to its receptor and suppresses serum IGF-1 levels.
- ***Use :*** Acromegaly.

## PROLACTIN :

- ***Physiological functions :*** Growth & development of breast, growth and development of ductal and lobular epithelium, induce lactation after birth of baby, increased prolactin levels suppress normal menstrual cycle.

### Hyperprolactinemia :

- ***Females :*** Galactorrhea, amenorrhea and Infertility.
- ***Males :*** Loss of libido, Infertility.
- ***Drug causing hyperprolactinemia :*** Chlorpromazine, haloperidol, metoclopramide, reserpine, alpha methyl dopa.
- ***Treatment of hyperprolactinemia :*** Dopaminergic agonists like Bromocriptine, Cabergoline and Pergolide are used.

### Bromocriptine :

- ***Uses :*** Hyperprolactinemia, acromegaly, parkinsonism, hepatic coma and suppression of lactation.
- ***Dose :*** Start 1.25 mg HS and after 1 week 1.25 mg can be added in morning. Can be increased to 5 mg BD.
- ***Adverse effects :*** Nausea, vomiting, postural hypotension, nasal decongestion, digital vasospasm and CNS effects : hallucinations, night mares, insomnia.

### Pergolide :

- Ergot derivative. Cheapest Dopamine agonist.
- ***Dose :*** 0.025 mg increased to 0.25 mg gradually.

### Cabergoline :

- Ergot derivative. Long half life of 65 hours, hence given twice weekly. Higher affinity and selectivity to $D_2$ receptors.

- ***Use :*** Preferred for hyperprolactinemia and acromegaly.
- ***Dose :*** 0.25 mg twice weekly.

## GONADOTROPINS (FSH & LH) :

- They control activity of the gonads.
- **Functions of FSH :** ***In females :*** Induces follicular growth, development of ovum and secretion of estrogen. ***In males :*** spermatogenesis.
- **Functions of LH :** ***In females :*** Ripening of graffian follicles, triggers ovulation, regulation of menstrual cycle, promotion of estrogen and progesterone production and sustaining of corpus luteum. ***In male :*** stimulates testosterone secretion.
- **Disturbances of gonadotropin secretion :** Excess - Precocious puberty. Deficiency - Amenorrhea, infertility and oligospermia.
- **Preparations of gonadotropins :**
  - ***Menotropin :*** FSH + LH (Obtained from urine of postmenopausal women).
  - ***Urofollitropin :*** Pure FSH - Preferred in PCOD.
  - hCG (Obtained From Urine of Pregnant Females).
  - DNA recombinant FSH.
- **Uses :** Infertility in females, infertility in males, cryptorchidism, to aid Invitro fertilisation, regress AIDS related Kaposi's Sarcoma.
- **Adverse effects :** Ovarian hyperstimulation, multiple pregnancies, polycystic ovarian disease, pain in abdomen, edema, headache, allergic reactions.

### GnRH (gonadotropin releasing hormone) & its analogues :

**Gonadorelin :**

- It is a synthetic human GnRH.
- ***Uses :*** Diagnostic use - Used for testing pituitary gonadal axis in male or female hypogonadism. Infertility, cryptorchidism & delayed puberty.

**GnRH agonists :** Goserelin, Buserelin, Leuprolide, Nafereline and Triptoreline.

- These are more potent and longer acting than GnRH. They can be given SC, IM or nasal spray.
- ***Mechanism :*** They cause initial increase in LH & FSH. But, after 1-2 weeks cause decrease in FSH & LH secretion. They decrease estrogen and testosterone levels. In short, they cause pharmacological oophorectomy and orchiectomy.
- ***Uses :*** Precocious puberty, prostatic carcinoma, breast cancer and contraception.
- ***Adverse effects :*** Hot flushes, loss of libido, vaginal dryness, osteoporosis.

**GnRH antagonists :** Cetrorelix, Granirelix, Abarelix, Degarelix.

- Competitive antagonists of GnRH.
- ***Advantage :*** No initial increase in gonadotropins & do not cause histamine release.
- ***Uses :*** Endometriosis, uterine fibroids, advanced prostate cancer, in-vitro fertilisation.

## TSH and ACTH :

- Not much used clinically.

□□□□□

# 28 THYROID HORMONES AND THYROID INHIBITORS

**Anatomy of thyroid gland :**

- Situated over trachea. Has two lobes connected together by an isthmus.
- Thyroid gland is composed over a million cluster of follicles. Follicles are spherical & consists of follicular cells surrounding a central mass (colloid). The colloid contains Thyroglobulin (TGB) which is a glycoprotein and contains tyrosine.
- ***Regulation of synthesis :*** Thyroid gland is under control of pituitary via TSH (thyroid stimulating hormone) and hypothalamus via TRH (thyroid releasing hormone). The synthesis is controlled through negative feedback inhibition.
- ***Function :*** secrets thyroid hormones viz.
  1. $T_4$ (L-Thyroxine or tetraiodothyronine).
  2. $T_3$ (Liothyronine or triiodothyronine).
- Iodine and iodides are necessary for thyroid hormone synthesis.
- Sea fish, eggs, milk, iodinated salt are dietary sources of iodides and iodine.

**$T_3$ and $T_4$ :**

- Thyroid gland normally secretes mainly $T_4$. 70% of $T_3$ derived from $T_4$ in peripheral tissues.
- $T_4$ is converted to $T_3$ by 5-deiodinase enzyme.
- Both $T_4$ and $T_3$ are in bound form (TBG, pre albumin and albumin).
- Only 0.025% of $T_4$ and 0.35% of $T_3$ are free.
- Free hormone concentration best correlates with thyroid status.
- $T_3$ is 5 times more potent than $T_4$.
- $T_4$ is the major circulating hormone.
- $T_3$ - the major mediator of physiological effects.
- The term thyroid hormone is used to comprise both $T_4$ plus $T_3$.
- Both forms are available for oral use.

## THYROID HORMONE - BIOSYNTHESIS :

**6 steps of synthesis :**

1. Iodide uptake or trapping.
2. Oxidation.
3. Iodination.
4. Coupling.

5. Storage and release.
6. Peripheral conversion of $T_4$ to $T_3$.

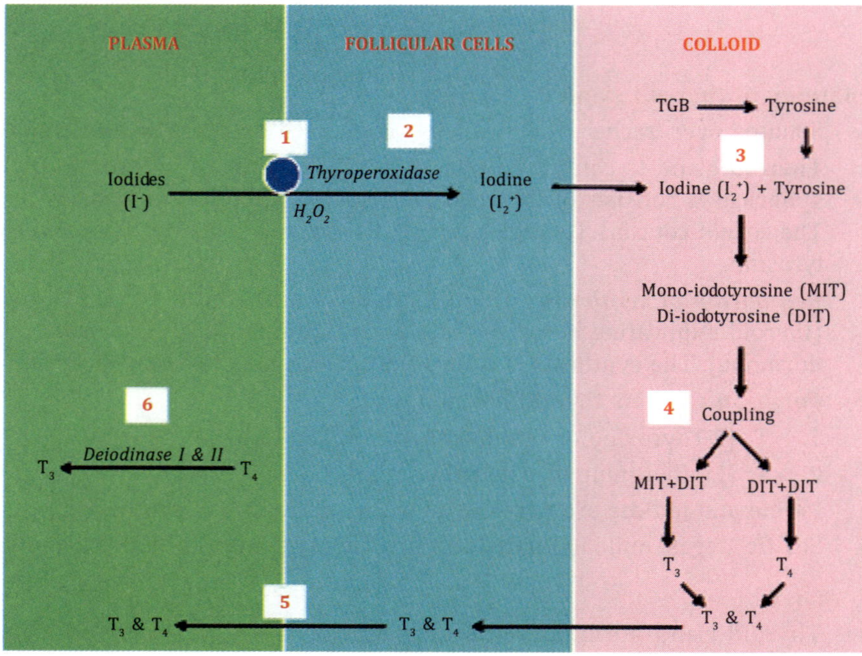


1. ***Uptake / trapping :*** Dietary iodides are taken up from the plasma in the follicular cells of thyroid by a transporter.
2. ***Oxidation :*** Here, iodides are converted to iodine by Thyroperoxidase enzyme and hydrogen peroxide. This iodine now gets transported to the colloid inside follicles.
3. ***Iodination of tyrosine :*** In colloid, the thyroglobulin (TBG) gives away its tyrosine which then combines with iodine to form monoiodotyrosine (MIT) and diiodotyrosine (DIT).
4. ***Coupling :*** Now, MIT combines with DIT to form tri-iodothyronine ($T_3$) and DIT combines with DIT to form tetraiodothyronine or thyroxine ($T_4$).
5. ***Synthesis and release :*** $T_3$ and $T_4$ are stored in thyroid and released as and when required into the plasma.
6. ***Peripheral conversion :*** In the periphery $T_4$ is converted to $T_3$ by Deiodinase I and II enzyme.

**Physiological actions of thyroid hormones :**

- To normalise growth and development, body temperature and energy levels.
- Increases BMR (basal metabolic rate) by promoting the consumption of cellular $O_2$ to produce ATP.

- Increased metabolism of carbohydrates, proteins and fats.
- ***Insufficiency :***
  1. Cretinism (infant & child).
  2. Myxedema (adult) and
  3. Hashimoto's thyroiditis (antibodies against TGB).
  4. Endemic goitre (Deficiency of iodine).
- ***Excess :*** Hyperthyroidism (Thyrotoxicosis).

### Cretinism :

- Endemic or sporadic.
- Endemic – extreme iodine deficiency.
- Sporadic – failure of thyroid to develop normally or defective hormone synthesis.
- Detectable at birth, may not be recognised until 3-5 months of age.
- ***Features :*** Dwarfism, mental retardation, short extremities, inactive, listless, puffy & expressionless face, enlarged tongue, skin yellow, dry & cool, bradycardia, low body temp., late teeth eruption, delayed closure of fontanelle, poor appetite, feeding slow, constipation, umbilical hernia.
- Iodine replacement institution prior to pregnancy till end of $2^{nd}$ trimester.

### Myxedema :

- Hypothyroid condition, results from the accumulation of increased amount of hyaluronic acid and chondroitin sulphate in the dermis.
- ***Symptoms :*** Thickening of skin, bradycardia, swollen lips, puffiness around the eyes, hoarse voice, lethargy, mental problems, dry skin, weight gain, constipation, brittle hair and cold intolerance.

### Uses of thyroid hormone :

- As replacement therapy in deficiency states.
- Available as L-thyroxine sod. 100, 50, 25 mcg tablets.
- $T_4$-consistent potency and prolonged duration of action.
- $T_3$ for quicker onset of action as in myxedema coma or preparation of a patient for $I^{131}$ therapy in thyroid cancer.

### Myxedema Coma :

- Serious medical emergency, mortality rate high (60%) despite early diagnosis and treatment.
- Pulmonary infections, CVA, CHF precipitate coma.
- ***Features :*** profound hypothermia, respiratory depression, unconscious, bradycardia, delayed reflexes, dry skin.
- ***Treatment :***
  - Ventilatory support.

- Rewarming the patient.
- Correct hyponatremia.
- I.V. steroid.
- I.V. $T_4$ (200–300 μg) bolus.
- I.V. $T_4$ (100 μg) after 24 hrs.
- Oral $T_4$ (500 μg) < 50 years plus Inj. $T_3$ I.V. 10 μg 8 hourly till patient is conscious.

### Endemic goitre :

- Occurs in areas having low levels of iodine in food and water.
- Thyroid gland increases in size to compensate for increasing the production of $T_3$ and $T_4$.
- Can be controlled by maintaining adequate iodine intake through salt.
- In severe deficiency, if hypothyroidism is there, levothyroxine is given till euthyroid status is reached.

### Hyperthyroidism (Thyrotoxicosis) :

***Hyperthyroidism can be due to Graves' disease or toxic nodular goitre :***

| Graves' disease | Toxic nodular goitre |
|---|---|
| • Autoimmune.<br>• TSH receptor stimulation antibodies.<br>• These antibodies mimic the action of TSH on thyroid.<br>• Excess production of $T_3$ & $T_4$. | • Adenomas of thyroid.<br>• Single or multipe (multinodular goitre). |

### Signs & Symptoms :

- Skin is flushed, warm and moist.
- Increased BMR.
- Heat intolerance.
- Muscle weakness and wasting.
- Tachycardia, increased cardiac output, angina, arrhythmia and heart failure.

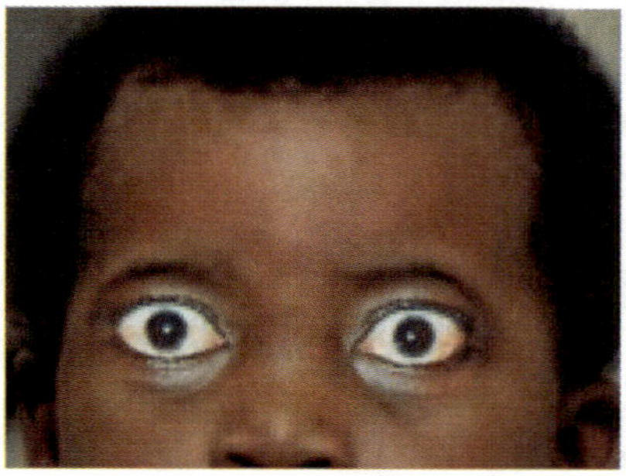

Exophthalmos

- Weight loss.
- Insomnia, anxiety, palpitations and fine tremors.
- Diarrhea.
- Exophthalmos (especially in Graves').

## THYROID INHIBITORS (ANTITHYROID DRUGS) :

- ***Inhibit Hormone synthesis (Thioamides) :*** Propylthiouracil, Carbimazole, Methimazole.
- ***Inhibits Hormone release :*** Iodine, Iodides of Na and K, Organic Iodide.
- ***Iodinated contrast media :*** Oral - Ipodate and Ipanoic acid, I.V. – Diatrizoate.
- ***Inhibit iodine uptake or trapping :*** Thiocyanates and perchlorates.
- ***Destroy Thyroid tissue :*** Radioactive Iodine ($I^{131}$, $I^{125}$, $I^{123}$).
- ***Symptomatic treatment :*** β blocker (Propranolol).

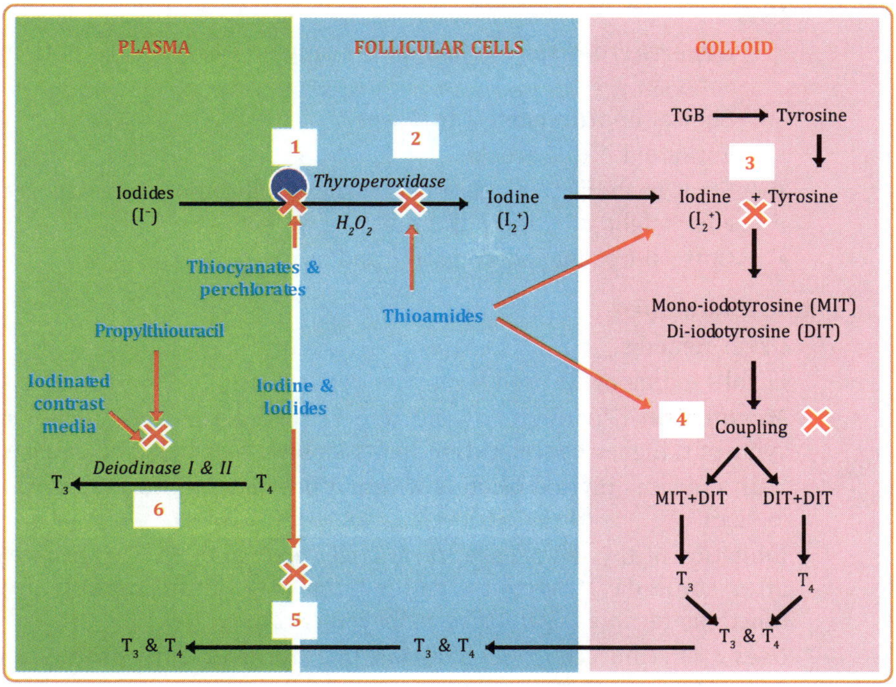


### Thioamides :

- Reduce formation of thyroid hormone.
- ***Mechanism :***
  1. Inhibit oxidation (inhibit thyroperoxidase).
  2. Inhibit iodination.
  3. Inhibit coupling.

- Propylthiouracil inhibits peripheral conversion of $T_4$ to $T_3$.

| Propylthiouracil | Carbimazole |
|---|---|
| • Less potent | • 5 times more potent |
| • Highly Plasma bound | • Less bound |
| • Less Placenta and milk entry (DOC in hyperthyroidism in pregnancy) | • High entry |
| • T½ 1-2 hrs | • 6-10 Hrs |
| • No active metabolite | • Active metabolite - methimazole |
| • Multiple dosing | • Single dose |
| • Inhibits $T_4$ to $T_3$ | • No $T_4$ to $T_3$ inhibition |

- ***Adverse effects :*** Agranulocytosis, Thrombocytopenia, Acute hepatic necrosis, Cholestatic hepatitis, Vasculitis, Lupus-like syndrome, teratogenicity (except propylthiouracil), rashes, urticaria, arthralgia, fever, anorexia, nausea, taste and smell abnormalities.
- ***Uses :***
  - ***Hyperthyroidism :*** Principal therapy and to prepare patient for surgery.
  - Clinical improvement 2 to 4 week.
  - Euthyroid 4 to 6 week.
  - Guide to therapy-decrease nervousness, palpitation, increase strength and weight gain and pulse rate.
  - Optimal treatment-decreased gland size.

**Iodine and iodides :**

- Oldest remedy.
- Lugol's iodine or KI used.
- ***Mechanism :*** Though iodides are required for thyroid hormone synthesis, higher concentration limits its own transport and release.
- It also reduces thyroid blood flow (gland becomes less vascular & shrinks in size).
- Inhibition of thyroid release (*thyroid constipation or wolff chaikoff effect*) after some days thyroid escapes from this inhibition and thyroid functions resumes again (*Escape phenomenon*).
- ***Uses :*** Thyroid crisis, preparation for thyroidectomy, prophylaxis of endemic cretinism and as antiseptic on skin.
- ***Adverse effects :*** Iodism (metallic taste, hypersalivation, running eyes and nose, sore throat, cough, diarrhea, skin rashes), Prolonged use-goitre and myxedema, flaring of acne.

**Radioactive Iodine ($I^{131}$, $I^{125}$, $I^{123}$) :**

- Swallowed $I^{131}$ trapped and conc. in thyroid follicles.
- Gamma and Beta radiation (beta rays destroy thyroid tissue).

- Used in diffuse toxic goitre (Thyrotoxicosis/Graves' disease), toxic nodular goitre, thyroid carcinoma.
- Contraindications - pregnancy, lactation, children.
- Danger of thyroid carcinoma.

**Iodinated contrast media :**

- Oral - Ipodate and Ipanoic acid and IV – Diatrizoate.
- ***Mechanism :*** inhibit Deiodinase I & II enzyme.
- Lower doses are needed than contrast radiography.

**β Blockers :**

- In hyperthyroidism there is increased tissue sensitivity to catecholamines which leads to palpitation, tremor, nervousness, and sweating. β blockers reduce these symptoms. They do not alter course of disease and thyroid function tests.
- ***Used in :***
    - Preoperative therapy with Iodine.
    - Awaiting response to carbimazole.
    - Propranolol 20–80 mg 6-8 Hrly.

## THYROID STORM OR THYROID CRISIS :

- A sudden exacerbation of symptoms of thyrotoxicosis, characterised by hyperthermia, sweating, severe tachycardia, extreme nervous excitability, diarrhea, vomiting, confusion, coma and death.
- Life-threatening emergency.
- Large amount of hormone into circulation occurs.
- Precipitated by infection, trauma, toxemia of pregnancy, surgery.
- **Treatment :**
    - Inj. Propranolol IV, slow, 1 mg / min. followed by 40-80 mg oral every 8 Hrly.
    - ***Propylthiouracil :*** large doses 300-400 mg 4-6 Hrly.
    - Potassium Iodide 600 mg to 1 g orally in first 24 hr to inhibit hormone release or Ipanoic acid/ipodate (iodinated contrast media).
    - Hydrocortisone 100 mg 8 Hrly IV followed by oral prednisolone.
    - ***Hyperthermia :*** cooling and aspirin.
    - Antibiotics and rehydration.

# 29 ANTI-DIABETIC DRUGS

Diabetes is a metabolic disorder characterised by hyperglycemia due to inadequate insulin secretion (type I) or due to reduced insulin activity (type II). It is also associated with various microvascular and macrovascular complications. Microvascular complications : Retinopathy, nephropathy and neuropathy. Macrovascular complications : cardiovascular diseases, cerebrovascular diseases, peripheral vascular diseases and diabetic foot.

### Clinical features : 3Ps

**P**olydypsia (increased thirst), **P**olyuria (increased urination) & **P**olyphagia (increased food intake).

### Diagnosis :

| | Normal | Prediabetes | Diabetes |
|---|---|---|---|
| **Fasting sugar** | < 100 mg/dL | 101-125 mg/dL | > 126 mg/dL |
| **Post-meal sugar** | > 140 mg/dL | 140-200 mg/dL | > 200 mg/dL |
| **HbA1c** | > 5.7% | 5.7-6.4% | > 6.5% |

### Classification of Diabetes mellitus :

- Type 1 (IDDM – Insulin dependent diabetes mellitus).
- Type 2 (NIDDM – Non-insulin dependent diabetes mellitus).
- Other specific types :
  - Gestational (in pregnancy).
  - Drug induced (*e.g.* steroids).

### Characteristics :

| Characteristic | Type 1 DM | Type 2 DM |
|---|---|---|
| **Age of onset** | Childhood / adolescence | > age 40 |
| **Rate of onset** | Abrupt | Gradual |
| **Etiology** | Autoimmune, heredity, viral | Heredity, sedentary lifestyle |
| **Islet cell antibodies** | Yes | No |
| **Body weight** | Thin, under-nourished | Obese |
| **Insulin** | Marked ↓;<br>Insulin T/t mandatory | ↓ or ↑ insulin; Diet / exercise /drugs / insulin (not necessary initially) |

| Characteristic | Type 1 DM | Type 2 DM |
|---|---|---|
| **Symptoms** | 3Ps, weight loss | Asymptomatic or 3Ps |
| **Ketoacidosis** | Common | Uncommon |

## Treatment :

### *Aims of therapy :*

- Control symptoms with non-pharmacological & pharmacological means, maintain the optimum body weight, correct the metabolic disturbances and prevent or delay the degenerative vascular complications.

### *Nonpharmacological Treatment :*

- Diet (low carbohydrate, low fat diet and high fibre diet), regular exercise, smoking cessation, reduce alcohol consumption, education, avoid stress.

### *Pharmacological Treatment :*

- Insulins.
- Oral antidiabetic drugs.

## CLASSIFICATION OF ANTIDIABETIC DRUGS :

### Insulins :

- ***Ultrashort acting (3-4 hrs) :*** Lispro, Aspart, Glulisine.
- ***Short acting (6-8 hrs) :*** Regular.
- ***Intermediate acting (16-20 hrs) :*** NPH (Neutral protamine hagedron), Lente.
- ***Long acting (16-24 hrs) :*** Glargine, Detemir.
- ***Ultralong acting (>24 hrs) :*** Degludec.

### Insulin analogues :

- Lispro, Aspart, Glulisine, Glargine, Detemir and Degludec.

### Oral Anti-Diabetic Agents :

- ***Biguanides :*** Phenformin, Metformin.
- ***Sulphonylureas :*** Glimepiride, Gliclazide, Glibenclamide, chlorpropamide.
- ***Thiazolidinediones :*** Pioglitazone, rosiglitazone.
- ***α Glucosidase inhibitors :*** Acarbose, Voglibose, miglitol.
- ***Dopamine D-2 receptor agonist :*** Bromocriptine.
- ***Incretin mimetics (GLP-1 receptor agonist) :*** Liraglutide, exenatide.
- ***Meglitinides :*** Repaglinide, nateglinide.
- ***Amylin analogues :*** Pramlinitide.
- ***Bile acid sequestrants :*** Colesevelam.
- ***DPP-4 inhibitors :*** Vildagliptin, teneligliptin, sitagliptin.
- ***SGLT-2 inhibitors :*** Canagliflozin, dapagliflozin, remogliflozin.
- ***Dual PPAR-α and PPAR-γ receptor agonist :*** Saroglitazar, aleglitazar.

## INSULINS :

### Sources of insulin :

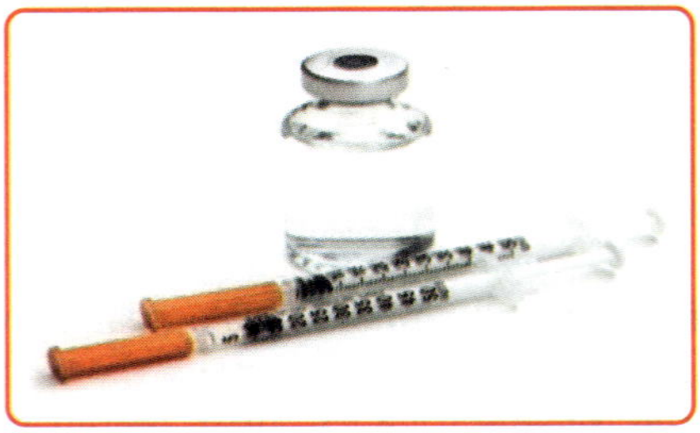

### Actions :

The main action of insulin is reduction of blood glucose levels. It is accomplished by following actions :

- ***Liver*** – Inhibits glycogenolysis, inhibits gluconeogenesis and promotes glycogen synthesis.
- ***Fat*** – Increases glucose uptake, increases storage of triglycerides and inhibits lipolysis.
- ***Muscle*** – Increases protein synthesis, increases glycogen synthesis and inhibits protein breakdown.

### Insulin administration :

- All insulin preparations are administered subcutaneously. However, in emergency situations and hospitalised patients, it can be given as i.v or i.v. infusions under strict blood sugar monitoring.

### Indications for insulin therapy :

- All patients of type 1 diabetes.
- Type 2 diabetes patients who are underweight, onset before 30-35 years, long standing diabetes, all diabetics with complications, during surgery, pregnancy, diabetic ketoacidosis, diabetic coma or pre-coma and failure of oral anti-diabetic therapy.

### Adverse effects :

- Hypoglycemia (symptoms – sweating, palpitations, tremors, anxiety, headache, hunger, fatigue, coma and death).
- Lipodystrophy of fat at injection site.
- Allergic reactions (Local itching, redness, pain, urticaria, anaphylaxis).
- Edema.

### Insulin analogues :

- These insulins are prepared by recombinant DNA technology by altering the sequence or position of amino acid in the insulin.
- ***Advantages of insulin analogues :*** Greater stability, improved pharmacokinetics, less immunogenicity, lower incidence of hypoglycaemia & better glucose control.

## BIGUANIDES :

- *E.g.* Metformin and phenformin.
- **Mechanism of action :** ↓ hepatic gluconeogenesis, ↑ glucose utilisation in muscle and fat, ↓ intestinal absorption of glucose.
- **Dose :** 500 mg BID orally with breakfast and dinner.
- **Non-diabetic uses of metformin :** Polycystic ovarian disease (PCOD) and Insulin resistance.
- **Adverse Effects :** Abdominal pain, anorexia, metallic taste, nausea, diarrhea, tiredness, lactic acidosis (more common with phenformin), vitamin $B_{12}$ deficiency with high dose of metformin.

## SULPHONYLUREAS :

- *E.g.* Glimepiride, Gliclazide, Glibenclamide, chlorpropamide.
- **Mechanism of action :** At least 30% β cells should be functional. Act on sulphonylurea receptors on β cell membrane. ↓ Conductance of $K^+$ channels. ↑ $Ca^{2+}$ influx. This causes degranulation of β cells and release of insulin.
- **Adverse effects :** Hypoglycemia (Commonest with chlorpropamide), hypersensitivity, rashes, photosensitivity, purpura, leucopenia, rarely agranulocytosis, nausea, vomiting, flatulence, diarrhea, headache, paraesthesia, weight gain.

## GLICLAZIDE :

- Less weight gain.
- Has anti-platelet action also.
- Both, gliclazide and glimepiride are having additional anti-oxidant effect also.

## THIAZOLIDINEDIONES :

- *E.g.* Pioglitazone, rosiglitazone.
- They are also called as insulin sensitisers.
- Primarily used to supplement Sulphonylurea / metformin in cases of insulin resistance.
- **Mechanism of action :** Selective agonists for nuclear PPAR- (peroxisome proliferator activated receptor – gamma). ↑ transcription of insulin responsive genes.
- **Adverse effects :** Hepatotoxicity, edema, weight gain, headache, myalgia, cardiac side effects.

## α-GLUCOSIDASE INHIBITORS :

- *E.g.* Acarbose, Voglibose, miglitol.
- **Mechanism of action :** Inhibit starch breakdown by inhibiting α-glucosidase. Delays carbohydrate absorption. Lowers post prandial hyperglycemia.
- **Adverse Effects :** Flatulence, diarrhea, abdominal pain.

## DOPAMINE $D_2$ RECEPTOR AGONIST :

- *E.g.* Bromocriptine.
- **Mechanism of action :** The mechanism is not completely understood. However, studies reveal suppression of hepatic gluconeogenesis by dopamine induced modulation. Has no effect on insulin secretion or insulin sensitivity.
- **Adverse Effects :** Nausea, dizziness, headache and vomiting.

## INCRETIN MIMETICS (GLP-1 RECEPTOR AGONIST) :

- *E.g.* Liraglutide, exenatide.
- **Mechanism of action :** Incretin is a group of hormones that includes glucagon like peptide-1 (GLP-1) and glucose dependent insulinotropic polypeptide (GIP) that are released after meals from the GIT and stimulates glucose dependent insulin secretion from pancreas. GLP-1 receptor agonists stimulate insulin secretion from β cells of pancreas, decreased glucagon release and slow the rate of nutrient absorption by slowing gastric emptying. They also reduce appetite by acting on the hypothalamus (used for weight loss).
- **Adverse effects :** Nausea, anorexia, diarrhea and rarely necrotising pancreatitis.

## MEGLITINIDES :

- *E.g.* Repaglinide, nateglinide.
- **Mechanism of action :** They are insulin secretion enhancers (insulin secretagogues). Their mode of action is similar to sulphonylureas. They have rapid onset of action, therefore taken shortly before a meal.
- **Advantages over sulphonylureas :** Meglitinides causes less weight gain. They are less allergenic than sulphonylureas.
- **Adverse effects :** Hypoglycemia.

## AMYLIN ANALOGUES :

- *E.g.* Pramlinitide.
- **Mechanism of action :** Amylin is a peptide secreted from pancreatic β cells along with insulin. The role of amylin is to inhibit glucagon secretion, delay gastric emptying and suppresses appetite. Pramlinitide acts as agonist at these amylin receptors. It is taken subcutaneously before meals.
- **Adverse effects :** Nausea, diarrhea and headache.

## BILE ACID SEQUESTRANTS :

- *E.g.* Colesevelam.
- **Mechanism of action :** Colesevelam is a bile acid binding resin which is used as a cholesterol lowering agent which has recently been approved for diabetes mellitus. The exact mechanism is not completely understood, however, it modulates the enterohepatic circulation of bile which affects glucose metabolism. It also increases secretion of GLP-1.

## DPP-4 INHIBITORS (DIPEPTIDYL PEPTIDASE - 4 INHIBITORS) :

- *E.g.* Vildagliptin, teneligliptin, sitagliptin.
- **Mechanism of action :** DPP-4 inhibitors selectively inhibits Dipeptidyl peptidase-4 enzyme that inactivates GLP-1. As a result GLP-1 levels are increased. This results in increased insulin secretion, decreased glucagon release, delayed gastric emptying and suppression of appetite and weight.
- **Adverse effects :** Nasopharyngitis (because substance P is also a substrate for DPP-4 whose levels gets elevated) and GI disturbances.

## SGLT-2 INHIBITORS (SODIUM-GLUCOSE COTRANSPORTER-2 INHIBITORS) :

- *E.g.* Canagliflozin, dapagliflozin, remogliflozin.
- **Mechanism of action :** Kidneys continuously filters glucose through glomerulus & nearly all of this glucose *i.e.* reabsorbed back from the proximal tubule by a transporter called as sodium-glucose cotransporter-2 (SGLT-2). Inhibiting SGLT-2 decreases glucose reabsorption & increases its excretion in urine.
- **Advantages :** Weight loss, no hypoglycemia, improves insulin resistance, beneficial for hypertension also due to its diuretic effect.
- **Adverse effects :** Increased risk of urinary tract infections (both bacterial and fungal) due to glucosuria, euglycemic ketoacidosis, increased risks of lower limb amputations are also reported.

## DUAL PPAR-α AND PPAR-γ RECEPTOR AGONIST :

- *E.g.* saroglitazar, aleglitazar.
- Dual PPAR-α and PPAR-γ (peroxisome proliferator activated receptor alpha and gamma) receptor agonist.
- **Mechanism of action :** Agonist action at PPAR-α targets lipids levels which improves dyslipidemia and agonist action at PPAR-γ improves peripheral glucose sensitivity and glycemic index in diabetes.
- **Adverse effects :** Weight gain, heart failure and bone fractures.

## DIABETIC KETOACIDOSIS :

- It is a serious complication of diabetes mellitus especially type I diabetes. It's a medical emergency.
- The condition develops when the diabetic patient's pancreas can't produce enough insulin. Insulin plays important role in helping glucose enter our cells. Without enough insulin, our body begins to break down fat as fuel for energy. This process causes increased production of ketone bodies, which leads to diabetic ketoacidosis if untreated.

### Clinical features :

- Excessive thirst, frequent urination, nausea and vomiting, abdominal pain, weakness or fatigue, shortness of breath, fruity scent of breath, tachycardia, confusion, dehydration, Kussmaul's breathing, coma and death.

## Treatment :

### *Primary measures :*

- Hospitalise the patient, maintain all vital parameters, monitor blood sugar, arterial blood gas monitoring, serum electrolyte levels and maintain hydration.

### *Pharmacotherapy :*

- Inj. Short acting Insulin (regular) 0.5 U/kg IV infusion till glucose levels fall to 250 mg/dl, then rate is adjusted according to plasma glucose levels.
- I.V normal saline at 1 L in first 30 min, then 1 L in next 1 hr, then 1 L in next 2 hrs, 1 L in next 6 hours and further correction as per need.
- Inj. KCl (Potassium chloride) 10-20 meq/L IV drip for correcting hypokalemia.
- Inj. Sodium bicarbonate 50 meq IV infusion for acidosis. (If pH is less than 6.8).
- Inj. Phosphate, when in lower range.
- Inj. Ceftriaxone 1 gm IV 8 hrly to prevent infections.

## NON KETOTIC HYPEROSMOLAR COMA :

- More common in elderly type 2 cases. Very high mortality.

### Principles of management :

- Faster fluid replacement with ½ NS.
- Alkali not required.
- Prophylactic heparin therapy.

## RECENT ADVANCES :

### Newer insulin delivery devices :

- Pen devices, Jet injectors, Insulin pumps.
- ***Inhaled insulins :*** EXUBERRA and AFFREZZA.

### Future Prospects :

- Islet cell transplant, stem cell therapy, gene therapy.

❑❑❑❑❑

# 30 CORTICOSTEROIDS

These are the hormones secreted by adrenal glands and are important for various metabolic functions. Their analogues are used in practice and are one of the most commonly used drugs worldwide.

### Synthesis and regulation :

These are synthesised by adrenal glands. Adrenal glands are under control of pituitary gland through ACTH and pituitary gland is under control of hypothalamus

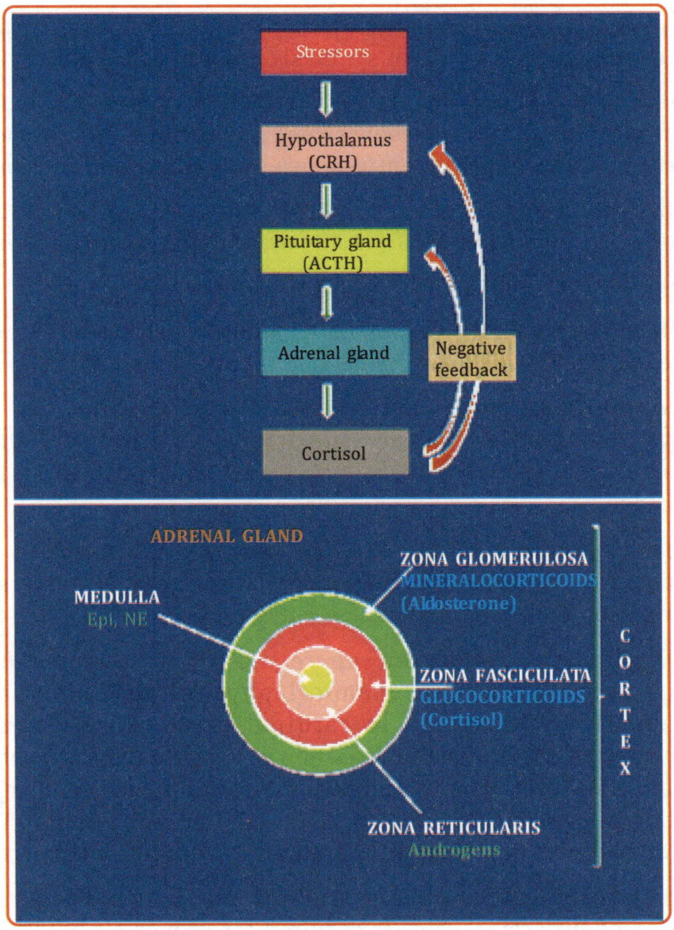

via CRH. The synthesis and release of these hormones are controlled by negative feedback mechanism.

The adrenal is mainly divided into two parts : outer cortex and inner medulla. Medulla synthesises catecholamines namely epinephrine (adrenaline) and nor-epinephrine (nor-adrenaline). The cortex is further divided into 3 parts; outer one is zona glomerulosa which synthesises mineralocorticoids (aldosterone), the middle part is called zona fasciculata which synthesises Glucocorticoids (cortisol) and the inner part is called as zona reticularis which synthesises androgens.

**Pharmacological actions :**

- ***Carbohydrate metabolism (Hyperglycemia) :*** Decreased peripheral utilisation of glucose, increased hepatic gluconeogenesis, mobilisation of amino acids for gluconeogenesis and increased glycogen deposition in liver.
- ***Protein metabolism (Catabolic effect) :*** Mobilisation of amino acids for gluconeogenesis, inhibit protein synthesis and muscle weakness and wasting.
- ***Fat Metabolism :*** Causes lipolysis and redistribution of fats (mobilisation of fat from peripheral stores towards central locations). Deposition of fats in face, neck and shoulder – moon face, fish mouth and buffalo hump.
- ***Calcium Balance :*** Decrease absorption of $Ca^{+2}$ in GIT and increased excretion – calcium depletion. Loss of osteoid – osteopenia and osteoporosis.
- ***CNS :*** Euphoria, Insomnia, anxiety, depression and seizures.
- ***CVS :*** Increase response of vascular smooth muscles to catecholamines, increase cardiac output. This results in hypertension.
- ***Hematopoietic system :*** Increases RBC, Platelets and neutrophils but decreases lymphocyte, eosinophil and basophils. In presence of malignancy of lymphatic cells – lytic actions are significant (apoptosis) – used in lymphomas.
- ***Immunosuppressive & anti-allergic actions :*** Suppresses all types of hypersensitivity & allergic phenomenon. Causes greater suppression of CMI (graft rejection & delayed hypersensitivity).
- ***Anti-inflammatory and immunosuppressive effects :*** Suppress inflammatory response to all pathogens, chemical, physical and immune mediated, hypersensitivity. Reduction in cardinal signs of inflammation. Anti-inflammatory effects are due to reduction of arachidonic acid metabolites like PG, LT and PAF synthesis by inhibiting Phospholipase $A_2$. They also block production of cytokines (IL-1, IL-4, IL-6 and TNF-α), reduction in activation of T-cells, suppress fibroblast proliferation and inhibits chemotaxis.
- ***Lungs :*** Development and maturation of fetal lungs (They stimulate the production of surfactant which is required for proper air breathing).
- ***GIT :*** They increase secretion of pepsin and gastric acid. They also suppress the immune response against H. pylori. This may lead to peptic ulcer.

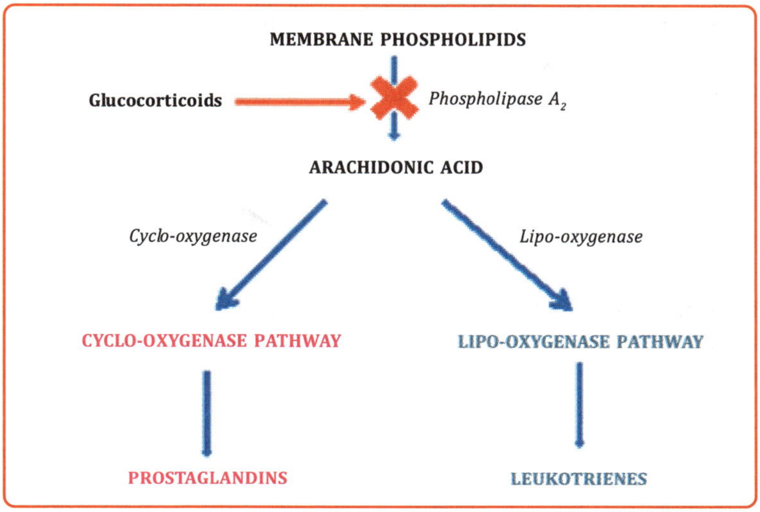


### Mechanism of action at cellular level :

- Glucocorticoids bind to cytoplasmic glucocorticoid receptor and form a complex.
- This complex translocates to the nucleus and binds to GRE (glucocorticoid response element).
- This causes transcription of specific mRNA causing regulation of protein synthesis.

## DEFICIENCY AND EXCESS OF CORTICOSTEROIDS :

| Deficiency (Addison's disease) | Excess (Cushing's syndrome) |
|---|---|
| • Hypotension<br>• Hyperkalemia<br>• Hyponatremia<br>• Weight loss<br>• Pigmentation | • Moon face<br>• Buffalo hump<br>• Increased abdominal Fat<br>• Muscle wasting<br>• Thinning of skin<br>• Purple striae<br>• Osteoporosis |

## CLASSIFICATION OF CORTICOSTEROIDS :

### Glucocorticoids (Based on Duration of action) :

- ***Short acting (>12 hr) :*** Hydrocortisone, Cortisone.
- ***Intermediate acting (12-36 hr) :*** Prednisolone, Methylprednisolone and Triamcinolone.
- ***Long acting (>36 hr) :*** Betamethasone, Dexamethasone.

### Glucocorticoids (Based on route) :

- ***Oral :*** Betamethasone, Prednisolone, Methylpredisolone.

- ***Injectables :*** Dexamethasone, Methylprednisolone, Hydrocortisone and Triamcinolone.
- ***Topical :*** Betamethasone, Clobetasol, Mometasone.
- ***Inhalation :*** Beclomethasone, Budesonide, Fluticasone.

**MINERALOCORTICOIDS :**

- Aldosteron, Fludrocortisone, Desoxycorticosterone.

**Uses :**

- ***Replacement Therapy :*** Acute adrenal insufficiency (Addisonian crisis), chronic adrenal insufficiency (Addison's disease), congenital adrenal hyperplasia. Glucocorticoid (*e.g.* hydrocortisone) is used along with a mineralocorticoid (*e.g.* fludrocortisone).
- ***Anti-inflammatory Uses :*** For suppression of inflammatory response in - Rheumatoid arthritis, osteoarthritis (also use as intra-articular injection), Rheumatic Heart disease and Gout.
- ***Allergic Disorders :*** In anaphylaxis, angioneurotic edema and serum sickness etc. – Adrenaline is the choice. Seasonal allergies, bee sting, drug allergies.
- ***Bronchial Asthma :*** In severe asthma attacks : I.V hydrocortisone. In chronic asthma :
  - Inhaled - beclomethasone, budesonide, fluticasone.
  - Oral steroids – prednisolone etc.
- ***Ocular Diseases :*** Allergic conjunctivitis, iritis and keratitis etc. Dexamethasone eye drops.
- ***Skin Diseases :*** Topical forms are widely used in many eczematous skin diseases like psoriasis etc. Systemic therapy are also required and may be life saving in Pemphigus vulgaris and Stevens-Johnson syndrome.
- ***GIT :*** Inflammatory conditions like Ulcerative colitis and Crohn's disease.
- ***Renal and collagen diseases :*** Nephrotic syndrome, SLE, sarcoidosis, glomerulo-nephritis, vascular disorders : Polyarteritis nodosa.
- ***Organ Transplant :*** Combined with other drugs like cyclosporin, azathioprine.
- ***Malignancy :*** Acute lymphatic leukemia, Hodgkin's and other lymphomas.
- ***Cerebral edema :*** It helps in reducing raised intra-cranial pressure *e.g.* raised ICP in brain tumors.
- ***Other uses :*** Hypercalcemia, myaesthenia gravis, stimulation of lung maturation in premature babies, Keloids, certain infective conditions but under adequate antibiotic cover : TB meningitis, severe lepra reaction and pneumocystis carinii pneumonia in AIDS patient and Thyroid storm (inhibit TRH secretion from hypothalamus which in turn decreases TSH).

## Adverse Effects :

- Altered fat distribution (Cushingoid features), $Na^+$ and water retention, hypertension, osteoporosis and avascular necrosis (*E.g.* AVN of head of femur), hyperglycemia, peptic ulcer, cataract and glaucoma, myopathy and muscle wasting, susceptibility to infections, delayed wound healing, **CNS :** euphoria, insomnia, anxiety and depression, growth retardation in children, teratogenic effects : intrauterine growth retardation can occur with prolong use, others : Acne, thinning of skin, purple striae over thighs and abdomen, hirsutism, menstrual irregularities, dyslipidemia, pancreatitis and weight gain.

**NOTE :**
- ☞ Suppression of hypothalamo-pituitary-adrenal (HPA) axis occurs on long term use or with larger doses of corticosteroids.
- ☞ In such cases, abrupt withdrawal of corticosteroids can result in precipitation of symptoms for which the corticosteroid was used and also, if subjected to stress, the patients can also land into acute adrenal insufficiency.
- ☞ In such patients corticosteroids should be discontinued by gradual tapering of the doses over the period of time.

## Contraindications :

- Peptic ulcer, hypertension, diabetes mellitus, viral and fungal infections, tuberculosis, osteoporosis, epilepsy and psychosis, CHF and renal failure.

## DEFLAZOCORT :

- Low potency glucocorticoid.
- Intermediate acting (Duration of action is 12-36 hours).
- Good efficacy.
- **Advantages :** Lower incidence of side effects such as osteoporosis, glucose intolerance and cushings syndrome.
- **Dose :** 1 mg, 6 mg and 30 mg.

❑❑❑❑❑

# 31 ANDROGENS, ANTI-ANDROGENS, ANABOLIC STEROIDS AND DRUGS FOR ERECTILE DYSFUNCTION

## ANDROGENS :

Androgens are the substances which cause development of secondary sex characters in the males. They are secreted by the testes.

### Classification :

#### *Natural Androgens :*

- **From Testes :** Testosterone, Dihydrotestosterone.
- **From Adrenal cortex :** Dehydroepiandrosterone, Androstenedione.

#### *Synthetic Androgens :*

- Testosterone propionate and Testosterone enanthate, Methyltestosterone, Fluoxymesterone.
- **Orally effective :** Testosterone undecanoate and Mesterolone.

### Characteristics :

- Testosterone is converted by 5-$\alpha$-reductase to the more potent, dihydrotestosterone (DHT), which is responsible for many of the responses to testosterone in the urogenital tract (*e.g.* prostate gland hyperplasia).
- It binds to and activates androgen receptor (AR) which is present in many tissues including reproductive tissue, skeletal muscle, brain, kidney etc.

### Pharmacological Actions :

- ***Androgenic Effects :*** In the fetus, testosterone promotes development of male reproductive tract; internal genitalia, vas deferens, epididymis and external genitalia (sex differentiation). During puberty, testosterone promotes development of primary sexual characteristics (*e.g.* enlargement of penis, scrotum and testes), secondary sexual characteristics (*e.g.* male body shape, axillary/pubic hair, deeper pitch of voice, thickening of skin). Adulthood : Baldness, benign hypertrophy of prostate, prostatic cancer.
- ***Testes :*** Promotion of spermatogenesis and maturation of sperm. Moderately high dose causes testicular atrophy by inhibiting Gonadotropin secretion.
- ***Anabolic effects :*** Pubertal spurt of growth at puberty in both boys and girls, bone growth (thickness and length), estrogen synthesised from

testosterone leads to fusion of epiphysis of bones and mineralisation, muscle building, positive nitrogen balance, minerals and water balance; increase in weight, increase in appetite and acceleration of erythropoiesis.

### Uses of Androgenic Effects :

***Androgen replacement therapy (ART) :*** In androgen insufficiency, especially seen in primary hypothalamic, pituitary and testicular disorders, hypopituitarism, AIDS related muscle wasting, hereditary angioneurotic edema, ageing.

### Adverse Effects :

***Virilisation :*** especially in women receiving relatively high doses for prolonged periods, such as in Ca breast, cholestatic jaundice, priapism (sustained erection), oligospermia, edema, precocious puberty and short stature, acne, hepatic carcinoma and gynecomastia.

## ANTIANDROGENS :

### Examples :

- **Danazol, Cyproterone acetate, Flutamide, Finasteride, Dutasteride.**

### Danazol :

- Weak androgenic, anabolic, progestational & glucocorticoid action. Also Labelled as impeded/attenuated androgen. It is orally effective.
- ***Mechanism of action :*** Suppression of Gonadotropins (FSH and LH) secretion from Pituitary which results in inhibition of testicular/ovarian function. This also results in endometrial atrophy and amenorrhea.
- ***Use :*** Endometriosis, fibrocystic breast disease, menorrhagia, hereditary angioneurotic edema, gynecomastia.
- ***Adverse effects :*** Amenorrhea, androgenic effects like decreased breast size, hirsutism, weight gain etc. Hot flashes, night sweating, cramps and loss of libido in men.

### Cyproterone acetate :

- Direct antiandrogenic action.
- ***Mechanism of action :*** Progesterone like activity : inhibits LH causing antiandrogenic action. Competes with DHT for intracellular receptor.
- ***Uses :*** Precocious puberty in boys, inappropriate sexual behavior in men, virilisation in women.

### Flutamide :

- It is nonsteroidal and have no hormonal activity but has antiandrogenic action.
- ***Mechanism of action :*** It causes competitive block of androgen action. Increased LH secretion by blocking feedback inhibition. Plasma testosterone level may increase to overcome direct antiandrogenic effect

- ***Uses :*** Cancer of prostate along with GnRH agonist, female hirsutism
- ***Adverse effects :*** Gynecomastia, breast tenderness and also liver damage

**Finasteride :**

- ***Mechanism of action :***

  It is competitive inhibitor of 5-α-reductase. This inhibits the conversion of Testosterone to the more potent, dihydrotestosterone (DHT), which is responsible for many of the responses to testosterone in the urogenital tract (*e.g.* prostate gland hyperplasia). Mainly acts on urogenital tract (prostate); DHT level lowered but not plasma Testosterone level.

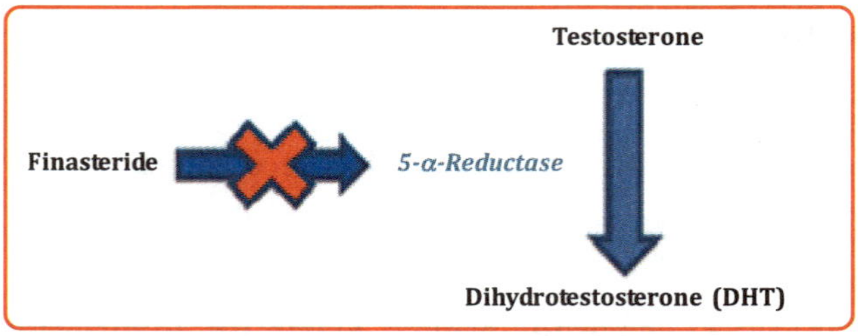


- ***Uses :*** Benign prostatic hypertrophy *i.e.* BHP (decrease in prostate volume, improved urinary flow, reversal of disease progression), Carcinoma of prostate and male pattern baldness (1 mg) *i.e.* androgenic alopecia.
- ***Doses :*** 5 mg OD (BHP) or 1 mg OD in baldness.
- ***Adverse effects :*** Loss of libido, impotence, decreased ejaculation.

**Dutasteride :**

- It is a newer inhibitor of 5 α-reductase with uses and adverse effects similar to Finasteride.
- Both Finasteride and Dutasteride are used in combination with Tamsulosin (selective $\alpha_{1A}$ receptor antagonist) in BHP and Ca prostate.

## ANABOLIC STEROIDS :

**Examples :**

- **Nandrolone propionate, Nandrolone decanoate, Stanazolol, Oxymetholone.**

**Characteristics :**

- Synthetic androgens with higher anabolic but lower androgenic activity (1:3 ratio). Similar anabolic effect, same receptors and same androgenic effects like that of androgens.

**Uses :**

- Used in catabolic states like acute illness, severe trauma, major surgery, renal insufficiency, osteoporosis, suboptimal growth in boys, anemia : hemolytic and malignancy associated, performance enhancement by athletes (Sports abuse).

## DRUGS FOR ERECTILE DYSFUNCTION :

- *PDE-5 (Phosphodiesterase-5) Inhibitors :* **Sildenafil, Tadalafil, Verdenafil.**
- *Prostaglandin :* **Alprostadil.**
- *Others :* **Phentolamine, Papaverin.**
- *Implants :* **Penis pumps, Penile implants.**

### Sildenafil :

- *Mechanism of action :* Inhibits PDE5 in the corpus cavernosa of the penis. Whenever there is sexual stimulation, the endothelial cells release NO (Nitric oxide). This stimulate formation of cyclic-GMP (cGMP), which causes smooth muscle relaxation of corpora cavernosa and increases blood supply of penis, which results in penile erection.
- *Dose :* 50 mg 1 hour before sexual activity.
- *Brand name :* VIAGRA.
- *Use :* Erectile dysfunction. Other Uses : Pulmonary hypertension.
- Ketoconazole, erythromycin etc. increases its level due to CYP3A4 inhibition.

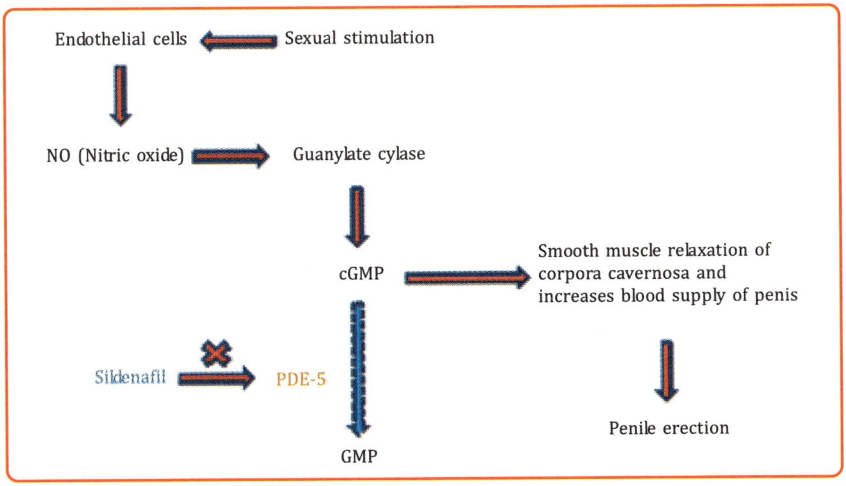


- *Adverse effects :* Headache, flushing, dyspepsia, myalgia, loose motion, color vision impairment (due to inhibition of PDE-6 in retina). Fall in BP and precipitation of acute myocardial infarction, especially in patients taking Nitrates for angina (It potentiates nitrate's hypotension activity).

### Tadalafil and Verdenafil :

- They are newer congeners with similar pharmacological properties.

### Alprostadil :

- It is a prostaglandin analogue, which has to be taken as self injection in the penis before intercourse.

- This results in non-compliance of the patients and also is painful.
- Alprostadil urethral suppositories are also available now.

**Phentolamine and papaverine :**

- These also need to be taken as intra-penile injections.
- These are not used nowadays due to availability of better drugs like sildenafil.
- Prolong erection and priapism are a possibility with these drugs.
- They are also painful and repeated use causes fibrosis.

**NOTE :** Most of the time the erectile dysfunction is due to psychiatric causes like anxiety, stress and depression. Proper treatment of these conditions and counselling will give better results rather than erectile dysfunction drugs.

❑❑❑❑❑

# 32 ESTROGENS, PROGESTINS AND CONTRACEPTIVES

**Contraception :**

It includes all measures temporary or permanent designed to prevent pregnancy due to coital act.

**Ideal Contraceptive :**

- Highly effective, safe, easily acceptable, cheap, simple to use, minimal motivation and has non contraceptive benefit.

**Method of contraception :**

- ***Temporary :*** Barrier method (Condoms), natural contraception, IUCD, Hormonal contraceptives.
- ***Permanent :*** Female and male sterilisation.

## HORMONAL CONTRACEPTIVES CLASSIFICATION :

**Oral contraceptives :**

- ***Combination pills*** – Monophasic, Biphasic and Triphasic.
- ***Mini pills*** – Progestin only pills.
- ***Post coital or morning after pills*** – Emergency contraception.
- ***Centchroman (non-hormonal contraceptive)*** – Ormeloxifen.

**Injectable contraceptives :**

- DMPA (Depot medroxyprogesterone acetate).
- Estradiol cypionate + medroxyprogesterone acetate.

**Hormonal contraceptives in males :**

- Testosterone undecanoate.
- Gossypol (obtained from cotton seed oil).

**Recent hormonal methods :**

- Levonorgestrel subcutaneous implant (NORPLANT).
- Levonorgestrel intrauterine inserts.

## ORAL CONTRACEPTIVES :

### Combination pills :

- It's a combination of estrogen + progesterone. It has 99-99.5% success rate.

- Various combinations are given below :

| Sr. No. | Estrogen | Progesterone |
|---|---|---|
| 1 | Ethinyl estradiol 50 μg | Norgestrel 0.5 mg |
| 2 | Ethinyl estradiol 50 μg | Levonorgestrel 0.25 mg |
| 3 | Ethinyl estradiol 30 μg | Levonorgestrel 0.15 mg |
| 4 | Ethinyl estradiol 30 μg | Desogestrel 0.15 mg |
| 5 | Mestranol 50 μg | Norethindrone 0.5 mg |

- ***Monophasic pills :***
  - Each tablet contains a fixed amount of estrogen and progestin.
  - The first pill is taken on the 5th day after the start of menses. Thereafter, one pill is to be taken each day for 21 days. Next 7 days are pill free period.
  - The next cycle of pills again starts at 5th day of next menstrual cycle.
- ***Biphasic pills :*** Each tablet contains a fixed amount of estrogen, while the amount of progestin increases in the second half of the cycle.
- ***Triphasic pills :*** The amount of estrogen may be fixed or variable, while the amount of progestin increases in 3 equal phases.

### *Mechanism of action :*

- Prevents ovulation by inhibiting gonadotropin (FSH, LH) secretion via effect on both pituitary and hypothalamus (mainly estrogenic effect). Progesterone ensures withdrawal bleeding after the pills are stopped. It also increases the viscosity of cervical mucus making the environment hostile for the sperms.

### *Adverse effects :*

- ***Mild adverse effects (no need to withdraw OC pills) :*** Some OC pills users will have minor side-effects during the first 3 cycles. These side-effects may lead to discontinuation of the combined OC pills. These are : Abnormal menstrual bleeding, nausea, weight gain, breast tenderness and headache.
- ***Adverse effects that appear later :*** Chloasma, pruritus vulvae, carbohydrate intolerance and mood swings.
- ***Serious adverse effects (need to withdraw OC pills) :*** Leg vein and pulmonary thrombosis, coronary and cerebral thrombosis, hypertension, benign hepatomas, gallstones, increased incidence of breast cancer and cervical cancer.

### *Contraindications :*

- Less than 6 weeks postpartum if breastfeeding, pregnancy, smoker over the age of 35 years of age, hypertension, current or past history of venous thrombo-embolism, ischemic heart disease, history of cerebrovascular accident, complicated valvular heart disease, migraine headache, breast and cervical cancer, diabetes with retinopathy/nephropathy/neuropathy, cirrhosis and liver tumor (adenoma or hepatoma).

***Benefits of OC pills :***

- Decreased risk of ovarian cancer, decreased risk of uterine cancer, decreased incidence of acne, menses become regular, decrease incidence of uterine fibroids and decrease incidence of ectopic pregnancy.

## Minipills (progestin only pills) :

- Pills are prescribed soon after delivery and continued without interruption. Success rate is lower than combined pills (98.3%). *E.g.* Norgestrel (75 μg) or Norethindrone (350 μg).
- ***Mechanism of action :*** Progestins place the endometrium prematurely to the secretory phase and increases the viscosity of cervical mucus making the environment hostile for the sperms. Used in cases where estrogen is contraindicated.
- ***Adverse effects :*** Acne, hirsutism and amenorrhea.

## Post coital or morning after pills (emergency contraceptive pill) :

- High dose estrogen and / or high dose of progesterone are quite effective in emergency contraception.
- ***Indication :*** Unprotected coitus like in condom rupture or rape.
- ***Regimes used :***
  1. *Levonorgestrel (75 μg)* alone – within 72 hrs. a second tablet is taken 12 hours after the first tablet. ***E.g.* i-pill**
  2. *Levonorgestrel 25 μg + Ethinyl estradiol 50 μg* – two such tablets taken within 72 hours and next 2 tablets after 12 hours.
  3. *Mifepristone 600 mg* single dose within 72 hours.
  4. *Ulipristal (selective progesterone receptor modulator)* in a single oral dose of 30 mg within 120 hours or 5 days.

## Centchroman (non-hormonal contraceptive) :

- It is a non-steroidal estrogen antagonist or SERM (selective estrogen receptor modulator) named ormeloxifene. It is developed at CDRI (central drug research institute, Lucknow) and distributed in national family welfare programme under the brand name SAHELI.
- ***Dosing :*** It is taken twice a week for first 3 months and then once a week. The first tablet is taken on first day of menstrual cycle.
- ***Mechanism :*** It acts as potent antagonist at estrogen receptors and suppresses proliferative phase. It also accelerates ovum transport.
- ***Benefit :*** Unlike hormonal contraceptives, centchroman does not cause weight gain, hypertension, breakthrough bleeding, thromboembolic episodes, cancers and does not have adverse effects on lipid profile.

## SELECTIVE ESTROGEN RECEPTOR MODULATORS (SERMs) :

- SERMs are synthetic agents whose agonist or antagonist activities on estrogen receptors (OR) are tissue selective.
- They produce beneficial estrogenic effects in certain organs / tissues like brain, bones and liver and prevent certain deleterious estrogenic effects in certain organs / tissues like breast and endometrium.
- **Examples :** Clomiphene, tamoxifen, raloxifene, ormeloxifene.

### Clomiphene :

- Used as Clomiphene Citrate. It is pure antagonist of estrogen receptor.
- ***Mechanism :*** Blocks estrogenic feedback inhibition of pituitary and induces Gn secretion. Increase in amount of secretion of FSH/LH at each secretory pulse. Creates favorable atmosphere (ovarian stimulation) for ovulation in ovaries.
- ***Dosage :*** 50 mg OD from 5$^{th}$ day onwards for 5 days. Continued for 2-3 cycles. Conception occurs within 4-6 cycles. If not then, dose increased.
- ***Use :*** Used in women with unexplained infertility or anovulatory infertility. It is also used in male infertility.
- ***Other Uses :*** Assisted reproduction (to develop multiple eggs) and Artificial insemination (irregular ovulation).
- ***Adverse effects :*** Multiple pregnancy, ovarian enlargement and polycystic ovaries.

### Tamoxifen :

- ***Actions :*** Is a competitive antagonist to estrogen at receptors in the breast and blood vessels but having agonist action on bone and liver.
- ***Uses :*** Hormonal treatment of ER +ve breast carcinoma, osteoporosis, improves lipid profile and thus lowers coronary artery disease.
- ***Adverse effects :*** Hot flushes, chances of DVT and endometrial carcinomas.
- ***Dose :*** Dose is 10 to 20 mg BD.

### Ormeloxifene (centchroman) :

- Already covered above.

### Raloxifene :

- Is estrogen antagonist of breast and endometrium while partial agonist of bone and CVS. Used primarily in post menopausal osteoporosis. Unlike tamoxifene, there is no risk of endometrial cancer.

❑❑❑❑❑

# 33 DRUGS ACTING ON UTERUS

## Uterine Stimulants (Oxytocics) & Relaxants (Tocolytics)

### UTERINE STIMULANTS (Oxytocic Drugs / Abortifacients) :

- These drugs stimulate the uterus and increases its contractility during labor or abortion.

**Drugs :**

- ***Posterior pituitary hormones :*** Oxytocin, Desamino oxytocin, Carbetocin.
- ***Ergot alkaloids :*** Ergometrine (Ergovonine), Methylergometrine.
- ***Prostaglandins :*** $PGE_2$ (Dinoprostone), $PGF_{2\alpha}$ (Dinoprost), 15-methyl $PGF_{2\alpha}$ (Carboprost), Misoprostol.
- ***Others :*** Ethacridine.

### Posterior pituitary hormones : Oxytocin

- Derived from terms Oxys + tokos *i.e.* quick + birth.
- Oxytocin is a posterior pituitary hormone.

**Actions :**

- ***Uterus :*** Increases the force and frequency of uterine contractions. Contraction of upper segment & relaxation of lower segment of uterus results in expulsion of fetus. Nonpregnant uterus is having resistance to oxytocin. The action of oxytocin is mediated by G-protein coupled oxytocin receptors on the uterus. There is depolarisation of muscle fibres and influx of calcium. These oxytocin receptors are increased during later part of pregnancy.
- ***Breast :*** Oxytocin contracts myoepithelium of mammary alveoli and forces milk into bigger milk sinusoids. It mediates the milk letdown reflex which is initiated by suckling.
- ***CVS :*** Higher doses causes fall in BP, reflex tachycardia and flushing.
- ***Renal :*** Higher doses cause decrease in urine output, pulmonary edema etc.

**Uses :**

- ***Induction of labor :*** Induction or stimulation of labor is needed in cases of premature rupture of membranes, post-maturity, toxemia of pregnancy, placental insufficiency. It is usually given by slow IV infusion 5 IU in 500 ml of saline.
- ***Uterine inertia :*** It is absence of effective uterine contractions during labor.

- ***Post partum hemorrhage (PPH) :*** Especially useful in hypertensive women where ergometrine is contraindicated. Action - It acts by forcefully contracting uterine muscle which compresses the blood vessels passing through it to stop hemorrhage.
- ***Breast engorgement :*** Due to insufficient milk ejection reflex. Intranasal spray few minute before suckling is used.
- ***Oxytocin challenge test :*** To assess fetal well being / utero-placental adequacy. IV infusion till uterus contracts about every 4 min and at the same time fetal heart rate is measured. If there is increased heart rate, it suggests uteroplacental flow is insufficient need immediate cesarean delivery.

**Adverse effects :**

- Fetal distress, placental abruption or uterine rupture, high concentration causes excessive fluid retention, hyponatremia, heart failure, seizures, bolus injection causes hypotension.

## Desamino-oxytocin :

- Buccal formulation of oxytocin. Action is similar to oxytocin.

## Carbetocin :

- It is a long acting analogue of oxytocin that is launched in the recent past and is used for control of PPH and prevention of uterine atony after cesarean section.

## Ergot alkaloids : *Ergometrine (Ergovonine), Methylergometrine*

- Ergometrine is derived from fungus Claviceps purpurea and Methylergometrine is a semi-synthetic derivative.
- Methyl ergometrine is more potent & preferred than ergometrine.
- They increase the strength, duration and frequency of uterine contraction of both upper & lower segment. Contraction involves the fundus, body and cervix.
- **Mechanism :** They have agonistic activity on 5-$HT_2$ & $\alpha_1$-adrenergic receptor present on uterine myometrium.
- **Actions :**
  - ***Uterus :*** Increases the force and frequency of uterine contractions. The lower segment of uterus is also involved. There is risk of fetal distress, compression, asphyxia and death.
  - ***CVS :*** No change in BP seen at doses used in OBGY.
  - ***CNS :*** No effects are seen at therapeutic doses. High dose causes interactions with adrenergic, serotonergic and dopaminergic receptors.
  - ***GIT :*** Direct stimulating action on emetic, increases peristalsis.

- **Uses :**
  - ***PPH :*** Prophylaxis and treatment of PPH (0.2 to 0.3 mg I.M. or 0.2 mg i.v.). Mechanism - cause sustained tonic uterine contraction. The uterine blood vessels are compressed by myometrial & bleeding stops.
  - ***To prevent uterine atony :*** After cesarean or instrumental delivery.
  - To ensure normal involution of uterus.
- **Adverse effects :** GI side effects and increase in BP is seen less frequently. High doses causes decrease in milk secretion. Overdose of ergometrine causes prolonged vasospasm, gangrene of finger & toes due to vasoconstriction effect.
- **Contraindications :** During pregnancy and before 3rd stage of labor, patients with hypertension, pre-eclampsia, eclampsia, porphyria, vascular diseases and collagen diseases, threatened spontaneous abortions, liver and kidney diseases, presence of sepsis may cause gangrene.

### Prostaglandins :

- They are autocoids.
- **Actions :** They increase tone & amplitude of uterine contractions. Also sensitise the uterus to oxytocin and also causes oxytocin release. They also promote ripening of cervix (Cervical priming). They also act as Luteolytic agents (causes structural and functional degradation of the corpus luteum).
- **Uses :**
  - ***Therapeutic abortion :*** 2nd trimester pregnancy termination. Administered vaginally as pessaries. Carboprost analogue of $PGF_{2\alpha}$ given as I.M. Misoprostol is given orally or I.V. combined with mifepristone (anti-progestine).
  - ***Cervical priming :*** Dinoprostone (cervical gels, suppositories and oral tablets) before delivery.
  - ***Post-partum Hemorrhage :*** PG analogue like carboprost is given I.M.
  - ***Induction and augmentation of term labor :*** Dinoprostone is preferred.

### Ethacridine :

- It is an alternative abortifacient used less frequently.
- It is mainly used for 2nd trimester medical termination of pregnancy.
- Used as extra-amniotic infusion.

## UTERINE RELAXANTS (TOCOLYTICS) :

- These are the drugs that relax the uterus and prevent contractions. Most commonly, they are used in preventing and treating premature labor and premature uterine contractions.

**Drugs :**

- ***$\beta_2$ adrenergic agonists :*** Ritodrine, Isoxsuprine, Salbutamol and Terbutaline.
- ***Calcium channel blockers :*** Nifedipine.
- ***Magnesium sulphate.***
- ***Miscellaneous :*** Nitrates, Progesterone, Indomethacin.
- ***Oxytocin antagonist :*** Atosiban.

## $\beta_2$ adrenergic agonists :

- ***Mechanism of action :***

**Bind to $\beta_2$ receptor on myometrium**

↓

**Activate adenyle cyclase activity**

↓

**↑cAMP levels - activate cAMP dependent protein kinase**

↓

**↓ intracellular $Ca^{+2}$**

↓

**(Uterine muscle relaxation)**

- ***Ritodrine :*** Selective $\beta_2$ adrenergic agonist specifically developed as a uterine relaxant. Adverse effects are pulmonary edema, hypotension, tachycardia hyperglycemia, hypokalemia.
- ***Isoxsuprine :*** Indicated in premature labor, habitual abortion, threatened abortion, dysmenorrhea. Adverse effects are rashes, nausea, vomiting, dizziness and hypotension.
- ***Salbutamol and terbutaline :*** Can be used as alternatives.
- ***Uses :*** Premature labor.

## Calcium channel blockers :

- ***Mechanism of action :*** It acts via impairing the entry of $Ca^{+2}$ into myometrial cells via voltage dependent channels & thereby inhibit contractility.
- ***Uses :*** Premature labor (Nifedipine is used 10 mg orally, repeated after 20-30 min and followed by 10 mg 6 hourly).
- ***Adverse effects :*** Hypotension, tachycardia.

## Magnesium sulphate :

- ***Mechanism of action :*** They compete with $Ca^{+2}$ ions for entry into the myometrium through voltage sensitive and ligand gated $Ca^{+2}$ channels. It suppresses uterine contractions.

- ***Uses :*** Prevention and treatment of seizures in pre-eclampsia and eclampsia, premature labor (Sometimes used when β-adrenergic agonists are contraindicated).
- ***Route :*** IV.
- ***Adverse effects :*** Life threatening respiratory depression and cardiotoxicity.
- It is monitored by 3 parameters : Patellar reflex, Respiratory rate and Urinary output.

## Nitrates :

- Potent vasodilator and smooth muscle relaxant, Nitroglycerine and other nitrates used to treat myocardial ischemia. Used for inhibition of preterm labor.
- ***Adverse effect :*** Maternal hypotension.

## Progesterone :

- Not used clinically as tocolytic but, used for the treatment of threatened abortion.

## Indomethacin :

- Used to delay preterm labor, but not that effective.
- ***Mechanism of action :*** Inhibiting the Prostaglandin synthesis.
- ***Adverse effects :*** Premature closure of fetal ductus arteriosus, chances of intraventricular hemorrhage in new born.

## Oxytocin receptor antagonist : Atosiban.

- Oxytocin receptor blocker.
- ***Mechanism of action :*** Increases uterine relaxation by competitively blocks the oxytocin receptor.
- ***Route :*** IV-infusion.
- ***Adverse effects :*** Nausea, vomiting, hypotension, skin rashes.

# 34 VITAMIN-D, PARATHYROID HORMONE, CALCITONIN & DRUGS AFFECTING CALCIUM BALANCE

## CALCIUM :

### Physiological Roles :

- Excitability of nerves and muscles and regulates permeability of cell membranes. Also integrity of cell membranes.
- $Ca^{++}$ essential for excitation and coupling of all types of muscles.
- Excitation and secretion of endocrine and exocrine glands and release of neuro-transmitters from nerve endings.
- Intracellular messenger for hormones, autacoids and transmitters.
- Impulse generation and conduction in heart.
- Coagulation of Blood.
- Structural function of Bone and Teeth – hydroxyapatite.

### Calcium Preparations :

- *Calcium chloride :* water soluble, but irritant - tissue necrosis on IM or IV on extravasation. Orally also irritant.
- *Calcium gluconate (9% Ca) :* 0.5 gm/1 gm tabs and 10% injections – a sense of warmth is produced on I.V. injection.
- Calcium lactate.
- Calcium dibasic phosphate.
- Calcium chloride.
- Calcium carbonate (has also been used as antacid).
- *Calcium citrate :* more bioavailability, less chances of renal calculi but more costly.

### Uses :

- *Tetany :* Severe cases - Calcium gluconate 10 to 20 ml IV over 10 minutes followed by 50 to 100 ml of Ca gluconate solution over 6 Hrs followed by oral calcium.
- *Dietary supplement :* growing children, pregnant, lactating and menopausal etc.
- *Osteoporosis :* Prevention and treatment of osteoporosis along with vitamin D / hormone replacement therapy / SERMS / Bisphosphonates – to ensure $Ca^{++}$ deficiency does not occur.
- In dermatoses, paraesthesia and weakness.
- As antacids.

## VITAMIN - D :

- Mainly $D_3$ (cholecalciferol) and $D_2$ (calciferol).
- Both are equally active.
- Calcitriol (active form of $D_3$) is more important physiologically.
- Released from liver in blood and binds to specific Vit D binding globulin.

### Synthesis :

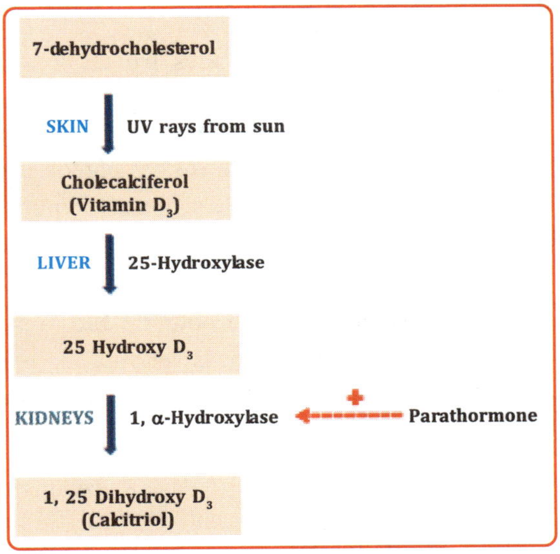


### Sources :

- Milk & milk products, spinach, fish, fortified foods. But, main source is sunlight.

### Plasma levels :

- *Normal :* > 30 ng/ml.
- *Insufficiency :* 10-30 ng/ml.
- *Deficiency :* > 10 ng/ml.
- *Severe deficiency :* > 5 ng/ml.
- *Toxicity :* > 80 ng/ml.

### Recommended daily allowance :

- *Children and healthy adults :* 400 IU/day. Old age, pregnancy and lactation : 800 IU/day.

### Actions :

- Enhancement of absorption of $Ca^{+2}$ and $PO^4$ from intestine. By increasing the synthesis of calcium channels and a carrier calcium binding protein named calbindin.
- Also enhances tubular reabsorption of Calcium from kidneys.
- Vitamin D induces RANK-L receptors on osteoblasts and increases osteoblasts mediated activation of osteoclasts. It also promotes differentiation of osteoclasts precursors.

### Units and preparations :

- 1 mcg of Cholecalciferol = 40 IU of vit. D.
- *Calciferol ($D_2$) :* oily solutions in gelatin capsules – 25000/50000 IU caps.
- *Cholecalciferol ($D_3$) :* 3 lakh IU/ 6 lakh IU IM injections – given 3 to 4 week's intervals. 60000 IU granules or tablet given orally weekly.
- *Calcitriol :* 0.25 to 1 mcg orally on alternate days.
- *Alphacalcidol :* Prodrug – rapidly hydrolysed to calcitriol in liver. Equally active to Calcitriol on long term use. **Dose** – 1-2 mcg/day.

### Deficiency states :

- Rickets in small children.
- Osteomalacia in adults, and
- Osteoporosis.

### Features of rickets :

- ***Osseous changes :***
  - *Head :* craniotabes, frontal bossing, box like skull, delayed closure of anterior fontanelle.
  - *Teeth :* delayed eruption, with abnormal order.
  - *Chest :* rachitic rosary, pigeon chest, funnel-shaped chest.
  - *Spinal column :* scoliosis, kyphosis, and lordosis.
  - *Extremities :* bowlegs (genu varum).
  - Rachitic dwarfism.
- ***Muscular system :*** potbelly, late in standing and walking.
- Motor development is delayed.
- Other nervous and mental symptoms.

### Uses :

- Prophylaxis (400 IU/day) & treatment (3000-4000 IU/day) of rickets & osteomalacia : alternatively Oral/IM injection 3-6 lac IU every 2-6 month.
- Metabolic rickets, Vit D dependent rickets, renal rickets.
- *Vit, D resistant rickets :* $PO^4$ with high doses of Calcitriol.
- Senile or postmenopausal osteoporosis.
- *Hypoparathyroidism :* calcitriol/alphacalcitriol.
- Fanconi like syndrome.
- *Calcipotriol :* Vitamin D analogue used topically in psoriasis.

## PARATHYROID HORMONE (PTH) :

- Also called as parathormone.
- Secreted by parathyroid gland.
- Hypocalcemia is a principal factor regulating PTH synthesis & release.

### Actions :

- ***Bone :*** PTH increases resorption of calcium from bone by increasing the activity and number of osteoblasts. Interestingly both resorption and bone formation are enhanced by PTH, but the net effect of excess of PTH is bone resorption. PTH in low and intermittent doses increases bone formation without causing bone resorption. This finding has led to recent use of low dose with intermittent dosing of recombinant PTH (Teriperatide) in treatment of osteoporosis.
- ***Kidneys :*** PTH increases calcium resorption from kidneys and promote

phosphate excretion. PTH in kidney also stimulates conversion of 25 (OH) $D_3$ to 1,25, $(OH)_2$ $D_3$ by stimulating 1, α Hydroxylase enzyme.

- ***Intestine :*** PTH has no direct effect on intestine. But, indirectly it does have action. As we have seen above that PTH helps in converting 25 (OH) $D_3$ to 1,25, $(OH)_2$ $D_3$ (Calcitriol, which is the active form) in kidneys. Now this active vitamin D promotes absorption of calcium from intestine.

### Use :

- ***Osteoporosis :*** PTH in low and intermittent doses increases bone formation without causing bone resorption. This finding has led to recent use of low dose with intermittent dosing of recombinant PTH **(Teriperatide)** in treatment of osteoporosis.

## CALCITONIN :

- Calcitonin acts to decrease plasma $Ca^{2+}$ levels, while PTH and vitamin D act to increase plasma $Ca^{2+}$, only calcitonin causes a decrease in plasma $Ca^{2+}$.
- Calcitonin is synthesised and secreted by the parafollicular cells of the thyroid gland. It has 32-amino acid peptide with a molecular weight of about 3400.
- The primary stimulus for Calcitonin secretion is increased plasma calcium levels.

### Actions :

- It has actions opposite to that of PTH.
- Inhibit bone resorption by direct action on Osteoclasts.
- Also inhibits the proximal tubular resorption of calcium and phosphate by direct action on kidney.

### Calcitonin Preparations :

- Porcine (Natural) calcitonin : It is antigenic.
- Synthetic human calcitonin : 1 IU = 4 μg of standard preparation.
- Synthetic salmon calcitonin : More commonly used because it is more potent due to slower metabolism.
- Calcitonin is given by SC/IM routes.
- Salmon calcitonin is also available as nasal spray.
- Adverse effects are nausea, flushing, tingling, bad taste etc.

### Uses :

- Hypercalcemia states *e.g.* associated with neoplasia.
- Paget's disease of bone.
- Postmenopausal osteoporosis & corticosteroid induced osteoporosis : Salmon calcitonin is used as nasal spray along with Vit. D supplements 200 IU/day.

## BISPHOSPHONATES (BPNS) :

- Non-hormonal agent in $Ca^{+2}$ homoeostasis which has recently attracted considerable attention. Prevents osteoporosis and useful in metabolic bone diseases and hyper-calcemia.

### Classification of BPNs :

- ***First-generation*** : Etidronate, clodronate and tiludronate.
- ***Second-generation*** : Alendronate, pamidronate and ibandronate.
- ***Third generation*** : Risedronate, zolendronate and oxidronate.

### Mechanism of action :

- Inhibit osteoclasts mediated resorption of bone by binding to the hydroxyapatite crystals of bone.
- BPNs are endocytosed in the osteoclasts and cause apoptosis of osteoclasts. The number of osteoclasts are thus reduced.

### Uses :

- Osteoporosis – age related, steroid induced and idiopathic osteoporosis.
- Prevention and treatment of post-menopausal osteoporosis.
- Paget's disease.
- Hypercalcemia of Malignancy.
- Osteolytic Bone Metastasis.
- Zolendronate is given parenterally.

### Adverse effects :

- Gastric erosion, retrosternal pain, reflux esophagitis and flatulence (therefore advised given : to take BPNs empty stomach with glass of water and do not allow to lie down or eat till 30 minutes.
- Other adverse effect is osteonecrosis of jaw.

## OSTEOPOROSIS :

- A systemic skeletal disease characterised by low bone mass and microarchitectural deterioration of bone tissue, with a consequent increase in bone fragility and susceptibility to fracture.

### Types :

- ***Primary osteoporosis :*** Postmenopausal : ↓ estrogen results in ↑ osteoclastic activity without ↑ osteoblastic activity. Most common fractures : vertebral, hip and wrist fractures. Age related : In later decades of life. Also called senile osteoporosis.
- ***Secondary Osteoporosis :*** Acromegaly, Addison's disease, Hyperparathyroidism, Amyloidosis, Lymphoma and leukemia, Multiple myeloma, Multiple sclerosis.
- ***Drug induced osteoporosis :*** Aluminium, Anticonvulsants, Excessive thyroxine, Glucocorticoids, GnRH agonists, Heparin and Lithium.

## Drugs used for osteoporosis :

- Bisphosphonates, Calcitonin, Vitamin D, Recombinant Parathormone *i.e.* r-PTH (Teriperatide), Hormone replacement therapy, Selective estrogen receptor modulators and Strontium ranelate.

### *Bisphosphonates, Calcitonin, vitamin D, r-PTH :*

Already covered in this chapter.

### *Hormone replacement therapy (estrogen replacement therapy – ERT) :*

- **Mechanism :**
  - ↓es osteoclast activity.
  - Acts on osteoblast to ↓ production of IL-6.
  - Interferes with recruitment of osteoclast precursors.
- **Dose :** Estrogen : 0.625 mg od, Progesterone 2.5 mg qd (if uterus present).
- **Advantages :** Increases bone density and decreases risk of fracture, relief of hot flashes, vaginal dryness, decreases LDL, increases HDL, relatively inexpensive.
- **Disadvantages :** ↑ bone loss after stopping, ↑ risk of uterine ca, ↑ risk of thromboembolic events, Possible ↑ risk of breast cancer.
- **Adverse effects :** Breast tenderness, breakthrough bleeding, ↑ risk of coronary events in women with known coronary artery disease.

### *Selective Estrogen Receptor Modulators (SERMs) :*

- **Raloxifene :** partial agonist in bone and CVS but an antagonist in endometrium and breast (for details refer estrogen, progestin and contraceptives chapter).
- **Dose :** Raloxifene 60 mg od.
- **Advantages :** Increases bone density and decreases fracture risk, no stimulation of breast or endometrial tissue, no need for progestin in women with uterus, decreases LDL.
- **Disadvantages :** Increased risk of thromboembolic events, doesn't treat post- menopausal symptoms, may increase hot flashes.

### *Strontium ranelate :*

- Oral strontium ranelate is an alternative oral treatment, belonging to a class of drugs called dual action bone agents.
- Proven efficacy, especially in the prevention of vertebral fractures.
- **Mechanism of action :** ↑ collagen & noncollagen protein synthesis, enhances preosteoblast differentiation, ↓ osteoclast function.
- **Dosage :** 2 g orally daily.
- **Adverse effects :** Risk of thromboembolism.

# DRUGS ACTING ON CENTRAL NERVOUS SYSTEM (CNS)

# 35 GENERAL ANESTHETICS

## GENERAL ANESTHESIA :

General anesthesia is the loss of response to & perception of all external stimuli. General anesthetics are the drugs which causes reversible loss of all the sensations and consciousness.

### Components of General Anesthesia :

- Unconsciousness (Hypnosis), analgesia and muscle relaxation.

### Phases of Anesthesia :

- ***Induction :*** putting the patient to sleep.
- ***Maintenance :*** keeping the patient asleep.
- ***Emergence :*** waking the patient up.

### Stages of Anesthesia :

- ***Stage 1 : Analgesia :*** Decreased awareness of pain, amnesia.
- ***Stage 2 : Delirium :*** Delirium & excitation, enhanced reflexes, retching, incontinence, irregular respiration.
- ***Stage 3 : Surgical Anesthesia :*** Unconscious, no pain reflexes, regular respiration, BP is maintained.
- ***Stage 4 : Medullary Depression :*** Respiratory & CVS depression requiring ventilation & pharmacologic support.

## CLASSIFICATION OF GENERAL ANESTHETICS :

### Intravenous anesthetics :

- ***Inducing agents :*** Thiopentone sodium, Propofol, Etomidate.
- ***Slower acting :*** Diazepam, Lorazepam, Midazolam.
- ***Dissociative anesthesia :*** Ketamine.
- ***Opioid analgesia :*** Fentanyl.

### Inhalational anesthetics :

- ***Gas :*** Nitrous oxide.
- ***Liquid :*** Ether, Halothane, Enflurane, Desflurane, Isoflurane, Sevoflurane.

### Mechanisms of Action :

1. ***Enhanced GABA effect on $GABA_A$ Receptors :*** Inhaled anesthetics, Etomidate, Barbiturates, Benzodiazepines, Propofol.

2. ***Activate K channels (hyperpolarise) :*** Nitrous oxide, ketamine.
3. ***Inhibit NMDA (glutamate) receptors :*** Nitrous oxide, ketamine.

## Intravenous anesthetics :

### *Barbiturates :*

- Thiopental is highly lipid soluble & can produce unconsciousness & surgical anesthesia in < 1 min.
- ***Mechanism of action :*** see in chapter on sedative-hypnotics.
- Actions are terminated by redistribution.
- With single bolus - emergence from GA occurs in ~ 10 mins.
- Hepatic metabolism is required for elimination.
- ***Uses :*** Induction of anesthesia & short procedures.

### *Benzodiazepines :*

- Midazolam > Diazepam & Lorazepam.
- ***Mechanism of action :*** See in chapter on sedative-hypnotics.
- Used to produce anxiolysis, amnesia & sedation prior to induction of GA.
- Effects are reversed with flumazenil.
- ***Uses :*** Pre-anesthetic medication, induction of anesthesia, Conscious sedation, commonly used for short diagnostic or endoscopic procedures.

### *Propofol :*

- Produces anesthesia as rapidly as I.V. barbiturate but recovery is more rapid. Patients are able to ambulate sooner & patients *"feel better"* in the post-op period compared to other I.V. anesthetics. Antiemetic effects (patients with - risk of nausea), marked hypotension. Commonly used as component of *"balanced anesthesia"* for maintenance of anesthesia following induction of anesthesia.
- ***Uses :*** Conscious sedation, Induction agent of anesthesia, Maintenance of anesthesia, Antiemetic.

### *Opioids (Fentanyl) :*

- ***Mechanism :*** Discussed in detail in opioids chapter.
- General anesthetics do not produce effective analgesia (except for ketamine).
- Given before surgery to minimise hemodynamic changes produced by painful stimuli. This reduces GA requirements.
- High doses can cause chest wall rigidity & post-op respiratory depression.
- ***Uses :*** Used for post-op analgesia, supplement anesthetic in balanced anesthesia.

### *Ketamine :*

- A *"dissociative anesthetic"* that produces a cataleptic state that includes intense analgesia, amnesia, eyes open, involuntary limb movement, unresponsive to commands or pain.

- Increases heart rate, blood pressure and causes brochodilatation.
- Can be used in shock states (hypotensive) or patients at risk for bronchospasm.
- ***Uses :*** Used in children & young adults for short procedures.
- ***Adverse Effects :*** Nystagmus, pupillary dilation, salivation, hallucinations & vivid dreams.

## Inhaled anesthetics :

***Nitrous Oxide :***

- Incomplete anesthetic.
- Good analgesia, no metabolism, rapid onset & recovery.
- Used along with other anesthetic; fast induction & recovery.

***Halothane :***

- The first halogenated inhalational anesthetic.
- Not pungent (use for induction especially in children).
- Medium rate of onset & recovery. Sensitises the heart to adrenaline.
- Although inexpensive, its use has declined.
- ***Adverse effects :*** Malignant hyperthermia, halothane induced hepatitis.

***Desflurane :***

- Most rapid onset of action & recovery. Widely used for outpatient surgery
- Irritating to the airway in awake patients & causes coughing, salivation & bronchospasm (poor induction agent).
- Used for maintenance of anesthesia.

***Sevoflurane :***

- Relatively rapid onset of action & recovery. Widely used for outpatient surgery.
- Not irritating to the airway.
- Useful induction agent, particularly in children.

***Isoflurane :***

- Medium rate of onset & recovery. Used for induction & maintenance of anesthesia. Isoflurane *"was"* the most commonly used inhalational GA in the US.
- Has been largely replaced by Desflurane

## PRE-ANESTHETIC MEDICATION :

*"It is the term applied to the administration of drugs prior to general anesthesia so as to make anesthesia safer for the patient".*

### Aim :

- Relief of anxiety & apprehension preoperatively & facilitate smooth induction.

- Amnesia for pre- & post-operative events.
- Potentiate action of anesthetics, so lesser doses is needed.
- Ensures comfort to the patient & to minimise adverse effects of anesthesia.
- Antiemetic effect extending to post-operative period.
- Decrease secretions & vagal stimulation caused by anesthetics.
- Decrease acidity, to prevent reflux & aspiration pneumonia.

### Drugs used for pre-anesthetic medication :

1. ***Anti-anxiety drugs :***
   - Provide relief from apprehension & anxiety.
   - Provides post-operative amnesia.
   - **Drugs : Diazepam** (5-10 mg oral), **Lorazepam** (2 mg I.M.).

2. ***Opioid analgesics :***
   - Provide sedation, pre & post-operative analgesia, reduction in anesthetic dose.
   - **Drugs : Morphine** (8-12 mg I.M.) or **Pethidine** (50-100 mg I.M.) used one hour before surgery. **Fentanyl** (50-100 mg I.M. or I.V.) preferred nowadays (just before induction of anesthesia).

3. ***Anticholinergics :***
   - Reduces salivary & bronchial secretions, vagal bradycardia, and hypotension.
   - **Drugs : Atropine** (0.5 mg I.M.) or **Hyoscine** (0.5 mg I.M.) one hour before surgery. **Glycopyrrolate** used nowadays, Reason - no central action, acts rapidly, longer acting, potent antisecretory agent, prevents vagal bradycardia effectively.

4. ***Antiemetics :***
   - Drugs that reduce nausea and vomiting due to anesthesia drugs. Also prevents aspiration of gastric contents in lungs.
   - **Drugs : Metoclopramide** (10 mg I.M.) used as antiemetic & as prokinetic gastric emptying agent prior to emergency surgery. **Domperidone** (10 mg oral) more preferred (does not produce extrapyramidal side effects). **Ondansetron** (4-8 mg I.V.), a $5HT_3$ receptor antagonist, found effective in preventing post-anesthetic nausea & vomiting.

5. ***Drugs reducing acid secretion :***
   - **Drugs : Ranitidine** (150-300 mg oral) given night before & in morning reduces risk of gastric regurgitation & aspiration pneumonia. Proton pump inhibitors like **Omeprazole** (20 mg) or **Pantoprazole** (40 mg) is preferred nowadays.

# 36 ETHYL AND METHYL ALCOHOLS (Ethanol and Methanol)

Ethanol is traditionally called as alcohol. Importance in medicine is due to abuse or misuse. Ethanol has effect on many systems in the body. It has also got effect on the development of fetus. It is manufactured by Fermentation of Sugar, starches and other carbohydrates. But, the major source of commercial alcohol is molasses (obtained from sugarcane industry from which no more sugar can be crystallised).

## MEDICALLY USED ALCOHOLS :

1. Absolute Alcohol – 99% w/w of ethanol.
2. Rectified Spirit – 90% w/w of ethanol.
3. Denaturated alcohol : It is ethanol to which some substance like methanol, camphor, aniline dyes are added. This makes it unfit for human consumption.

## MECHANISM OF ACTION OF ALCOHOL :

- Ethanol enhances action of GABA on $GABA_A$ receptor similar to actions of benzodiazepines (GABA-BZD-$Cl^-$ channel).
- Inhibition of NMDA excitatory amino acid receptor.
- Pleasure and alcohol dependence is due to dopamine and endorphins.

## PHARMACOKINETICS OF ALCOHOL :

- Rapidly absorbed from GIT. Rapidly distributed. Crosses BBB as well as placenta. 95% metabolised and 5% excreted through breath, urine and sweat. Alcohol excreted in breath can reveal amount of alcohol in blood (medico-legal purposes). Alcohol is also an enzyme inducer.

## METABOLISM OF ALCOHOL :

Ethanol is first metabolised to acetaldehyde with the help of enzyme alcohol dehydrogenase and then again metabolised to acetic acid by enzyme aldehyde dehydrogenase.

**ETHANOL**
↓ *Alcohol dehydrogenase*
**ACETALDEHYDE**
↓ *Aldehyde dehydrogenase*
**ACETIC ACID**

## PHARMACOLOGICAL ACTIONS :

- **Local :** Rubefacient and counterirritant to skin, irritant to soft skin and mucous membrane, pain, inflammation and necrosis on s/c injection, astringent (precipitates surface protein) and antiseptic (precipitates bacterial protein). Antiseptic action increases with concentration from 20–70%, remains constant from 70-90 and decreases above that. No action on spores.

- **CNS :** Depressant action – dose dependent manner :

| Plasma concentration | Effects |
|---|---|
| 30 - 60 mg/dl | Decreased anxiety, euphoria, loss of self restraint and caution and altered mood and feelings. |
| 80 -150 mg/dl | Mental clouding, impaired co-ordination, disorganisation of thought, impairment of memory and drowsiness. |
| 150 - 200 mg/dl | Sloppy, Slurring of speech, loss of judgement and inhibition. |
| 200 - 300 mg/dl | Stupor and unconsciousness. |

- **CVS :** Small doses cause cutaneous vasodilatation, flushing. Medium dose causes tachycardia and mild rise in BP and higher dose causes vasodilatation due to direct vascular smooth muscle dilatation and vasomotor centre depression (fall in BP).
- **RS :** Stimulation of respiration by irritation of pharyngeal and buccal mucosa. Central depressant action.
- **Blood :** Mild to moderate drinking increases HDL-cholesterol level.
- **GIT :** Low doses stimulate GI secretion. Higher doses inhibit GI secretion. Gastritis, vomiting, reflux and acute pancreatitis. Liver – Alcoholic Cirrhosis.
- **Kidney :** Diuresis – this is due to increased water ingestion with drinks and inhibition of ADH by alcohol.
- **Uterus :** Relaxation of uterine muscles.
- **Endocrine :** Low dose – adrenaline release and hyperglycemia. High dose – hypoglycemia due to hepatic depletion of glycogen and inhibition of gluconeogenesis.
- **Sex :** Aphrodisiac action.

## ADVERSE EFFECTS OF ALCOHOL :

- Nausea, Vomiting, hangover and traffic accidents, CNS depressant effect, depression of inhibitory control, vasodilatation, warm, flushed, reddish skin, decreased memory & concentration, poor judgement, decreased reflexes and emotional outbursts, teratogenicity (Fetal alcohol syndrome : growth retardation, facial malformations and reduced intelligence).

## ACUTE ALCOHOL INTOXICATION :

### Clinical features :

- Hypotension, hypoglycemia, respiratory depression, coma and death due to respiratory depression or aspiration of vomit.

## CHRONIC ALCOHOLISM :

Chronic alcoholism has following features :

- **Craving :** A strong need, or compulsion to drink.

- **Loss of control :** The inability to limit one's drinking on any given occasion.
- **Tolerance :** The need to drink greater amounts of alcohol for getting high.
- **Physical dependence :** Withdrawal symptoms such as nausea, sweating, tremors, hyperexcitability, psychosis, seizures and **delirium tremens** (confusion, agitation, aggressiveness and hallucinations) occur when alcohol use is stopped after a period of heavy drinking.
- **Neurotoxicity :** Ataxia, dementia, neuropathies and Wernicke-Korsakoff syndrome.
- **Wernicke-Korsakoff syndrome** is due to thiamine (Vit. B1) deficiency seen in chronic heavy drinkers and is characterised by ataxia, confusion and paralysis of extraocular muscles.
- **GIT :** Chronic Gastritis, Intestinal mucosal damage : Lack of absorption leading to nutritional deficiencies especially water soluble vitamins, Microsomal enzyme induction, Chronic pancreatitis, Fatty infiltration of liver and Liver cirrhosis (scarring of liver).
- **CVS :** Hypertension, ventricular hypertrophy, cardiomyopathy, CHF arrhythmias and stroke.
- **Hormonal :** Impotence, gynecomastia and infertility.

## TREATMENT OF ACUTE ALCOHOL TOXICITY :

- Gastric lavage.
- Maintain patent airway.
- Fluid and electrolyte balance.
- Glucose infusion.
- Inj. Thiamine IV or IM.
- Hemodialysis.

## TREATMENT OF WITHDRAWAL SYMPTOMS.

- **Chlordizepoxide and diazepam** - Long acting BZD.
- **Clonidine** – central $\alpha_2$ agonist.
- **Propranolol** – $\beta$ blocker.

## TREATMENT OF ALCOHOL DEPENDENCE :

### Disulfiram :

- Aldehyde dehydrogenase inhibitor.
- Disulfiram inhibits Aldehyde dehydrogenase. Thus, acetaldehyde is not converted to acetic acid. This leads to rise in concentration of aldehyde in blood and leads to distressing aldehyde syndrome.
- ***Symptoms (Alcohol+Disulfiram) :*** flushing, burning sensation, throbbing

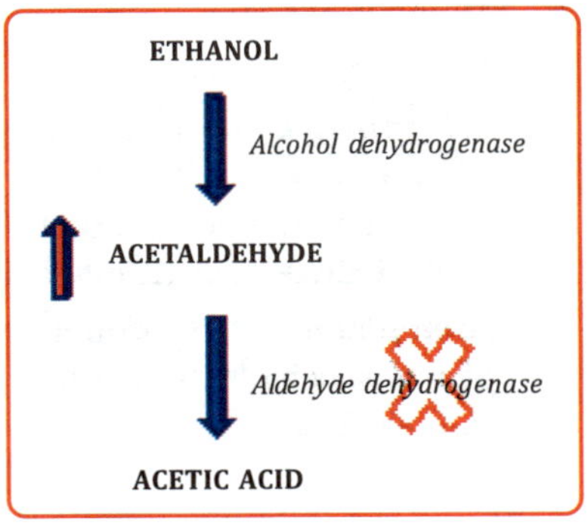

headache, perspiration, dizziness, vomiting, loose stools, visual disturbance, mental confusion, fainting and circulatory collapse.

- Available as 250 mg tablets.

## OTHER DRUGS FOR ALCOHOL DEPENDENCE :

These drugs reduce craving for alcohol in patients :

- **Naltrexone** (50 mg) – Long acting Opioid antagonist.
- **Acamprosate** – NMDA receptor antagonist, GABAa agonist.
- **Topiramate** – anticonvulsant.
- **Ondansetron** – 5-$HT_3$ antagonist.
- **Fluoxetine** - SSRIs.

## USES OF ETHANOL :

- Antiseptic, rubefacient and counterirritant, antiperspirant and aftershave, appetite stimulant and carminative : 30–60 ml of 7-10%, neuralgias : severe cancer pain – injection round the nerve, as astringent (precipitates protein) and methanol Poisoning.

## METHANOL POISONING :

- Methanol is used as industrial solvent & also to adulterate ethanol to make it unfit for drinking. Poisoning is common due to unscrupulous mixing with alcoholic beverages and accidental. Methanol is metabolised similarly like ethanol.

  Methanol is first metabolised to formaldehyde with the help of enzyme alcohol dehydrogenase and then again metabolised to formic acid by enzyme aldehyde dehydrogenase.

**METHANOL**

↓ *Alcohol dehydrogenase*

**FORMALDEHYDE**

↓ *Aldehyde dehydrogenase*

**FORMIC ACID**

### Clinical features :

vomiting, epigastric pain, dyspnea, bradycardia, acidosis, hypotension, retinal damage and Death. These symptoms are mainly due to ***formic acid.***

### Treatment :

- Maintain vitals.
- ***For acidosis :*** Sodium bicarbonate.
- ***Ethanol :*** ethanol has higher affinity for alcohol dehydrogenase than methanol. Ethanol becomes the substrate for alcohol dehydrogenase and saturates it. There is no alcohol dehydrogenase left to metabolise methanol to formaldehyde and formic acid. Thus, the toxic symptoms are prevented.
- ***Fomepizole :*** It is alcohol dehydrogenase inhibitor which prevents formation of formaldehyde and formic acid (toxic metabolites).
- Hemodialysis.

37

# SEDATIVE-HYPNOTIC DRUGS (Benzodiazepines and Barbiturates)

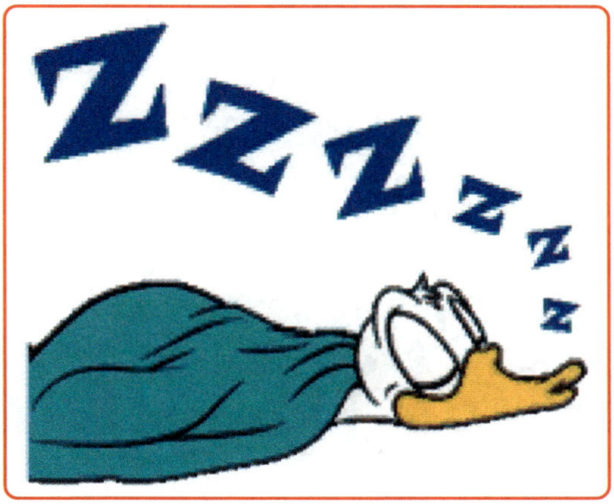


**Sedation** means decreased alertness without inducing sleep. **Hypnosis** means a state that resembles natural sleep but the person can be aroused by strong stimuli such as pin prick or sound of alarm clock. The drugs which reduce anxiety are also called as anxiolytics. Sedatives and hypnotics produce many therapeutically desirable effects such as anxiolysis, sedation and sleep, muscle relaxation and anticonvulsant action. They produce various levels of CNS depression.

## CLASSIFICATION :

- **Benzodiazepines (BZD) :**
  - ***Short acting :*** Triazolam, midazolam, oxazepam.
  - ***Intermediate acting :*** Alprazolam, Lorazepam, nitrazepam.
  - ***Long acting :*** Diazepam, clonazepam, chlordiazepoxide.
- **Barbiturates :**
  - ***Ultrashort acting :*** Thiopentone, methohexital.
  - ***Short acting :*** Pentobarbitone, Amobarbitone.
  - ***Long acting :*** Phenobarbitone, Mephobarbitone.
- **Non-benzodiazepines (Z-hypnotics) :**
  - Zolpidem, Zopiclone, Zaleplon.
- **Atypical anxiolytics :**
  - Buspirone, Ipsapirone.

- **Non-sedating anxiolytic :**
  - Propranolol (β blocker).

## Benzodiazepines :

***Mechanism of Action :***

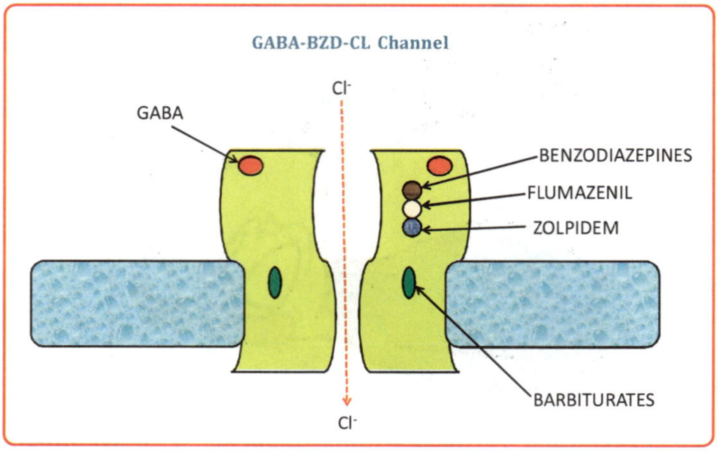


Benzodizepines increase the activity of GABA by acting on GABA-BZD-$Cl^-$ (GABA- Benzodiazepine-chloride) channel complex. Increases the frequency of $Cl^-$ channel opening and causes hyperpolarization.

***Effects :***

Usually, ***CNS depression :***

- Sedation.
- Hypnosis.
- Anxiolysis.
- Amnesia.
- Anticonvulsant.
- Muscle relaxation.

***Uses :***

- Insomnia.
- Anxiolytic.
- Anesthetic.
- ***Pre-anesthetic medication :*** Diazepam, lorazepam, midazolam.
- ***Muscle relaxant :*** Diazepam.
- ***Anticonvulsant :*** Diazepam, lorazepam.
- Prevents stress ulcer.
- Alcohol withdrawal.

*Adverse effects :*

- Drowsiness, fatigue, lethargy.
- Vertigo, dizziness, disorientation.
- Anterograde amnesia.
- Rebound insomnia.
- ***Nightmare :*** Nitrazepam.
- Withdrawal syndrome.
- Tolerance, dependence and abuse potential.

*Flumazenil :*

- Antagonist of BZD (Refer picture above).
- Reverses all effects of BZD.
- Used in overdose and toxicity of BZD.

## Barbiturates :

- Barbiturates are derivatives of barbituric acid.
- They have been largely replaced by BZDs.

*Mechanism of Action :*

- Like BZDs, they also increase the activity of GABA by acting on GABA-BZD-$Cl^-$ (GABA- Benzodiazepine-chloride) channel complex but, the binding site is different than that of BZD. Increases the duration of $Cl^-$ channel opening and causes hyperpolarisation.

*Barbiturates – Clinical Effects :*

- ***CNS :*** Produce all degrees of CNS depression. May produce paradoxical excitement with increased reaction to painful stimuli. They are not analgesics. Anxiolysis usually accompanied by significant sedation. Little use for these drugs as anxiolytics. Anticonvulsant properties also accompanied by sedation.
- ***RS :*** Depresses respiratory drive and rhythmicity.
- ***CVS :*** Dose dependent effects.
- ***Kidney :*** Decrease renal blood flow (thiopental).
- ***Liver :*** Hepatic microsomal enzymes induction CYP 450.

*Uses :*

- ***As sedative-hypnotic :*** replaced by BZD nowadays.
- ***As anticonvulsants :*** long acting like phenobarbitone.
- Tetanus.
- ***General anesthesia :*** ultra short acting like thiopentone.
- ***Narcoanalysis :*** Thiopentone is used.
- Treatment of neonatal jaundice as barbiturates increase the activity of hepatic microsomal enzymes and bilirubin gets conjugated faster and excreted through bile.

### *Adverse drug reactions :*

- Hangover (after effects).
- Allergic reactions (swelling of lips, eyelids, cheeks).
- Enzyme induction and drug interactions.
- Respiratory depression.
- Porphyria (enhance porphyrin synthesis).
- Tolerance.
- Drug automatism (loss of short term memory) – patient forgets that he has taken the barbiturate and again takes it repeatedly leading to toxicity.
- Drug dependence.
- Withdrawal symptoms.

### *Acute barbiturate poisoning :*

- ***Clinical features :*** CNS depression, Respiratory depression and CVS collapse.
- ***Treatment :***
    - Hospitalisation.
    - Monitor airway, breathing, circulation.
    - Gastric lavage.
    - Forced alkaline diuresis (Alkalinisation).
    - IV fluids.
    - No specific barbiturate antagonist is available.
    - Dialysis and hemoperfusion.

## Difference between benzodiazepine and barbiturates :

| Benzodiazepines | Barbiturates |
|---|---|
| Binds to Benzodiazepine binding site of GABA-BZD-Cl receptor complex | Binds to barbiturate binding site of GABA-BZD-Cl receptor complex |
| Do not affect REM sleep | Affect REM sleep |
| No drug automation | Drug automation |
| Wide therapeutic index | Narrow therapeutic index |
| Low abuse potential | High abuse potential |
| Not enzyme inducers | Enzyme inducers |

## Z hypnotics :

- *E.g.* Zolpidem, Zopiclone, Zaleplon.
- Structurally unrelated to each other and to benzodiazepines.
- Therapeutic efficacy of Z hypnotics is due to agonist effects on the benzodiazepine site of the $GABA_A$ receptor.
- Two types of benzodiazepine receptors are there : BZ-1 and BZ-2.
- BZ-1 is responsible for antianxiety, sedative and hypnotic action and BZ-2 receptor is responsible for muscle relaxation.

- BZD acts on both BZ-1 and BZ-2 receptors causing antianxiety, sedative, hypnotic and muscle relaxation effect.
- Z hypnotics selectively acts on BZ-1 receptor only and not BZ-2 receptor and thus, causes antianxiety, sedative and hypnotic action without causing muscle relaxation.
- Actions are blocked by BZD receptor antagonist like Flumazenil.
- Are effective in relieving sleep-onset insomnia. Have been approved by the FDA for use for up to 7-10 days at a time.
- Sustained hypnotic efficacy without occurrence of rebound insomnia on abrupt discontinuation.

## Atypical Anxiolytics :

- *E.g.* Buspirone.
- Does not interact directly with GABAergic systems.
- Anxiolytic effects due to partial agonist at 5-$HT_{1A}$ receptors.
- Relieves anxiety without causing marked sedative, hypnotic, or euphoric effects.
- No anticonvulsant or muscle relaxant properties.
- The anxiolytic effects of buspirone may take more than a week.
- Unsuitable for management of acute anxiety states.
- No rebound anxiety or withdrawal signs on abrupt discontinuance.
- Buspirone has minimal abuse liability.
- The drug is used in generalised anxiety states.

## Non-sedating anxiolytic :

Propranolol (β blocker). Reduces sympathetic symptoms. More effective in anxiety, apprehensions, worry, performance anxiety, tremors, hyperthyroidism induced palpitations and anxiety.

# 38 ANTI-EPILEPTIC DRUGS

**Important terms :**

- ***Seizures :*** Transient alteration of sensation, awareness or behaviour due to disordered, abnormal firing of brain neurons.
- ***Epilepsy :*** Recurrent episodes of such seizures is epilepsy.
- ***Status Epilepticus :*** Epileptic seizures occurring repeatedly with no recovery of consciousness in between.

**Types of epilepsy :**

- ***Generalized epilepsy :*** Generalised tonic clonic, absence, myoclonic and atonic.
- ***Partial epilepsy :*** Simple and complex.

**Causes :**

- Genetic/hereditary, birth trauma, meningitis/brain abscess, hypocalcemia, hypoglycemia, Vit. $B_6$ deficiency and withdrawal of many drugs.

**Why seizures occur ?**

- Inhibition of inhibitory neurons or excitation of excitatory neurons.

**Antiepileptics act by restoration of normal neuronal activity *i.e.* :**

- Activation of inhibitory neurons or inhibition of excitatory neurons.

## CLASSIFICATION OF ANTIEPILEPTIC DRUGS :

- ***Hydantoins :*** Phenytoin, Fosphenytoin.
- ***Barbiturates :*** Phenobarbitone, Mephobarbitone.
- ***Benzodiazepines :*** Diazepam, Clonazepam, Lorazepam.
- ***Iminostilbene :*** Carbamazepine.
- ***Succimide :*** Ethosuxsimide.
- ***GABA transaminase inhibitors :*** Valproic acid (Valproate).
- ***GABA analogues :*** Gabapentin, Pregabalin.
- ***Newer drugs :*** Topiramate, Lamotrigine, Vigabatrin, Levetiracetam.

**Classification based on mechanism :**

- ***Inhibition of $Na^+$ channels :*** Carbamazepine, Phenytoin, Topiramate, Valproate.
- ***Inhibition of glutamate neurons :*** Topiramate, Lamotrigine.

- ***Enhancing GABA action :*** Benzodiazepines, Barbiturates, Valproate, Gabapentin, Pregabalin.
- ***Blockage of 'T' type $Ca^{+2}$ channels :*** Ethosuxsimide, Valproate.

## Phenytoin :

- ***Mechanism of action :*** Inhibition of $Na^+$ channel.
- It follows zero order kinetics. Plasma monitoring needed. It is an enzyme inducer.
- It should not be used in absence seizures.
- ***Fosphenytoin*** is a prodrug and used IV as a substitute for phenytoin. It is better tolerated than phenytoin.
- ***Uses of Phenytoin :*** Generalised tonic clonic seizures, partial seizures, status epilepticus, cardiac arrhythmia due to digitalis.
- ***Adverse effects :*** Ataxia, vertigo, nystagmus, gum hypertrophy, megaloblastic anemia, osteomalacia, hirsutism, vitamin K deficiency, if used in pregnancy; fetal hydantoin syndrome (cleft lip, cleft palate, congenital heart disease, growth restrictions, mental retardation).

## Barbiturates (Phenobarbitone, Mephobarbitone) :

- ***Mechanism of action :*** Increases the activity of GABA by acting on GABA-BZD-Cl channel complex. They increase the duration of Cl channel opening and causes hyper-polarisation.
- Phenobarbitone is an enzyme inducer.
- ***Uses :*** Partial seizures, generalised tonic clonic seizures, prophylaxis after febrile seizures.
- ***Adverse effects :*** Long term administration cause behavioral abnormalities, impaired learning and memory. It is contraindicated in porphyria.

GABA-BZD-CL CHANNEL

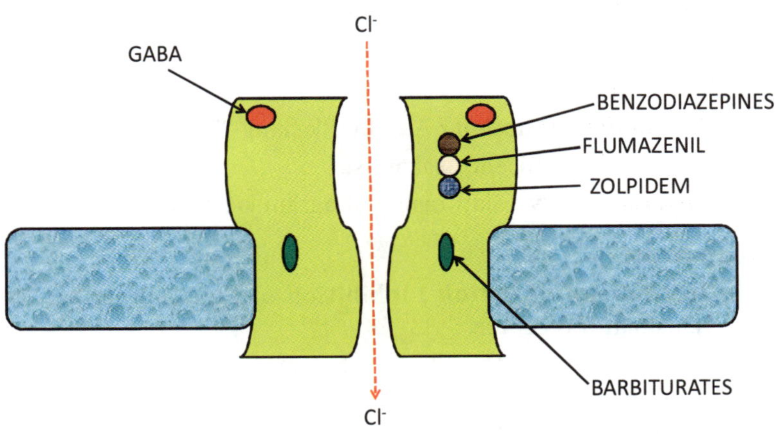

## Carbamazepine :

- ***Mechanism of action :*** Inhibition of $Na^+$ channel.
- Metabolised in liver to toxic epoxide derivative. It is an enzyme inducer.
- ***Auto-induction :*** Increases its own metabolism.
- ***Oxcarbazepine :*** It is analogue of carbamazepine but better safety and less enzyme induction as compared to carbamazepine.
- ***Uses :*** Partial / Generalised tonic clonic seizures, trigeminal neuralgia, bipolar disorder, neuropathic pain.
- ***Adverse effects :*** Sedation, ataxia, vertigo, diplopia, agranulocytosis, liver toxicity, water retention (Antidiuretic effect by ↑ ADH action), allergic reaction, rashes and teratogenicity (chances are low but, can cause craniofacial abnormalities).

## Valproate (Valproic acid) :

- It is also called as "Broad spectrum antiepileptic" because it is nearly used in all types of epilepsy. It is an enzyme inhibitor.
- ***Mechanism of action :*** Inhibition of $Na^+$ channel, blockage of 'T' type $Ca^{+2}$ channels and inhibition of degradation of GABA by transaminase.
- ***Uses of Valproate :*** Generalised tonic clonic and partial seizures, absence seizures, myoclonic seizures, bipolar disorder and migraine.
- ***Adverse effects :*** Nausea, weight gain, hepatotoxicity in children, neural tube defects and spina bifida in baby, if used in pregnancy.

## Benzodiazepines :

- ***Mechanism of action :*** Is similar to barbiturates *i.e.* increases the activity of GABA by acting on GABA-BZD-Cl (GABA- Benzodiazepine-chloride) channel complex but, the binding site is different to that of barbiturates.
- ***Uses :*** Clonazepam – Absence and Myoclonic seizures. Lorazepam, Diazepam – Status epilepticus.
- ***Adverse effects :*** Sedation and tolerance are the disadvantages on long term use.

## Ethosuxsimide :

- ***Mechanism of action :*** Acts by Blocking 'T' type $Ca^{+2}$ channels.
- **Use :** Used in absence seizures.
- ***Adverse effects :*** Skin rash and agranulocytosis are the adverse effects.

## Topiramate :

- ***Mechanism of action :*** Inhibition of $Na^+$ channel blocks the AMPA (glutamate) receptor.
- ***Use :*** Used for treatment of partial seizures.
- ***Adverse effects :*** Weight loss (Nowadays used in treatment of obesity), renal stones, blindness.

## Lamotrigine :

- ***Mechanism of action :*** Inhibition of $Na^+$ channel blocks the AMPA (glutamate) receptor.
- ***Use :*** Used in absence seizures, partial epilepsy.
- ***Adverse effects :*** Ataxia and SJS are adverse effects.

## Gabapentin & Pregabalin :

- ***Mechanism of action :*** Promotes the release of GABA.
- ***Use :*** Used for neuropathic pain, partial seizures, and chronic pain disorders.
- ***Adverse effects :*** Sedation, dizziness and peripheral edema are the side effects.

## Levetiracetam :

- ***Mechanism of action :*** It acts by reducing $Ca^{+2}$ currents in glutaminergic neurons.
- ***Use :*** Useful in partial, tonic-clonic and myoclonic epilepsy.
- ***Adverse effects :*** Somnolence, asthenia and ataxia are the adverse effects.

## STATUS EPILEPTICUS :

- Epileptic seizures occurring repeatedly with no recovery of consciousness in between are called as status epilepticus.

### Treatment :

***Primary measures :***

- Maintain patent airway, prevent tongue bite by mouth gag.
- Maintain adequate oxygen, BP, fluid and electrolytes.

***Pharmacotherapy :***

- Inj. Lorazepam 4 mg IV stat and repeated after 10 min if required. OR
- Inj. Diazepam 10 mg IV at 2 mg/min repeated once after 10 min. OR
- Inj. Fosphenytoin 100-150 mg/min IV infusion under ECG monitoring. OR
- Inj. Phenobarbitone 100 mg/min IV stat.
- Inj. Thiopentone (general anesthesia) should be given for refractory cases.

39

# ANTI-PARKINSON'S DRUGS

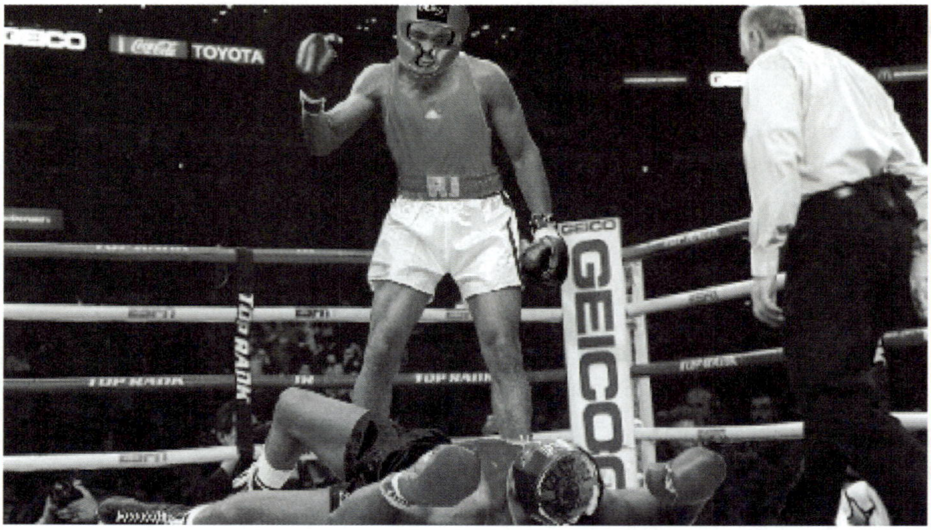


*"The greatest boxer of all time Mohammed Ali had Parkinson's disease"*

## PARKINSON'S DISEASE :

- **Parkinson's disease** (PD) is a progressive neurodegenerative disorder caused by *degeneration of substantia nigra*, and consequent loss of Dopamine (DA) containing neurons in the nigrostrial pathway.
- Two balanced systems are important in the extrapyramidal control of motor activity at substantia nigra; in the first *i.e.* the cholinergic system, the neurotransmitter is ACh, in the second *i.e.* the dopaminergic system the neurotransmitter is DA.

### Causes :

- Etiology is unknown. Genetic predisposition is likely. Free radicals & oxidative stress can be implicated.

### Clinical features :

- Pin rolling tremors, bradykinesia, mask like blank faces, muscle rigidity, stooping posture, shuffling gait, depression.

### Synthesis and metabolism of dopamine :

Phenylalanine
↓
Tyrosine
↓
DOPA
↓
Dopamine
COMT ↓ MAO
HVA and DOPAC

**COMT** : Catachol-O-Methyl Transferase, **MAO** : Monoamine oxidase, **HVA** : Homovanillic acid.

## CLASSIFICATION :

### Drugs acting on dopaminergic system :

- **Dopamine precursors :** Levodopa.
- **Peripheral decarboxylase inhibitors :** Carbidopa, Benserazide.
- **Dopamine agonists :** Bromocriptine, Pramipexole.
- **MAO-B inhibitors :** Selegiline, Rasagiline.
- **COMT inhibitors :** Entacapone, Tolcapone.
- **Dopamine facilitator :** Amantadine.

### Drugs acting on cholinergic system :

- **Central anticholinergics :** Benzhexol, Benztropine.

**NOTE :** Dopamine is not used for Parkinson disease therapy because, Dopamine doesn't cross the Blood Brain Barrier and we need dopamine in substantia nigra in CNS.

### Dopamine precursors :

#### *Levodopa :*

- ***Prodrug :*** It is metabolic precursor of dopamine.
- Levodopa can cross the blood-brain barrier while dopamine cannot.
- In CNS, it is enzymatically converted to dopamine by DOPA-decarboxylase.
- 1-3% of Levodopa actually enters the brain, primarily due to extracerebral metabolism of levodopa to dopamine by DOPA-decarboxylase.
- Extracerebral metabolism can be reduced by administering a **peripheral DOPA-decarboxylase inhibitor** (levodopa + carbidopa).

***Tab. Levodopa 100 mg + Carbidopa 25 mg :***

- Levodopa is a pro-drug and crosses blood-brain barrier where it is converted into a dopamine in the nigrostriatal pathway of brain which is required by the brain for proper functioning and relieves symptoms associated with Parkinson's disease. In the periphery levodopa is converted to dopamine by enzyme peripheral decarboxylase (DOPA-decarboxylase).
- Dopamine is unable to cross the blood brain barrier. Carbidopa inhibits decarboxylase enzyme which inhibits conversion of levodopa to dopamine and more levodopa is able to cross blood brain barrier where it is required in treatment of Parkinson's disease.
- By rationally combining levodopa with carbidopa, we can prevent sympathetic side effects of dopamine.

***Adverse effects :***

- ***Dyskinesias :*** occur in 80% of patients on long-term levodopa therapy.
- ***"On-off" Effect :*** Fluctuations in clinical response to levodopa.
  - Off : marked reduction of movements.
  - On : improved mobility.
  - It is thought to be related to fluctuations in levodopa plasma concentrations. Fluctuations can be managed by incorporating a dopamine receptor agonist or MAO-B inhibitor into pharmacotherapy.
- ***Acute side effects :*** Related to increased peripheral concentrations of dopamine like Nausea, Anorexia – treated with peripherally-acting dopamine antagonist (*i.e.*, Domperidone), Hypotension – particularly in patients on anti-hypertensives.
- ***Other common side effects :*** Confusion, insomnia, nightmares, schizophrenic-like syndrome (delusions and hallucinations due to enhanced CNS concentrations of dopamine).

## Dopamine Agonists :

- ***Bromocriptine :*** Selective $D_2$ receptor agonist.
- ***Pramipexole :*** Preferential affinity for $D_3$ receptor (also $D_2$ and $D_4$). Used primarily in patients with advanced Parkinson's disease. Possibly neuroprotective (scavenges free radicals).

## Monoamine Oxidase Inhibitors (MAOIs) : *Selegiline, Rasagiline.*

- Two types of MAO have been identified :
  - MAO-A : primarily metabolises NE and 5-HT.
  - MAO-B : primarily metabolises dopamine.
- Drugs are selective, irreversible inhibitors of MAO-B.
- ***Therapeutic Effectiveness :*** Effective in early Parkinson's disease (as monotherapy or in combination with levodopa).

- Enables reduction in levodopa dose or may smooth the "on-off" fluctuations associated with levodopa.
- ***Adverse Effects :*** Selectivity for brain MAO-B makes these drugs less likely to produce ADRs involving peripheral tyramine (*i.e.* cheese reaction).

**Catechol-O-Methyltransferase (COMT) Inhibitors :** *Tolcapone and Entacapone.*

- They inhibit peripheral metabolism of levodopa. They also reduce "on-off" fluctuations.
- Tolcapone blocks both central and peripheral COMT whereas entecapone blocks only peripheral COMT.
- ***Adverse Effects :*** They are due to increased plasma concentrations of levodopa. Dyskinesias, nausea, confusion, diarrhea, abdominal pain, orthostatic hypotension, sleep disorders and red urine discoloration. Tolcapone is potentially hepatotoxic.

**Dopamine facilitator :** *Amantadine.*

- Antiviral drug with anti-Parkinsonian properties.
- Mechanism of action is unclear. It potentiates dopaminergic function by modifying synthesis, release, or reuptake of dopamine.
- Therapeutic effectiveness : Less effective than levodopa or bromocriptine. Therapeutic benefits are short-lived.
- ***Adverse Effects :*** restlessness, depression, irritability, insomnia, agitation, excitement, hallucinations, confusion, overdose can cause acute toxic psychosis. Other adverse effects are headache, edema, postural hypotension, heart failure, GI disturbances.

**Central Anti-Cholinergics :** *Benzhexol, Benztropine.*

- Muscarinic cholinergic receptors which are localised in striatal neurons of CNS mediate cholinergic tremors and cause presynaptic inhibition of dopamine release.
- Therapeutic Effectiveness : Improve muscle rigidity and tremor.
- ***Adverse Effects :*** anticholinergic effects like dry mouth, decreased sweating, impaired vision, urinary retention, constipation, drowsiness, confusion.

## FOR STUDENTS WHO WANT TO SCORE MORE :

**Newer drugs :**

| *Drug* | *Action* |
|---|---|
| Safinamide | MAO-B inhibitor |
| Coenzyme Q-10, Vitamin E | Antioxidants |
| Rotigotine | Dopamine agonist |

# 40 ANTI-ALZHEIMER'S DRUGS

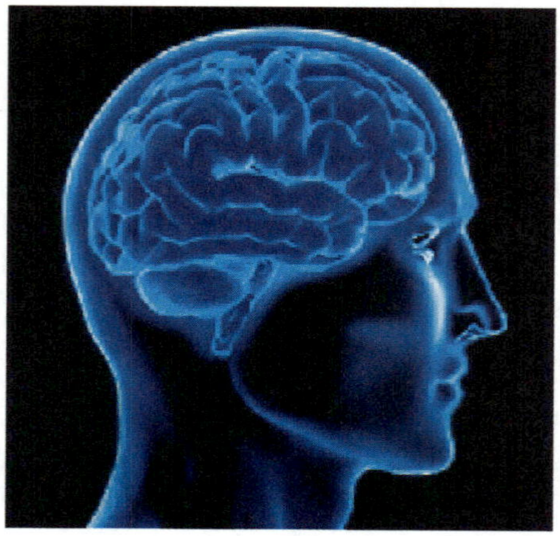

## ALZHEIMER'S DISEASE :

- Alzheimer's disease (AD) is a slowly progressive disease of the brain that is characterised by impairment of memory and eventually by disturbances in reasoning, planning, language, and perception.
- Many scientists believe that Alzheimer's disease results from an increase in the production or accumulation of a specific protein (beta-amyloid protein) in the brain that leads to nerve cell death.
- Generally, it is diagnosed in people over 65 years of age, although the less-prevalent early onset of Alzheimer's can occur much earlier.
- ***Pathological features :*** deposits of beta-amyloid protein in brain, neurofibrillary tangles and loss of cholinergic neurons.

### Causes :

- Advancing Age, female sex, family history, trauma, education, environmental factors : aluminium, mercury, viruses, and vascular diseases like stroke.

### Clinical features :

- Progressive loss of memory, loss of short term memory that precedes long term memory, reduced cognitive function, reduced verbal fluency, impairment of speech due to failure to arrange words; patient may go into vegetative state. Death as a result of complications of immobility *e.g.* pneumonia.

## CLASSIFICATION OF ANTI-ALZHEIMER'S DRUGS :

- **Acetylcholinesterase inhibitors.**

  Tacrine, Donepezil, Rivastigmine, Galantamine.

- **Nootropic agents (cognition enhancers).**

  Piracetam, Aniracetam, Oxiracetam.

- **NMDA receptor antagonists.**

  Memantine, Riluzole.

- **Newer drugs.**

  Antioxidants (vitamin E, selenium), Gingko biloba, Ginseng, Acetyl-L-carnitine (Ach analogue).

### Acetylcholinesterase inhibitors :

***Rivastigmine :***

- Used to delay or slow the symptoms of AD. Loses its effect over time. Used for mild to moderate AD. Can get in pill form or as a skin patch. Does not prevent or cure AD.

### Donepezil :

Used to delay or slow the symptoms of AD. Loses its effect over time. Used for mild, moderate and severe AD. Does not prevent or cure AD. It is a reversible inhibitor bind with higher affinity. It is more hydrophobic & has longer duration of action. Readily crosses the BBB to inhibit AChE in the CNS.

### Nootropic agents :

*E.g.* Piracetam, Aniracetam. These drugs modulate cholinergic and glutamate receptors. They enhance learning and memory. Also used in other forms of dementia and mental retardation.

### NMDA receptor antagonists :

They prevent glutamate induced neuronal excitotoxicity in AD. They are better tolerated and less toxic than cholinesterase inhibitors.

❑❑❑❑❑

# 41 ANTI-PSYCHOTIC DRUGS
## (Anti-Schizophrenia Drugs / Neuroleptics)

Psychosis is a thought disorder characterised by disturbances of reality and perception, impaired cognitive functioning, and inappropriate effect (mood).

### SCHIZOPHRENIA :

- ***Features of schizophrenia are :*** Visual hallucinations, auditory hallucinations, delusions, intense suspicion, feelings of persecution (paranoia) or control by external forces and depersonalisation.
- ***Positive Symptoms :*** Hallucinations, delusions, paranoia, aggressive behavior.
- ***Negative Symptoms :*** Apathy, social withdrawal, anhedonia, emotional blunting, cognitive deficits, extreme inattentiveness or lack of motivation, introvert behavior. These symptoms are progressive and non-responsive to medication.

### Psychosis Producing Drugs :

- Levodopa, CNS stimulants (Cocaine, Amphetamines), Apomorphine and Phencyclidine.

### Pathogenesis of Schizophrenia :

- There is usually genetic predisposition. Evidences point out towards the involvement of dopamine & 5-HT in the pathogenesis of schizophrenia.
- ***Dopamine theory :*** Many evidences show increased activity of the dopaminergic system in the symptomatology of schizophrenia like :
  - Antipsychotics reduce dopamine synaptic activity.
  - Antipsychotic drugs produce Parkinson-like symptoms.
  - Drugs that increase DA in the limbic system cause psychosis.
  - Drugs that reduce DA in the limbic system ($D_2$ antagonists) reduce psychosis.
  - Increased DA receptor density (Post-mortem, PET scans).
  - Changes in amount of homovanillic acid (HVA), a DA metabolite, in plasma, urine, and CSF.
- ***5-HT theory :*** Evidence that points towards the role of 5-HT are :
  - LSD, a central $5\text{-}HT_2$ receptor agonist produces hallucinations which are similar to those of psychosis.

- $5\text{-}HT_{2A}$ receptors modulate the release of DA in mesolimbic and striatal region.

### Antipsychotic drugs :

- They have also been termed ***neuroleptics***, because they suppress motor activity and emotionality. Schizophrenics must be treated with medications indefinitely, because the disease is lifelong and it is preferable to prevent the psychotic episodes than to treat them.

## CLASSIFICATION OF ANTIPSYCHOTICS :

### *Older drugs (Typical Antipsychotics) :*

- ***Phenothiazines :*** Chlorpromazine, Thioridazine, Fluphenazine, Trifluperazine.
- ***Thioxanthines :*** Thiothixene, Flupenthixol.
- ***Butyrophenones :*** Haloperidol, Droperidol, Benperidol.
- ***Miscellaneous :*** Pimozide, Loxapine.

### *Newer drugs (Atypical Antipsychotics) :*

- Clozapine, Olanzapine, Quetiapine, Risperidone, Ziprasidone, Aripiprazole etc.

### Mechanism of action :

- Old drugs are $D_2$ dopamine receptor antagonists.
- Newer drugs have higher affinities for $D_1$, 5-HT or a receptors.

### Clinical Problems with antipsychotic drugs include :

- Failure to control negative effect, significant toxicity : neurological, autonomic, endocrine & cardiac, poor concentration.

### Advantages of Newer or atypical antipsychotics :

- Unique receptor affinity, patients who are refractory to typical antipsychotics, more effective for negative symptoms, better tolerated and better safety profile, lower chances of extrapyramidal effects.

### Uses of anti-psychotics :

- Schizophrenia, drug induced psychosis, schizo-affective disorder (either depression or mania is associated), Huntington's disease, as antiemetics ($D_2$ blockade in CTZ), pre anesthetic medication and Intractable hiccups (chlorpromazine).

### Adverse effects :

- ***Central nervous system :*** Sedation, Psychomotor impairment, Tolerance (to the sedative and autonomic effect but not to antipsychotic effect) and Dependence.

- ***Neurological :*** Acute dystonia, akathisia, parkinsonism (Due to $D_2$ blockade in nigrostriatal pathway), neuroleptic malignant syndrome, rabbit syndrome (perioral tremors) and tardive dyskinesia. These are termed as Extrapyramidal side effects.

- ***Neuroleptic Malignant Syndrome :*** is a rare but serious and life threatening side effect of antipsychotics. Commonly seen with typical antipsychotics such as *haloperidol.*

  *Clinical features :* Hyperpyrexia, muscle rigidity, fluctuating BP, Increased myoglobin and Creatine kinase.

  *Treatment :* Discontinuation of the drug. Supportive therapy, antipyretics like paracetamol. Peripherally acting muscle relaxants such as dantrolene.

- ***Anticholinergic effects :*** Dry mouth, blurred vision, constipation etc.
- ***$\alpha$-adrenergic receptors blocking action :*** Orthostatic hypotension.
- ***Effects at $H_1$-histaminergic receptors :*** Sedation.
- ***Hyperprolactinemia :*** Blockade of $D_2$ receptors in lactotrophs in anterior pituitary leads to gynecomastia and galactorrhea.
- ***Increased appetite and weight gain*** (Blockade of $D_2$ receptors in medullary-periventricular pathway).
- ***Agranulocytosis :*** With clozapine.

❑❑❑❑❑

# 42 ANTIMANIAC DRUGS (Mood Stabilizing Drugs)

Mania is a psychiatric disorder characterised by excitement, racing thoughts, pressured speech and a little need for sleep. Mood swings between excitement and depression.

**Pathogenesis :**

- Exact not known, but ↓ Norepinephrine-Dopamine seem to exacerbate mania.

**Clinical features :**

- It is characterised by an elevated "high" mood, talkative, go on-and-on about the things they will do, increased self-esteem, auditory hallucinations, decrease need to sleep and lack of judgement.

## ANTI-MANIC DRUGS :

**Lithium :**

- Lithium remains the drug of choice for the treatment and prophylaxis of mania.

***Mechanism of action of Lithium :***

- Normally $IP_3$ and DAG serve as second messengers for α-adrenergic transmission.
- Such activity is markedly increased in mania.
- Lithium interferes with this second messenger system by blocking the conversion of $IP_2$ to $IP_1$ and $IP_1$ to inositol.
- Thus, reduces free inositol which is necessary for NE and DA transmission.

***Clinical significance :***

- Lithium has narrow therapeutic window (0.5-1.5 mEq/L).
- Therapeutic monitoring of blood levels is needed during treatment.

***Adverse effects :***

- Tremors.
- Subclinical hypothyroidism (↓ $T_3$ & $T_4$ secretion).
- Nephrogenic diabetes insipidus (inhibit ADH).
- Diarrhea.
- Edema ($Na^+$ retention).

### Newer drugs :

1. **Atypical Antipsychotics :** Olanzapine and Risperidone.
2. **Carbamazepine.**
3. **Valproic acid.**
4. **Newer Anticonvulsants :** Gabapentin, Lamotrigine, Topiramate.

These drugs are already covered in their respective chapters.

# 43 ANTI-DEPRESSANT DRUGS

Depression is a disorder of mood (and not of thought as seen in schizophrenia).

### Types of depression :

- Unipolar depression (only depression is present).
- Bipolar depression / Manic depressive psychosis (patient's symptoms fluctuates between depression and mania).
  (The above 2 are also called as endogenous major depression).
- Reactive depression (due to grief, sadness, relative's death, unemployment or illness).

### Clinical features :

- Feeling of misery, apathy and pessimism, low self esteem, feelings of guilt, loss of interest in pleasurable activities, indecisiveness, loss of motivation, retardation of thought and action, sleep disturbance and significant weight change, psychomotor agitation and suicidal ideation.

### Biogenic theory of depression :

- The exact cause of depression is unknown.
- Evidence implicates alterations in the firing patterns of a Norepinephrine (NE), Serotonin (5-HT) and sometimes dopamine (DA) in the CNS.
- ↓ **Activity of NE and 5-HT.**

### Treatment :

The treatment of depression is divided into :

- Psychotherapy.
- Pharmacotherapy.
- ECT.

Here, we would discuss only the pharmacotherapy or drug treatment. As we know that depression is due to lack of NE and 5–HT. Hence, the drugs that inhibit the reuptake of Norepinephrine (NE) and Serotonin (5-HT) will increase the quantity of NE and 5-HT in the synaptic cleft and will be helpful in treating depression.

- Norepinephrine (Noradrenaline) is released in the synaptic cleft of noradrenergic neuron. It then acts on the post-synaptic receptors to produce a response. Here, Norepinephrine meets two fate; it is taken back into the pre-synaptic neuron by a process called as reuptake and it is also metabolised by enzyme monoamine oxidase (MAO).

**Noradrenergic Transmission**

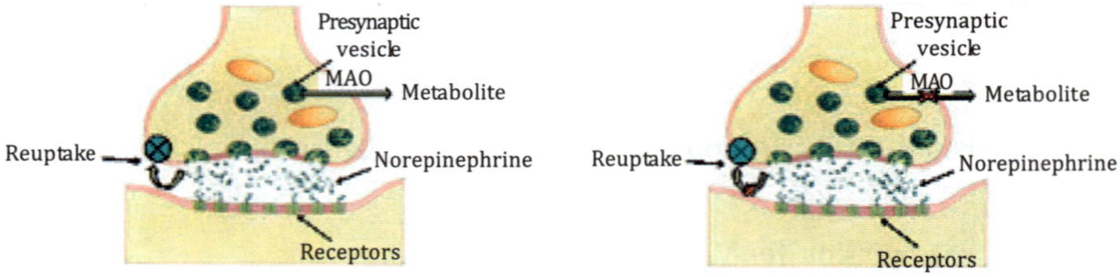


**Serotonergic (5-HT) Transmission**

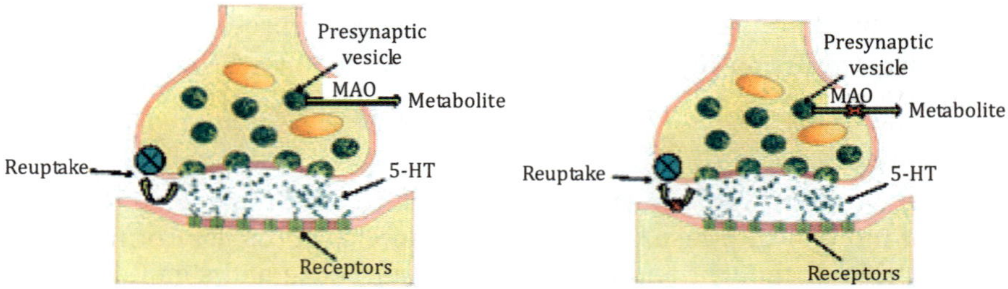


- If we inhibit the reuptake or inhibit the metabolism by MAO, the quantity of NE will increase in the synapse and symptoms of depression will reduce.
- Similarly, 5-HT (Serotonin) is released in the synaptic cleft of serotonergic neuron. It then acts on the post-synaptic receptors to produce a response. Here also, 5-HT meets two fate; it is taken back into the pre-synaptic neuron by a process called as reuptake and it is also metabolised by enzyme monoamine oxidase (MAO).
- If we inhibit the reuptake or inhibit the metabolism by MAO, the quantity of 5-HT will increase in the synapse and symptoms of depression will reduce.

## CLASSIFICATION :

- **Tricyclic anti-depressants (TCAs) :**
  - **Non-selective (NE + 5-HT reuptake inhibitor) :** Imipramine, Amitriptyline, Doxepin.
  - **Selective (NE reuptake inhibitor) :** Desipramine, Nortriptyline.
- **Selective serotonin-norepinehrine reuptake inhibitor (SNRI) :**
  - Venlafaxine, Duloxetine.
- **Selective serotonin reuptake inhibitors (SSRIs) :**
  - Fluoxetine, Fuvoxamine, Citalopram, Escitalopram, Sertraline, Paroxetine.
- **Atypical anti-depressants :**
  - Bupropion, Trazodone.

- **Antidepressant of natural origin :**
  - St. Johns wart.
- **Monoamine oxidase inhibitors (MAOIs) :**
  - **Non-selective (MAO-A & MAO-B) inhibitor :** Tranylcypromine.
  - **Selective MAO-A inhibitor :** Clorgylline, Moclobemide.
- **Tricyclic Antidepressants (TCAs) :**
  - Characteristic three ring nucleus.

**Mechanism of Action :**

- Inhibition of NE & 5-HT reuptake. They are called non-selective because these drugs also have effect on muscaranic (cholinergic) receptors, $H_1$ (histaminic) receptors and a-adrenergic receptors as well.
- ↑ NE and 5-HT in synapse.
- Takes up to 4 weeks for all TCA antidepressants to have an effect.

**Adverse Effects :**

- ***Anticholinergic side effects :*** dry mouth, constipation, blurred vision, mydriasis, urine retention.
- ***Antihistaminic side effects :*** Drowsiness, sedation and weight gain.
- ***α-1 blocking effect :*** postural hypotension.
- ***Cardiac toxicity :*** Palpitations, tachycardia (↑ NE in Heart), QT prolongation, arrhythmias.
- ***Sexual :*** Sexual dysfunction, including loss of libido, impaired erection and ejaculation.

## Selective serotonin-norepinephrine reuptake inhibitor (SNRI) :

**Mechanism of Action :**

- Inhibits reuptake of both NE and 5-HT.
- Lacks antihistaminic, anticholinergic and adrenergic blocking effects of TCAs.

**Adverse effects :**

- Similar to SSRIs.

## Selective serotonin reuptake inhibitors (SSRIs) :

They are most widely prescribed drugs for depression nowadays.

**Mechanism of action :**

- Specific serotonin uptake inhibitors, increase 5-HT by inhibiting reuptake.

**Major limitations of TCAs :**

- Frequent anticholinergic, antihistaminic, anti-adrenergic and cardiovascular side effects.
- Low safety margin.

- Lag time of 2-4 weeks before antidepressant action manifests.
- Significant number of patients respond incompletely and some do not respond.

**Advantages of SSRIs :**

- Produce less or no sedation.
- Do not interfere with cognitive or psychomotor function.
- No anticholinergic action.
- No CVS problems.
- No a blocking action – safe in elderly.
- No weight gain.
- Safer and good patient acceptability.

**Adverse effects :**

- Nausea, decreased libido and decreased sexual function.
- Serotonin syndrome (hyperthermia, muscle rigidity, myoclonus, rapid changes in mental status and vital signs).

## Atypical Antidepressants :

They have slightly different mechanism as compared to other anti-depressants, hence the name atypical.

**Bupropion :**

- Inhibitor of DA, NE and 5-HT reuptake (NDRI).
- Non-sedative, very little anticholinergic, CVS or sexual side effects.

**Trazodone :**

- 5-HT reuptake inhibitor, $\alpha_1$-blocker, 5-$HT_{2A}$ blocker.
- No anticholinergic action, No arrhythmia.
- ***Adverse effects :*** Priapism, Postural Hypotension.

## Antidepressants of natural origin :

- A natural antidepressant, St Johns wart (*Hypericum Perforatum*) containing *hypericin* and *hyperforin* as active principle having antidepressant and anti-anxiety property is available in many European countries.

## MAO Inhibitors :

**Mechanism of action :**

- Inhibit MAO enzymes.
- Decrease metabolism of NE, 5HT, DA.
- Increase availability of NE, 5HT, DA in the neurons.

**NOTE :** Always remember which type of monoamine oxidase *i.e.* MAO metabolises which biogenic amine. MAO-A metabolises → NE, 5-HT, Tyramine and MAO-B metabolises → DA. Therefore, MAO-A inhibitors are used in depression and MAO-B inhibitors are used in parkinson's disease.

**Cheese Reaction :**

This is seen in patient taking tyramine containing foods like cheese, curd, beer, banana and wine and simultaneously he is on MAO inhibitor.

- MAO inhibitors will also inhibit the metabolism of tyramine which is a sympathomimetic. This will lead to increased quantity of tyramine in the body.

**MAO inhibitors causes ↓ MAO-A**

⇓

**↑ Tyramine in the body**

⇓

**↑NE in circulation**

⇓

**Hypertensive crisis**

⇓

**Intracranial bleeding, myocardial infarction and other organ damage**

## Uses of Antidepressants :

- **Endogenous Major Depression :** The goal is to relieve symptoms of depression and restore normal social behavior.
  - 1st choice – SSRI (atypical ones also may be considered).
  - TCAs – in non-responsive cases.
  - MAO – A inhibitors in mild and moderate cases.
- **Obsessive Compulsive Disorder (OCD) and Phobic states :**
  - (SSRIs are useful).
  - Compulsive eating in Bulimia.
  - Body dysmorphic disorder.
  - Compulsive buying.
  - Kleptomania.
- **Anxiety Disorders :** Benzodiazepines like Alprazolam is usually preferred.
- **Neuropathic pain and chronic pain :** Amitriptyline, nortriptyline.
- **Attention Deficit Hyperactivity Disorder :** TCAs.
- Nocturnal enuresis in children.
- **Migraine :** Amitriptyline as prophylactic.
- **Nicotine dependence :** bupropion.

# 44 OPIOID AGONISTS AND ANTAGONISTS

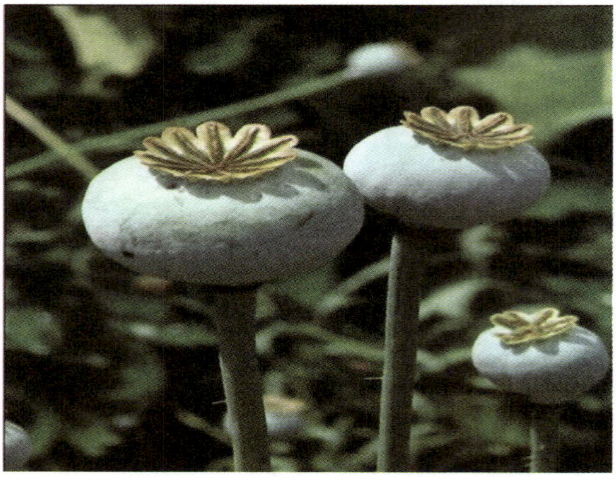

**Opium :** The dark brown, resinous material obtained from poppy (papaver somniferum).

## CLASSIFICATION :

### Based on their sources :

- ***Natural opium alkaloids :*** Morphine, Codeine.
- ***Semi synthetic opiates :*** Heroin, Pholcodeine.
- ***Synthetic opioid :*** Pethidine, Fentanyl, Methadone, Tramadol, Dextropropoxyphene.

### Based on mechanism of action :

- ***Opioid agonists :*** Pethidine, Fentanyl, Alfentanil, sufentanil, Methadone, Dextropropoxyphene.
- ***Opioid partial agonists :*** Buprenorphine, Pentazocine.
- ***Opioid antagonists :*** Naloxone, Naltrexone, Nalmefene.
- ***μ receptor agonist with other mode of action :*** Tramadol, Tapendalol.
- ***Opioids that lack analgesic activity and have other use :*** Loperamide, Noscapine, Diphenoxylate, Dextromethorphan.

## OPIOID RECEPTORS :

μ (mu), κ (kappa) and δ (delta).

**Effects of receptor stimulation :**

1. **μ (mu)** : Physical dependence.
   Euphoria.
   Analgesia (supraspinal).
   Respiratory depression.
2. **κ (kappa)** : Sedation.
   Analgesia (spinal).
   Miosis.
3. **δ (delta)** : Analgesia (spinal & supraspinal).
   **Re**lease of **g**rowth **h**ormone.

## PHARMACOKINETICS :

- Readily absorbed from GIT, nasal mucosa, lung, subcutaneous, IM and IV route.
- CNS is primary site of action (analgesia/sedation).
- Oral morphine not given due to erratic oral availability.

## PHARMACOLOGICAL ACTIONS : (MORPHINE) :

1. ***Analgesia :***
   - Raises the pain threshold at the spinal cord level, alters nociception in the brain.
   - Relieves all types of pain, but most effective against continuous dull aching pain.
2. ***Euphoria :***
   - Produces a powerful sense of contentment and well-being by stimulation of the ventral tegmentum. Relieves anxiety and fear.
3. ***Respiratory depression :***
   - Causes respiratory depression by reduction of the sensitivity of respiratory centre neurons to carbon dioxide.
4. ***Cough suppression :***
   - Causes suppression of cough reflex. Called as anti-tussives. Non-analgesic opioids like dextromethorphan, codeine and noscapine are effective anti-tussives. May allow accumulation of secretions and thus lead to airway obstruction thus, avoided in cough with expectoration.
5. ***Sedation :***
   - Drowsiness and clouding of judgement are frequently associated with opioids.
6. **Miosis :**
   - The pinpoint pupil is the characteristic of morphine use.

### 7. *Emesis :*

- Causes vomiting by stimulating the CTZ in the medulla but with no unpleasant sensations.

### 8. *Gastrointestinal effect :*

- Decreases motility of smooth muscle and increases sphincter tone, which causes constipation. This is the basis for their use in diarrhea. Increases pressure in the biliary tract, constriction of sphincter oddi and increases contraction of gall bladder, thus avoided in biliary colic.

### 9. *Tolerance :*

- Tolerance develops to nausea, analgesia, sedation, respiratory depression and euphoria but, not to miosis and constipation.

### 10. *Dependence :*

- Opioids produce physical dependence and it is a commonly abused drug. Withdrawal symptoms : Rhinorrhea, lacrimation, yawning, chills, gooseflesh, hyperventilation, hyperthermia, mydriasis, muscular aches, vomiting, diarrhea, anxiety and hostility.

## Uses :

### 1. *Analgesia :*

- Moderate to severe deep-seated visceral pain such as MI, renal colic, traumatic, post-operative and cancer pain.
- Relieves all types of pain, but most effective against continuous dull aching pain.
- Fentanyl patch is also available for cancer pain.

### 2. *Cardiac asthma :*

- Acute left ventricular heart failure induces pulmonary edema.
- Reduces anxiety, cardiac preload and afterload.
- Particularly useful for painful myocardial ischemia with pulmonary edema.

### 3. *Treatment of diarrhea :*

- Diphenoxylate (*Lomotil*) and loperamide (*Andial*) are commonly used for symptomatic treatment of diarrhea.

### 4. *Relief of cough :*

- Antitussives are used for dry cough or non-productive cough.
- Codeine, pholcodeine, dextromethorphan and noscapine are used.

### 5. *Pre-anesthetic medication :*

- Sedative, anxiolytic, and analgesic properties.
- For high-risk surgery administered systemically.

- Also used in epidural anesthesia.
- **Caution :** respiratory suppression.

### Adverse effects :

- Respiratory depression.
- Vomiting, constipation, biliary colic.
- Elevation of intracranial pressure (especially in head injury).
- Tolerance and dependence.
- Postural hypotension.
- Dysphoria.
- Urinary retention (especially in prostatic hypertrophy).

## ACUTE MORPHINE POISONING (Overdose/Toxicity) :

- May be accidental, suicidal or overdosing especially in addicts.
- **Clinical features :** Pin-point pupils, convulsions, cyanosis, coma, severe respiratory depression and death.
- **Treatment :** Supportive measures, respiratory support, gastric lavage with potassium permanganate, antidote – ***Naloxone or Naltrexone*** 0.4-0.8 mg IV repeatedly every 5 min till respiration recovers, then repeated every 1-3 hrs till morphine is cleared from the body.

## OPIOID ABUSE :

Covered in chapter of drug dependence and abuse.

### Contraindications :

1. Hypotension (causes postural hypotension).
2. Hypertrophy of prostate (causes urinary retention).
3. Bronchial asthma (worsens due to histamine release. Also due to cough suppressant action, mucus accumulates in the respiratory tract).
4. Biliary colic (causes biliary colic).
5. Head injury (Because opioids causes respiratory depression, this will increase $PCO_2$ which leads to cerebral vasodilation and consequential increase in cerebral blood flow and intracranial pressure and thus aggravate the head injury. Another reason is that opioids causes pin point pupil (miosis) which interferes with the management and prognosis as the treating doctor constantly checks the pupils in head injury patient).
6. Productive cough or cough with expectoration (Cough is a protective reflex of body to remove secretions and mucus from the respiratory tract. Due to cough suppressant action of opioids, mucus accumulates in the respiratory tract and is unable to clear, thus, opioids should only be given in dry cough and not in cough with expectoration).

# 45 DRUG DEPENDENCE AND ABUSE

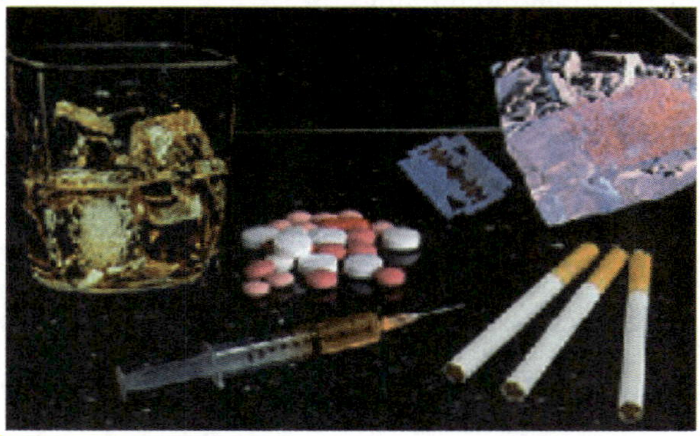

## COMMON TERMS :

- **Drug abuse :** Compulsive, excessive and self-damaging use of habit forming drugs or substances, leading to addiction or dependence, serious physiological injury (such as damage to kidneys, liver, heart) and/or psychological harm (such as dysfunctional behavior patterns, hallucinations, memory loss), or death. Also called as substance abuse.
- **Drug dependence :** When an individual persists in use of substance despite problems related to use of substance it is called as Drug Dependence. Compulsive and repetitive use may result in tolerance to the effect of the drug and withdrawal symptoms when use is reduced or stopped.
- **Drug seeking behavior :** Abused drugs and abused substances are known to increase demand of drug.
- **Misuse :** Indiscriminate use of drugs which is not a CNS stimulant or depressant is termed as misuse. ***E.g.*** Laxatives.
- **Addiction :** Chronic use of drug leads to drug addiction. Drug addiction is characterised by the following :
  - The person aims to consume drug at any circumstances.
  - Procurement of the drug becomes a must for the person.
  - Drug addiction leads to development of drug tolerance.
  - Tolerance increases the effective dose requirement
  - Addicted people must use the drugs regularly to avoid abstinence syndrome.

- Discontinuation of the drug leads to relapse.
- *E.g.* : Amphetamines, LSD, Cocaine, cannabis.

- **Habituation :** It is a state of mind of a drug abuser characterised by the following features :
  - There is no compulsion to consume the drug.
  - Tolerance, withdrawal symptoms are minimal.
  - Habituation is not harmful to society but it is problematic for an individual.
  - *E.g.* : Addiction to Tea, Coffee, Alcoholism, Energy Drinks, Tobacco in the form of Cigarettes or Chewing.

- **Detoxification :** It is one of the processes of drug dependence treatment. It involves administration of abused drug in reduced doses so that slow withdrawal is possible.

- **Craving :** Increased drug seeking property or wanting of drug or desire to procure the drug.

## WHY DO PEOPLE GET ADDICTED ?

- Peer pressure, relief of stress, increased energy, to relax, to relieve pain, to escape reality, to feel more self-esteem, for recreation, athletes and body-builders may take anabolic steroids to increase muscle mass and performance.

## NEGATIVE EFFECTS :

- Problems with work, school, family and society, legal difficulties (*e.g.* assault, theft), physically dangerous situations. *E.g.* using drugs while operating machinery or driving a car, transmission of diseases (*E.g.* HIV due to sharing needles), teratogenicity and various health issues.

## MECHANISM OF DRUG ABUSE AND DEPENDENCE :

- All dependence producing drugs activate the "reward-reinforcement pathway" called the mesolimbic dopaminergic pathway. These drugs increase the release of dopamine which is also called as a pleasure neurotransmitter.

**We will discuss clinically important drugs of abuse in this chapter.**

## NICOTINE :

Nicotine is obtained from Nicotiana tobaccum and is potent, toxic substance that exists in tobacco and is responsible for drug dependence. Consumed in various forms; smoked as cigars, cigarette, beedi, hookka, inhaled as snuff, chewed as jarda, khaini, gutka, maawa etc.

### Pharmacological actions :

- ***CNS :*** Nicotine stimulates CNS and causes alertness, attention, anorexia and improved memory. Apart from regions of brain, nicotine also stimulates respiratory centres and vomiting centers. It inhibits spinal reflexes which causes relaxation of skeletal muscle. Excess intake of nicotine causes seizures, coma and even death due to respiratory failure.

- *CVS :* Vasoconstriction, tachycardia, increased cardiac output and BP.
- *GIT :* Salivary secretions are increased. Nausea, vomiting. Excess stimulation of GIT delays healing of peptic ulcers, increased motor activity and diarrhea are noticed.

**Adverse effects :**

- ***Respiratory Problem :*** Chronic bronchitis, recurrent respiratory infections, COPD and cancer.
- ***CVS :*** Thrombosis, coronary heart diseases, hypertension and Peripheral vascular diseases.
- ***Reproductive system :*** Premature delivery, spontaneous abortion and placenta previa.
- ***Others :*** Teratogenicity (decreased birth weight, physical and mental abnormalities).

**Treatment of abuse :**

- Replacement therapy.
- Drug therapy.
- Counselling and education.

- ***Replacement Therapy :***
  - Nicotine chewing gum.
  - Nicotine transdermal patch.

- ***Drug Therapy :***

  These drugs reduce craving for tobacco products and also reduce withdrawal effects :
  - **Clonidine** (Central sympatholytic).
  - **Bupropion** (Atypical antidepressant).
  - **Nortriptyline** (Tricyclic antidepressants).
  - **Varenicline** (Partial agonist-antagonist at presynaptic NN receptors on dopaminergic neurons).

**ALCOHOL :**

- Already covered in ethyl and methyl alcohol chapter.

**OPIOIDS (also *see* chapter on opioids) :**

- An opioid is any psychoactive substance derived from poppy plant (papaver Somniferum). Opioids work by binding to opioid receptors, which are found principally in the central and peripheral nervous system and the gastrointestinal tract (details under the chapter of opioids). Commonly abused opioids are morphine, heroin, codeine, oxycodeine.

### Mechanism of action :

- Opioids act opioid receptors (μ, κ, δ). The inhibitory actions of opioids lead to depression. Prolonged exposure of opioids exerts an opposite effect. All these cellular effects not only decrease the inhibitory actions of opioids but also lead to development of tolerance, dependence and withdrawal symptoms.

### Dependence :

- Physical and psychological dependence develop in opioid drug abusers. Physical dependence develops to a greater extent that compared to psychological dependence. Sudden withdrawal of opioids may lead to death of individuals. The symptoms of physical dependence include dysphoria, GI upset, mydriasis, cough, hyperventilation, ocular discharge, diarrhea, yawning, hyperthermia, piloerection, aggressiveness and emesis. Psychological dependence is characterised by craving. Sudden withdrawal effects are termed as **noradrenergic storm** due to increased release of Noradrenaline (norepinephrine).

### Tolerance :

- Tolerance is developed to euphoria, respiratory depression, sedation and emetic actions but not to miosis and constipation. Cross tolerance to opioid agonists is also developed.

### Treatment :

- Replacement therapy.
- Drug therapy.
- Counseling and education.

- ***Replacement Therapy :***
  - Replacement therapy is found useful in treating opioid dependence.
  - Long acting agonist drugs like **Methadone** are administered in place of short acting drugs like Heroin. (receptors are occupied for longer duration and the patient is spared from withdrawal effects) Thereafter methadone is gradually tapered and withdrawn.
  - Another option is **Buprenorphine** which is partial opioid agonist.

- ***Drug Therapy :***
  - **Naltrexone (long acting opioid antagonist) :** Blocks pleasurable effects, given three times a week. Successful only if patient is detoxified and opioid fee for past 10 days otherwise withdrawal effects.
  - **Clonidine / lofexidine :** Centrally acting sympatholytic, reduces central NE outflow and reduces withdrawal effects.

### CANNABIS :

- Main active constituent is **∇9-tetrahydrocannabinol (THC)**.
- Derived from plant cannabis Indica and cannabis sativa.

- Used in following forms :
  1. ***Bhang :*** Dried leaves are dried, made a paste and used as a drink.
  2. ***Marijuana (Pot / weed / ganja) :*** Dried leaves and flowering tops. Smoked in pipes or rolled as cigarettes.
  3. ***Charas / hashish :*** Resinous exudate of flower and leaves.

**Actions :**

- Actions on CNS include both depressant and psychotomimetic (psychosis like) effects. Euphoria and a feeling of relaxation, with sharpened sensory awareness, increased talkativeness, increased appetite, laugh uncontrollably, cry, sedation. THC also shows analgesic and antiemetic activity. Peripheral actions include vasodilatation, reduction of intraocular pressure, tachycardia, reddening of conjunctiva and bronchodilatation. Actions are mediated through cannabinoid receptors (CB receptors).

**Dependence and abuse :**

- Cannabinoids are less liable than opiates, nicotine or alcohol to cause dependence but may have long term psychological effects.

**Drugs :**

- ***Nabilone and Dronabinol*** are THC analogue (CB1 receptor agonist) which has been developed for their antiemetic property (Cancer chemotherapy induced vomiting) and also stimulates appetite in AIDS patients.
- ***Rimonabant*** (CB1 receptor antagonist) was used for treatment of obesity as it suppresses appetite, but later banned because it caused depression and suicidal tendencies.

❑❑❑❑❑

# DRUGS ACTING ON CARDIOVASCULAR SYSTEM (CVS)

# 46 DRUGS ACTING ON THE RENIN-ANGIOTENSIN SYSTEM

## RENIN-ANGIOTENSIN SYSTEM :

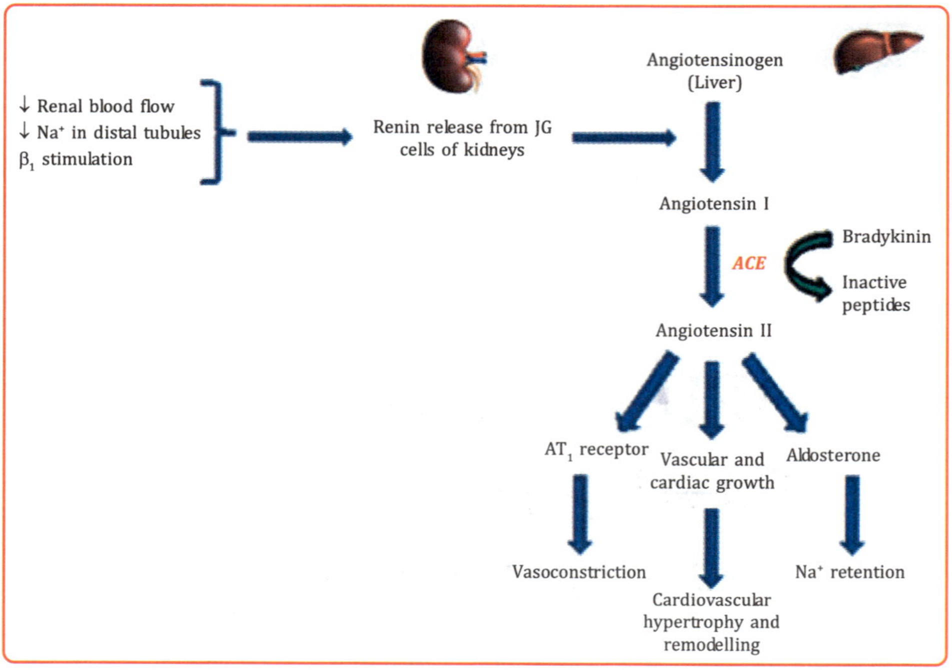


**ACE** : Antiotensin converting enzyme, **$AT_1$** : Angiotensin II receptor type 1

- Decreased renal perfusion, decreased sodium in distal tubules and $b_1$-adrenergic stimulation causes juxtaglomerular cells of the kidneys to release renin.
- Renin then converts angiotensinogen from the liver to Angiotensin I. This Angiotensin I is then converted to Angiotensin II with the help of ACE (angiotensin converting enzyme). ACE also converts bradykinin to inactive peptides.
- Angiotensin II causes vasoconstriction ($AT_1$ receptor mediated), vascular and cardiac growth (remodeling) and aldosterone secretion which enhances sodium absorption.
- Other Angiotensin II receptor is $AT_2$ receptor. Little is known about $AT_2$ receptor. However, fetal tissue development, anti-proliferative action,

apoptosis and vasodilation are some of the effects of Angiotensin II which are believed to be mediated by $AT_2$ receptor.

## DRUGS ACTING ON RENIN-ANGIOTENSIN SYSTEM :

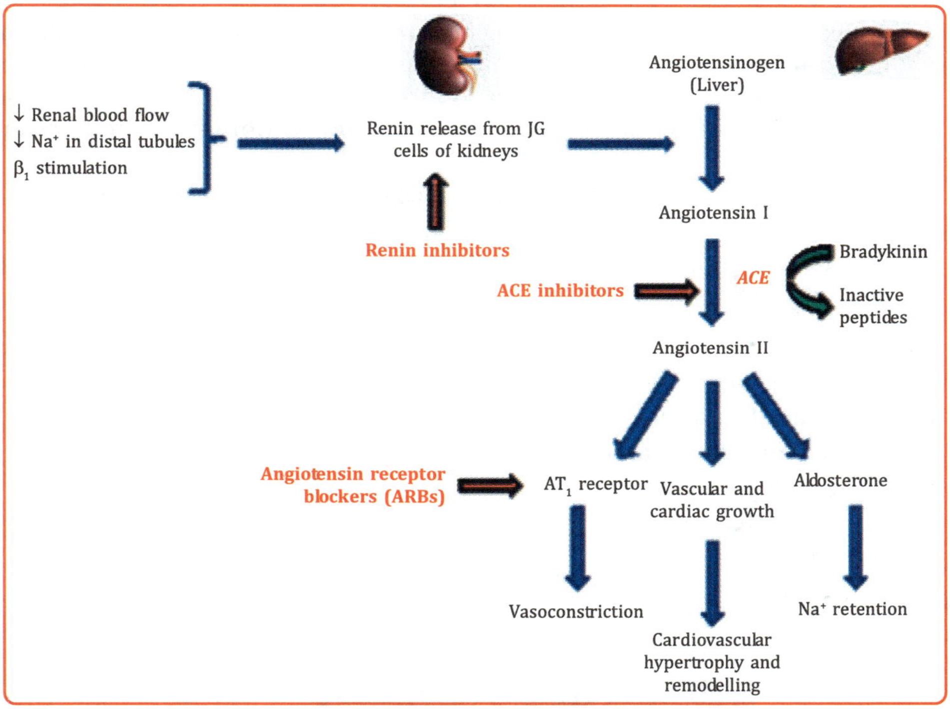


**ACE** : Antiotensin converting enzyme, **$AT_1$** : Angiotensin II receptor type 1

## RENIN INHIBITORS :

- **Drugs : Enalkiren, Remikiren and Aliskiren.**
- Enalkiren and Remikiren are orally active direct renin inhibitors. However, their clinical efficacy in patients of hypertension has been disappointing due to their poor availability.
- Aliskiren, which is a newer member of this group and which is also orally active is being increasingly used nowadays. It not only decreases renin activity but also neutralises the renin rise as a result of ACE inhibition (feedback rise) or $AT_1$ receptor blockade.
- **Use :** Hypertension.
- **Adverse effects :** Diarrhea and hyperkalemia.

## ACEI (ANGIOTENSIN CONVERTING ENZYME INHIBITORS) :

**Drugs :**

- **Captopril, Enalapril, Lisinopril, Benzapril, Ramipril, Perindopril, Quinapril, Trandolapril, Fosinopril.**

**NOTE :** Captopril and Ramipril are active by themselves. Others are inactive prodrugs which are converted to active metabolite inside the body. *E.g.* Enalapril is converted to active metabolite Enalaprilat.

### Mechanism of action : (refer diagram above)

- ACEIs inhibit the conversion of Angiotensin I to Angiotensin II. This results in inhibition of effects produced by Angiotensin II like vasoconstriction and also inhibits aldosterone which reduces sodium retention. Both effects help in reducing the blood pressure. There is also inhibition of cardiovascular hypertrophy and cardiac remodelling.
- There is also inhibition of bradykinin metabolism which leads to accumulation of bradykinin. Bradykinin also helps in reducing blood pressure by vasodilation. But, it is also responsible for the adverse effects like dry cough and angio-edema.

### Uses :

- Hypertension.
- Congestive heart failure.
- Acute myocardial infarction.
- Diabetic nephropathy.
- Diabetic retinopathy.
- Scleroderma renal crisis.
- Prophylaxis in high cardiovascular risk patients.

### Doses :

| ACEIs | Dose |
|---|---|
| Captopril | 25-50 mg BD |
| Enalapril | 2.5-40 mg OD |
| Lisinopril | 5-40 mg OD |
| Benzapril | 5-80 mg OD |
| Ramipril | 1.25-20 mg OD |
| Perindopril | 2-16 mg OD |
| Quinapril | 5-80 mg OD |
| Trandolapril | 1-8 mg OD |
| Fosinopril | 10-80 mg OD |

### Adverse effects :

- ***Hypotension :*** usually after 1$^{st}$ dose and especially in hyponatremia.
- ***Dry cough :*** due to accumulation of bradykinin in the bronchial mucosa. This adverse effect is not dose related. Once ACEIs are stopped, the cough disappears.
- ***Angio-edema :*** due to accumulation of bradykinin.
- ***Hyperkalemia :*** especially in patients of renal failure & patients taking

potassium sparing diuretics due to reduced Angiotensin II stimulated aldosterone secretion.

- ***Dysgeusia (altered taste sesation) :*** seen mostly with captopril.
- ***Acute renal failure :*** seen in patients with *bilateral renal artery stenosis.* Angiotensin II, by constricting the efferent arteriole, maintains adequate GFR even when renal blood supply is low. Inhibition of ACE can lead to renal failure as Angiotensin II is reduced.
- ***Teratogenicity :*** ACEIs are teratogenic especially if given in $2^{nd}$ and $3^{rd}$ trimester of pregnancy. They can cause fetal hypotension, anuria, renal failure, fetal malformations and neonatal death.
- ***Others :*** Skin rash, Neutropenia, proteinuria.

**Drug interactions :**

- NSAIDs may reduce the anti-hypertensive effects of ACEIs by blocking bradykinin mediated vasodilation.
- $K^+$ sparing diuretics or $K^+$ supplementation may aggravate ACEIs induced hyperkalemia.
- Antacids reduce bioavailability of ACEIs.
- ACEIs may elevate plasma levels of lithium and digoxin and may produce their toxicity.
- Diuretics synergise with hypotensive action of ACEIs by depleting $Na^+$ and raising renin levels. Therefore, in diuretic treated patient, the starting dose of ACEIs must be low.

## ARBS / ARAS (ANGIOTENSIN RECEPTOR BLOCKERS / ANGIOTENSIN RECEPTOR ANTAGONISTS) :

**Drugs :**

- **Losartan, Valsartan, Telmisartan, Olmesartan, Irbesartan, Candesartan, Azilsartan.**

**Mechanism of action : (refer diagram above)**

- ARBs block the Angiotensin II receptor $AT_1$. This leads to inhibition of the action mediated via $AT_1$ receptors such as vasoconstriction and also inhibits aldosterone which reduces sodium retention. Both effects help in reducing the blood pressure. There is also inhibition of cardiovascular hypertrophy and cardiac remodelling.
- Differentiating features of ARBs as compared to ACEIs :
    1. They do not metabolise bradykinin; no rise in bradykinin levels. Hence, incidence of cough is rare.
    2. ACEIs are not enough for total elimination of Angiotensin II because some Angiotensin II is also formed by alternative pathways. Whereas, ARBs block the $AT_1$ receptors regardless of from where the Angiotensin II is also synthesized.

3. Due to $AT_1$ receptor blockade, there is increase synthesis of Angiotensin II due to feedback inhibition. Now, this increased Angiotensin II will activate the $AT_2$ receptors resulting in vasodilatation.

**Uses :**

- Hypertension.
- Congestive heart failure.
- Acute myocardial infarction.
- Diabetic nephropathy.
- Diabetic retinopathy.
- Prophylaxis in high cardiovascular risk patients.

**Doses :**

| ARBs | Dose |
|---|---|
| Losartan | 50 mg OD |
| Valsartan | 80-300 mg OD |
| Telmisartan | 40-80 mg OD |
| Olmesartan | 20-40 mg OD |
| Irbesartan | 150-300 mg OD |
| Candesartan | 8 mg OD |
| Azilsartan | 40-80 mg OD |

**Adverse effects :**

Unlike ACEIs the incidence of dry cough, angio-edema and dysgeusia is rare with ARBs. However, following are the adverse effects seen with ARBs :

- ***Hypotension :*** Rarely.
- ***Hyperkalemia :*** Same like ACEIs.
- ***Acute renal failure :*** In patients with *bilateral renal artery stenosis* (same like ACEIs).
- ***Teratogenicity :*** Same like ACEIs.
- ***Others :*** Headache, dizziness, GI disturbances.

47

# DRUGS FOR CONGESTIVE HEART FAILURE

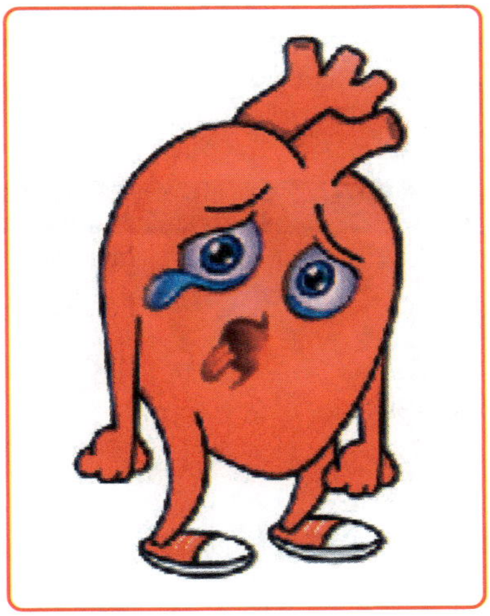

## WHAT IS HEART FAILURE ?

When the heart is unable to pump sufficient amount of blood to meet the metabolic requirements of the body, it is called as heart failure or CHF (congestive heart failure).

### Types of heart failure :

***On the basis of ejection Fraction :***

- Reduced ejection fraction (< 40-50%) – systolic heart failure.
- Preserved ejection fraction (> 40-50%) – diastolic heart failure.

***On the basis of time course :***

- Chronic.
- Acute.

***On the basis of Anatomy :***

- Left sided.
- Right sided.

***On the basis of output :***

- High output failure (when the output of heart is normal but the metabolic demands of the body are high). Seen in thyrotoxicosis, anemia, pregnancy.

- Low output failure (when the metabolic demands of the body are normal but the output of heart is low). This is the commonest type.

## WHAT IS PRELOAD AND AFTERLOAD ?

- ***Preload :*** It is the amount of ventricular stretch before contraction. It depends upon venous blood pressure and the rate of venous return.
- ***Afterload :*** It is the pressure against which the heart must work to eject blood during systole. It depends upon the peripheral resistance of arteries.

### Clinical Features :

| Left ventricular failure | Right ventricular failure |
|---|---|
| Dyspnea, Orthopnea | Increased venous pressure |
| Cough | Edema |
| Fatigue | Hepatomegaly |
| Decreased exercise tolerance | |
| Cardiomegaly | |

### Compensatory mechanisms :

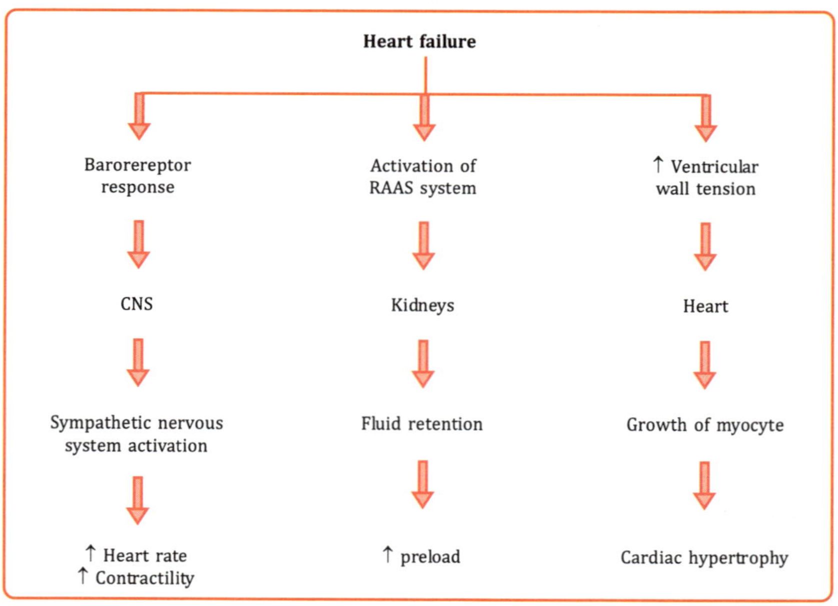


### Treatment of heart failure :

#### *Non-pharmacological treatment :*

- Hospitalise the patient in CCU.
- Propped up position to maintain airway.
- Fluid restriction (< 2 L/day).

- Salt restriction (< 2 g).
- Oxygen 5-8 liters/min.

## DRUGS FOR HEART FAILURE :

### Inotropic drugs :

- ***Cardiac glycosides :*** Digoxin, Digitoxin.
- ***β adrenergic agonists :*** Dopamine, Dobutamine.
- ***Phosphodiesterase inhibitors (Inodilators) :*** Inamrinone, Milrinone.

### Vasodilators :

- ***Arteriolar dilators :*** Hydralazine, Minoxidil.
- ***Venodilators :*** Nitrates.
- ***Arteriolar and venodilators :*** Sodium nitroprusside.

### Diuretics :

- ***Loop diuretics :*** Furosemide, torsemide.
- ***Thiazide diuretics :*** Hydrochlorothiazide.
- ***$K^+$ Sparing diuretics :*** Spironolactone.

### β Blockers :

- Metoprolol, Bisoprolol, Carvedilol etc.

### Angiotensin Converting Enzyme Inhibitors (ACEI) :

- Ramipril, Enalapril, Lisinopril etc.

### Angiotensin Receptor Antagonists (ARBs) :

- Telmesartan, Olmesartan, Candesartan etc.

## INOTROPIC AGENTS :

### Cardiac glycosides :

- Obtained from the leaves of *Digitalis lanata* **(Digoxin)**, *Digitalis purpura* **(Digitoxin)**, *Strophanthus gratus and Strophanthus kombe* **(Strophanthin and Ouabain).**

### Mechanism of action :

- **It inhibits sodium potassium ATPase ($Na^+/K^+$ ATPase)** enzyme. By inhibiting the $Na^+/K^+$-ATPase, cardiac glycosides cause intracellular $Na^+$ concentration to increase. This then leads to an accumulation of intracellular calcium via the $Na^+$- $Ca^{+2}$ exchanger. In the heart, increased intracellular calcium causes more calcium to be released by the sarcoplasmic reticulum, thereby making more calcium available to bind to troponin-C, which increases contractility of the heart and thus increases the cardiac output.

### Digitalisation :

- ***Slow digitalisation :*** 0.125 mg-0.25 mg daily (takes 7-10 days for steady state plasma concentration).

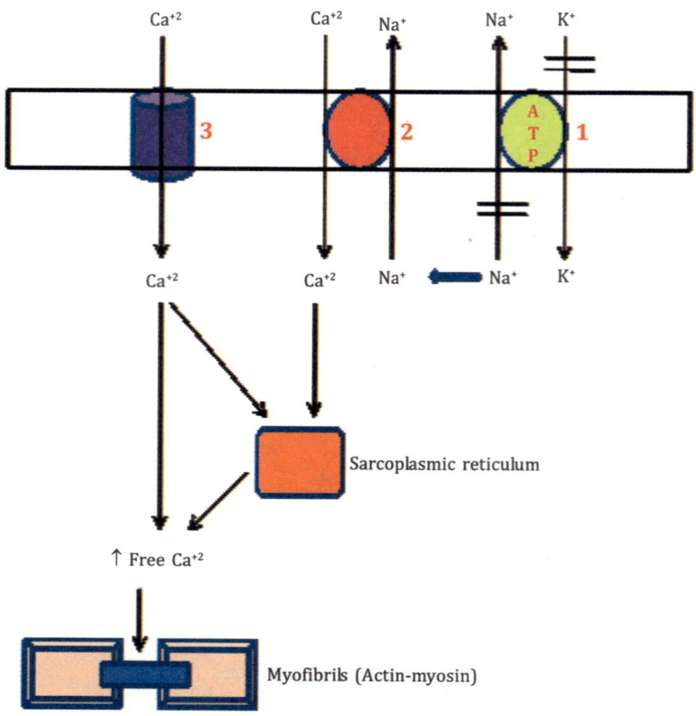


*1–$Na^+/K^+$ ATPase, 2–$Na^+$ – $Ca^{+2}$ exchanger, 3–L-type $Ca^{+2}$ channel*

- ***Rapid digitalisation :*** 0.5 mg-0.75 mg 8 hourly for 3 doses, then 0.25 mg daily.
- ***Signs of digitalisation :*** Nausea, vomiting, Bradycardia, diuresis and ECG changes (Sagging of ST wave and T wave inversion).

### Adverse effects :

- ***Cardiac :*** Bradycardia, heart block, SVT, VT, VF.
- ***GIT :*** Nausea, vomiting, anorexia, abdominal pain.
- ***Psychiatric :*** Fatigue, malaise, confusion, delirium, dizziness.
- ***Visual :*** Yellow / white vision, transient amblyopia.

### Uses :

- CHF patients with atrial fibrillation or atrial flutter.
- CHF patients refractory to ACE inhibitors / β blockers.
- PSVT.

### Toxicity of Digitalis :

- ***Features :*** Sinus bradycardia, first degree AV (atrio-ventricular) block, second / third degree AV block, ectopic beats, ventricular arrhythmias.

- ***Factors predisposing to toxicity*** : High dose, hypokalemia, hypomagnesaemia, hypercalcemia, old age, drugs like quinidine and verapamil.
- ***Management of digitalis toxicity*** :
  - Dose adjustment & monitoring.
  - Atropine for bradycardia and AV block.
  - Potassium supplementation.
  - Lidocaine / phenytoin for arrhythmias.
  - Digibind fab fragments (digitalis antibodies) : acts as antidote.

## β-ADRENERGIC & DOPAMINERGIC AGONISTS :

### Dopamine :

- ***Low dose (2-5 mcg/kg/min)*** : stimulates dopaminergic $D_1$ receptors; Vasodilation.
- ***Intermediate dose (5-10 mcg/kg/min)*** : stimulates dopaminergic $D_1$ and $\beta_1$-adrenergic receptors; Vasodilation and +ve Inotropic effect on heart.
- ***High dose (> 10 mcg/kg/min)*** : stimulates $\alpha_1$-adrenergic receptors; Vasoconstriction (This increases the afterload and beneficial effect of dopamine in CHF is lost).

### Dobutamine :

- Stimulates $\beta_1$ receptors on heart.
- Inotropic effect which leads to increased cardiac output.

### Role :

- Both drugs are used for short term support of circulation in advanced heart failure.
- Dopamine is used in CHF with compromised renal functions.

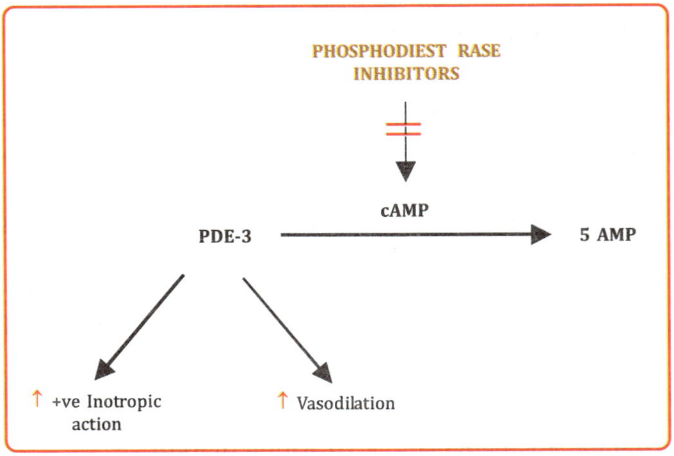

## PHOSPHODIESTERASE [PDE] INHIBITORS :

### Mechanism of Action :

- Phosphodiesterase inhibitors inhibit the enzyme phosphodiesterase-3 (PDE-3). This enzyme converts of cAMP to 5-AMP. This 5-AMP formed is inactive. But when Phosphodiesterase inhibitors are given, they prevent the conversion of cAMP to 5-AMP. Thus, more quantity of cAMP is now available which causes both contraction of heart (+ve inotropic effect) and vasodilation of blood vessels (reduces the preload and afterload). Hence, they are also called as inodilators (Ino-Inotropic and dilator- vasodilator).

### Adverse effects :

- ***Inamrinone :*** Thrombocytopenia, hepatotoxicity.
- ***Milrinone :*** Arrhythmias.

## VASODILATORS :

### Nitrates :

- Reduces both preload & after load.
- Also increases coronary blood flow.
- Available as tablets / sprays / ointments / IV.
- ***Adverse effect :*** flushing, headache, tolerance etc.
- More details are given in chapter on anti-anginal drugs.

### Sodium nitroprusside :

- Fall in peripheral resistance.
- ***Rapid onset :*** short duration; preferred in ICU settings.
- ***Adverse effect :*** Hypotension.

### Hydralazine :

- Direct relaxation of arteriolar smooth muscle.
- May involve fall in intracellular $Ca^{+2}$ levels.
- Causes reduction of afterload.

### Minoxidil :

- It is a powerful vasodilator with similar mechanism as that of hydralazine.
- Vasodilator effects are more marked and there is risk of cardiac ischemia and heart failure. Hence, rarely used nowadays.
- One of the side effects observed with minoxidil was hirsutism. This leads to the use of minoxidil in treating alopecia.
- It is applied topically in the dose of 2-10% and it promotes hair growth. It takes 4-6 months for hairs to grow. Once it is discontinued, hair fall starts again.

## DIURETICS :

- Almost all symptomatic patients treated with a diuretic.

- High ceiling diuretics (loop diuretics) are preferred.
- Low dose therapy is used for maintenance.
- They increase salt and water excretion & reduce blood volume.
- Reduce preload & venous pressure.
- Improve cardiac performance & relieve edema.
- Potassium sparing diuretics are weak diuretics; used to limit $K^+$ wasting by other diuretics.
- **More details in diuretics chapter.**

## β-BLOCKERS :

- Ideally speaking β Blockers should not be used in CCF.

### Reason for use :

- Prevents fatal cardiac arrhythmias.
- ↓ HR, ↓ Oxygen demand.
- Prevent remodelling.
- Anti-oxidant effect (Carvedilol).

## ACE INHIBITORS & ARBS :

### ACEIs :

- Angiotensin II causes vasoconstriction; $Na^+$/water retention (aldosterone), Catecholamine release; arrhythmias. Myocardial hypertrophy & remodelling.
- To prevent these effects we need ACE inhibitors.
- ***Adverse effects :*** cough, angio-edema etc.

### ARBs :

- More complete blockade of angiotensin II effects as blocks the receptor itself.
- Less risk of angio-edema & cough.
- However, both groups cause Teratogenicity, if used in pregnancy.

# 48 ANTI-ARRHYTHMIC DRUGS

## CARDIAC ARRHYTHMIAS :

- Any deviations from the normal pattern of cardiac rhythm are called as cardiac arrhythmias.

### Types of cardiac arrhythmias :

- ***Bradyarrhythmias :*** It is decreased automacity of heart. It may be due to failure of impulse generation at SA node or failure of impulse conduction through AV node.
- ***Tachyarrhythmias :*** It is increased automacity of heart. It may be due to after depolarisations or re-entry of impulse.

### Common types of cardiac arrhythmias seen are :

1. Various kinds of heart block (*e.g.* AV block) and asystole.
2. ***Atrial flutter :*** the heart beats faster than normal but regular.
3. ***Atrial fibrillation :*** the heart beats faster than normal but irregular.
4. ***PSVT (Paroxysmal supraventricular tachycardia) :*** is the episodes of rapid heart rate that starts in a part of the heart above the ventricles.
5. ***Extrasystoles :*** are premature ectopic beats.
6. Ventricular tachycardia (VT).
7. ***Torsades de pointes :*** It is a specific form of polymorphic ventricular tachycardia in patients with long QT interval and characterised by rapid irregular QRS complexes which appear to be twisting around ECG baseline.
8. ***Ventricular fibrillation (VF) :*** It is grossly irregular, rapid and life threatening heart rhythm where the electrophysiological activity of ventricles is chaotic and cardiac output almost stops.

### Action potential in heart :

***Non-nodal tissues (atria, ventricles, purkinje fibres) :***

The action potential of non-nodal tissues is divided into five phases :

- **Phase 0** : Rapid depolarisation (Due to $Na^+$ inflow).
- **Phase 1** : Early repolarisation (Due to $K^+$ outflow).
- **Phase 2** : Plateau phase (Due to $Ca^{+2}$ inflow and $K^+$ outflow).
- **Phase 3** : Rapid repolarisation (Due to $K^+$ outflow).
- **Phase 4** : Resting phase (Ion balance restored by $Na^+$-$K^+$ ATPase pump, outward $K^+$ current and $Na^+$- $Ca^{+2}$ ion exchanger).

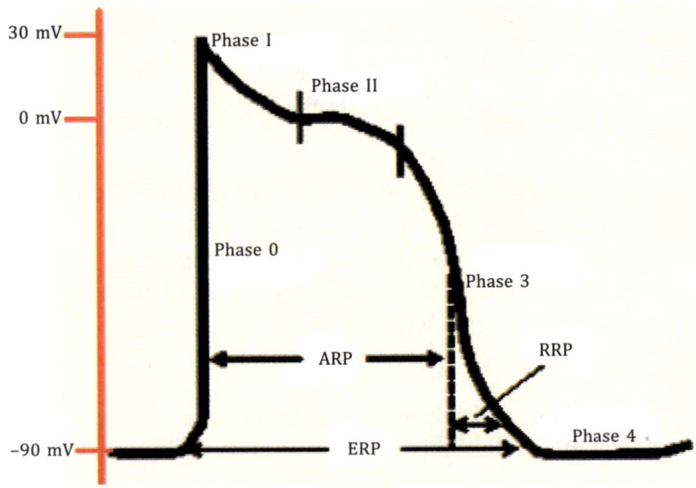


**ARP:** Absolute refractory period, **RRP:** Relative refractory period, **ERP:** Effective refractory period.

***Nodal tissues (SA node, AV node) :***

- Unlike the nodal tissues, the resting membrane potential is -60 mV & not -90 mV.
- Phases 0, 1, 2 and 3 are indistinguishable.
- Depolarisation is due to $Ca^{+2}$ inflow and not due to $Na^{+}$.
- Pacemaker cells (automatic cells) have unstable membrane potential so they can generate action potential spontaneously (automaticity).

## CLASSIFICATION OF ANTI-ARRHYTHMIC DRUGS :

- **Class I ($Na^{+}$ channel blockers) :**
  - **IA :** Quinidine, Procainamide, Disopyramide.
  - **IB :** Lidocaine, Phenytoin, Mexiletene.
  - **IC :** Flecainide, Encainide, Propafenone.
- **Class II (β-blockers) :**
  Propranolol, Metoprolol, Esmolol.
- **Class III ($K^{+}$ channel blockers) :**
  Amiodarone (also has class IA, II & IV actions), Bretylium, Sotalol (also has class II actions), Ibutilide, Dofetilide, Dronedarone, Vernakalant.
- **Class IV ($Ca^{+2}$ channel blockers) :**
  Verapamil, Diltiazem.
- **Miscellaneous :**
  Adenosine, Magnesium sulphate, Potassium, Digoxin, Atropine.

## CLASS I – Antiarrhythmics :

- All drugs in this group block $Na^+$ channels (same as that of local anesthetics). They bind more strongly to $Na^+$ channels when they are in activated state then in resting state.

### Class IA :

- They slow the rate of rise of phase 0 of action potential, increase the ERP and prolong the APD (action potential duration).
- **Uses :** Paroxysmal supraventricular tachycardia (PSVT), premature ventricular contractions (PVCs), premature atrial contractions (PACs) and ventricular tachycardia (VT).

### Quinidine :

- Quinidine is not commonly used nowadays due to chances of developing ventricular pro-arrhythmias and availability of better drugs.
- It has atropine like vagolytic action and increases AV conduction.
- ***Other actions :*** alpha blockade, decreased skeletal muscle contractility and uterine contractions, vomiting and diarrhea etc.
- ***Uses :*** It is a broad spectrum antiarrhythmics used for atrial fibrillation and flutter, prevention of PSVT and prevention of ventricular tachycardia.
- ***Adverse effects :*** diarrhea, proarrhythmia, sudden cardiac arrest or VF, cinchonism, angio-edema, vascular collapse and thrombocytopenia.
- ***Contraindications :*** AV block, CHF, digitalis toxicity, myasthenia gravis and persons like QT prolongation.

### Procainamide :

- It is a procaine derivative with identical action with quinidine except :
  - Minimal antivagal action.
  - Lesser suppression of ectopic automaticity.
  - Lesser depression of contractility and AV conduction.
  - No alpha blocking action.
- ***Uses :*** Mainly for monomorphic VTs and to prevent recurrences.
- ***Adverse effects :*** Hypersensitivity, flushing, hypertension, torsades de pointes and CNS symptoms (mental confusion, hallucinations).

### Disopyramide :

- It is an alternative to quinidine or procainamide but longer acting.
- It has both anticholinergic and direct depressant effects on SA node.
- It should be avoided in patients of benign prostatic hyperplasia and glaucoma.
- ***Adverse effects :*** Constipation, dry mouth, urinary retention, precipitation of heart failure, glaucoma and torsades de pointes.

### Class IB :

- They shorten phase 3 repolarisation, decreases ERP as well as APD.
- ***Uses :*** VT, PVCs, ventricular extrasystoles secondary to MI or cardiac surgery and digitalis induced arrhythmias.

**Lidocaine (Lignocaine) :**

- It is a popular antiarrhythmic and also local anesthetic (membrane stabilizing action).
- ***Adverse effects :*** Neurological; drowsiness, paresthesia, blurred vision, nystagmus and convulsions etc.

**Phenytoin :**

- It is anti-epileptic drug with actions similar to lignocaine and especially useful in digitalis induced arrhythmia.
- Not used much as it causes injuries to injected vein, produces hypotension & VF and shows inconsistent efficacy.

**Mexiletene :**

- It is an oral analogue of lidocaine.
- It is preferred for chronic treatment of ventricular arrhythmias associated with previous MI.
- ***Adverse effects :*** Tremors, nausea, bone marrow aplasia and pulmonary fibrosis.

### Class IC :

- These drugs markedly decrease the rate of phase 0 depolarisation in purkinje and ventricular fibers.
- This slows the conduction in all cardiac tissues with minimal effect on ERP and APD.
- ***Uses :*** PVCs, Ventricular tachyarrhythmias which are refractory to other drugs. They are also useful in supraventricular arrhythmias especially WPW syndrome.

**Flecainide and Encainide :**

- Flecainide is effective orally. These drugs are pro-arrhythmogenic.
- They are currently reserved for refractory ventricular arrhythmias.

**Propafenone :**

- It has got similarities with propranolol and is given orally.
- It has some beta-blocking action and decreases AV conduction.
- ***Adverse effects :*** Sinus bradycardia, bronchospasm, metallic taste, etc.

## CLASS II – Antiarrhythmics (β-Blockers) :

- They competitively block catecholamine induced stimulation of cardiac beta receptors and depress phase 4 depolarisation of pacemaker cells.

- They slow sinus as well as AV nodal conduction which results in decrease in HR and prolongation of PR interval.
- They increase the ERP and prolong the APD.
- ***Uses :*** propranolol, metoprolol are used for supraventricular arrhythmias like atrial flutter, and fibrillation, PSVT, tachyarrhythmias of hyperthyroidism, digitalis induced ventricular arrhythmias and PVCs. Esmolol is used for supraventricular tachycardia.
- Adverse effects and other details of beta blockers are covered in their respective chapter.

## CLASS III – Antiarrhythmics :

- They block the outward $K^+$ channels during phase 3 of action potential.
- They prolong the APD without affecting phase 0 of depolarisation. Instead, they prolong ERP.
- ***Uses :*** covered under individual drug below.

### Amiodarone :

- It is iodine containing anti-arrhythmic drug. Besides class III, it also has Class IA, Class II and Class IV properties. Hence, considered as broad spectrum anti-arrhythmic agent.
- ***Uses :*** Most tachyarrhythmic conditions (ventricular and supraventricular), recurrent VT and VF, WPW syndrome.
- ***Adverse effects :*** Photosensitisation (skin pigmentation), peripheral neuropathy, heart block, pulmonary alveolitis and fibrosis, corneal micro deposits and hypothyroidism (inhibits conversion of $T_4$ to $T_3$).

### Bretylium :

- It is an adrenergic neuron blocker which was used as antihypertensive agent.
- Its use declined due to poor bioavailability and tolerance. But, it was again introduced as an anti-arrhythmic drug.
- ***Uses :*** it is used only in ICU setups for managing refractory life threatening ventricular arrhythmias like VT and VF.
- ***Adverse effects :*** postural hypotension, parotid swelling and nausea.

### Sotalol :

- It is a non-selective beta blocker. It has got both Class II and Class III actions.
- ***Uses :*** same as that of amiodarone.

### Ibutilide and Dofetilide :

- It is a structural analogue of sotalol.
- Selective $K^+$ channel blockers, less adverse events.
- ***Uses :*** atrial flutter and fibrillation.
- ***Adverse effects :*** QT prolongation and torsades de pointes.

### Dronedarone :

- It is amiodarone like drug but without iodine atoms (no thyroid or pulmonary toxicity).
- ***Uses :*** treatment and recurrences of atrial fibrillation.

### Vernakalant :

- It is a mixed $K^+$ and $Na^+$ channel blocker.
- ***Uses :*** atrial fibrillation.

## CLASS IV – Antiarrhythmics ($Ca^{+2}$ channel blockers) :

- They block the activated L-type $Ca^{+2}$ channels in the heart which results in decrease in the rate of phase 4 depolarisation in SA node and AV node and slowed conduction through AV node. They also prolong ERP.
- Verapamil and diltiazem are commonly used.
- ***Uses :*** PSVT, control ventricular response in atrial flutter and fibrillation.
- ***Adverse effects :*** ankle edema, constipation etc.
- ***Contraindications :*** AV block, severe hypotension, CHF and WPW syndrome.

## Miscellaneous :

### Adenosine :

- It is a naturally occurring nucleoside present normally in all cells of the body.
- **Mechanism of action :** It stimulates adenosine ($A_1$) receptors and opens G-protein coupled $K^+$ channels and inhibits conduction in SA node, atria and AV node. It terminates re-entry circuit through AV node and restores normal sinus rhythm.
- It is usually given as rapid IV bolus injection in a dose of 3 mg.
- **Use :** PSVT (*drug of choice*)
- **Adverse effects :** Nausea, dyspnea, flushing, bronchospasm and headache.

### Magnesium sulphate :

- Its mechanism of action is unknown but may influence $Na^+/K^+$ ATPase, $Na^+$ channels, certain $K^+$ channels & $Ca^{+2}$ channels.
- **Use :** Digitalis induced arrhythmias if hypomagnesemia present, refractory ventricular tachyarrhythmias, Torsades de pointes.
- Overdose toxicity is detected by loss of deep tendon reflexes.

### Potassium :

- Both high levels and decreased levels of $K^+$ in the body are potential scenarios for causing arrhythmias.
- The goal is to normalise $K^+$ levels.

### Digoxin :

- **Mechanism of action :** inhibiting the cardiac $Na^+/K^+$-ATPase.
- **Uses :** CHF patients with atrial fibrillation or atrial flutter and PSVT.

### Atropine :

- It is anticholinergic drug.
- It decreases AV node ERP and increases conduction velocity in bundle of His.
- **Use :** It is used in AV block when it is due to vagal overactivity like in digitalis toxicity or MI.

❑❑❑❑❑

49

# ANTI-ANGINAL DRUGS AND DRUGS FOR MYOCARDIAL INFARCTION

## ANTI-ANGINAL DRUGS :

### Angina pectoris :

- It is the primary symptom of ischemic heart disease which is caused by an imbalance in the myocardial oxygen supply and demand relationship.
- It is a heavy pressing sub-sternal discomfort or pain, often radiating to left shoulder, flexor aspect of left arm, jaw or epigastrium.

### Types of Angina pectoris :

- ***Classical angina (Exertional angina) :*** Commonest type. There is atheromatous obstruction of coronary arteries. Symptoms occur when oxygen demand increases as with exertion, exercise or meals.
- ***Unstable angina :*** There is rupture of atherosclerotic plaque in the coronary arteries and formation of platelet thrombi at the site of rupture leading to narrowing of the lumen. There are recurrent attacks of angina with minimal exertion or even at rest.
- ***Prinzmetal angina (Variant angina) :*** There is transient spasm of localised portions of coronary arteries which leads to angina pain.

### Treatment :

***Non-pharmacological management :***

- Control of risk factors like : Smoking, hypertension, hyperlipidemia, obesity and diabetes.

## CLASSIFICATION ANTI-ANGINAL DRUGS :

- **Organic nitrates :**
  - ***Short acting :*** Glyceryl trinitrate (Nitroglycerine), Isosorbide dinitrate (sublingual).
  - ***Long acting :*** Isosorbide dinitrate (oral), Isosorbide mononitrate, Erythrityl tetranitrate, Pentaerythritol tetranitrate.
- **Calcium channel blockers :**
  - Verapamil, Diltiazem, Amlodipine, Nifedipine and others.
- **β-blockers :**
  - Propranolol, Atenolol, Metoprolol and others.

- **Potassium channel openers :**
  - Nicorandil.
- **Others :**
  - ***Cytoprotective drugs :*** Trimetazidine, Ranolazine.
  - ***Anti-platelet drugs :*** Aspirin, Clopidogrel, Prasugrel, Cilostazole, Dipyridamole.
  - ***Bradycardiac drugs :*** Ivabradine.
  - ***Lipid lowering drugs :*** Atorvastatin, Rosuvastatin etc.
  - ***Miscellaneous :*** Drug eluting stents.

## Organic Nitrates :

- Nitrates have low oral bioavailability due to first pass metabolism hence, sublingual route is preferred.
- Isosorbide mononitrate has no major first pass metabolism and therefore has negligible first pass effect. Therefore, it is effective orally.
- They are available as tablets, ointment, spray and injectable.

### Mechanism of action :

- Organic nitrates are converted to NO (nitric oxide) which activates cytosolic guanylyl cyclase. This increases the cyclic GMP. cGMP then causes dephosphorylation of myosin light chain kinase. There is also reduction in free cytosolic calcium. The net result of these effects is relaxation of smooth muscles (In context of angina pectoris, relaxation of vascular smooth muscles).

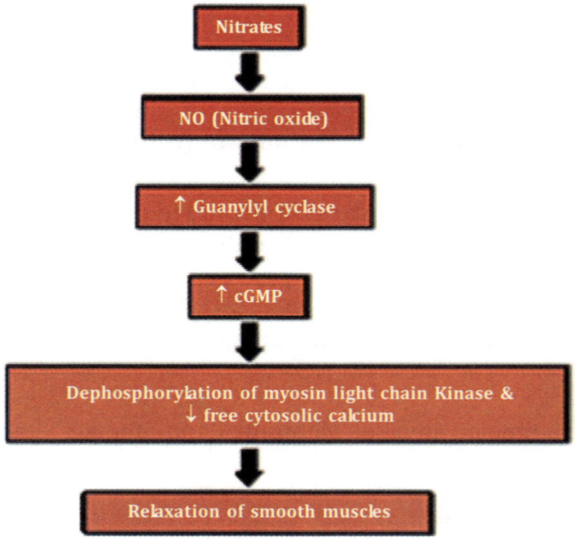

## Pharmacological effects :

### Vascular effects :

- ***Small doses :*** mainly dilates venous vessels. This decreases the pre-load and thus reduces oxygen demand by the heart. There is reduction in ventricular pressure, reduction in pressure on sub-endocardial vessels and redistribution of coronary blood flow to ischemic areas. Due to decrease venous pressure, there can be postural hypotension or syncope.

- ***Large doses :*** causes both arteriolar & venous dilatation. This decreases the pre-load as well as the afterload and thus reduces oxygen demand by the heart. Arteriolar dilatation of facial vessels causes flushing and meningeal vessels causes throbbing headache.

### Other effects :

- ***Smooth muscles :*** Bronchial, biliary, GIT, uterine smooth muscle relaxation. Nitrates can also cause penile erection.

- ***Platelets :*** Inhibition of platelet aggregation.

## Uses :

- ***Angina pectoris :*** Nitrates are used as sublingual (for acute attack), orally (for prophylaxis), 2% ointment topical application on chest (for nocturnal angina) and buccally (for short term prophylaxis).

- ***CCF :*** Reduces preload and afterload.

- ***Acute MI.***

- ***Cyanide poisoning :*** Cyanide chelates iron of cytochrome oxidase and cause tissue anoxia, coma and death. Nitrates convert hemoglobin to methemoglobin. The later traps cyanide and forms cyanomethemoglobin. Subsequently, sodium thiosulphate is given which reacts with cyanomethemoglobin to form sodium thiocyanate which gets excreted through urine.

- ***Other uses :*** Biliary colic, esophageal spasm.

## Adverse effects :

- ***Acute :*** Throbbing headache, flushing, tachycardia, postural hypotension, syncope.

- ***Tolerance :*** Tolerance occurs with use of nitrates. It can be overcome by providing nitrate free interval every day.

- ***Dependence :*** Sudden withdrawal of nitrates can cause coronary and peripheral vasospasm which can result in MI or sudden death. Withdrawal should be gradual.

- ***Methemoglobinemia :*** It can be treated with Methylene blue.

## Calcium Channel Blockers (CCBs) :

### Classification :

**Dihydropyridines (DHPs) :**

- ***Ultra-short acting :*** Clevidipine.
- ***Short acting :*** Nifedipine, Nicardipine, Nimodipine.
- ***Intermediate acting :*** Lacidipine, Cilnidipine, Lercanidipine.
- ***Long acting :*** Amlodipine, Benidipine, Felodipine.

**Non-dihydropyridines (Non-DHPs) :**

- ***Short acting :*** Verapamil, Diltiazem.
- ***Long acting :*** Bepiridil.

### Mechanism of action :

- CCBs block voltage dependent L-type $Ca^{+2}$ channels and thus reduce the frequency of opening of these channels in response to depolarisation.

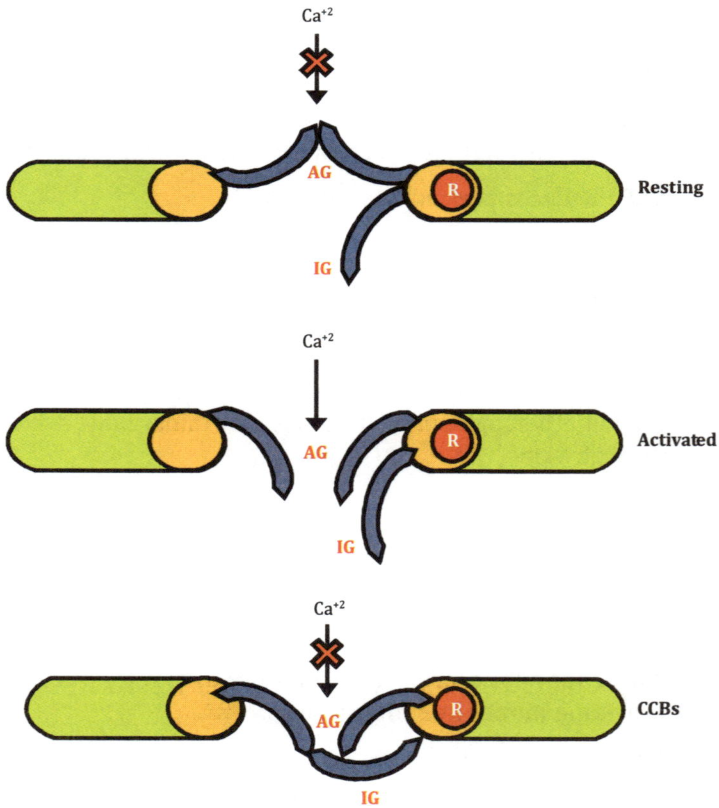


**AG :** Activation gate, **IG :** Inactivation gate, **R :** receptor for CCBs

This results in marked decrease in trans-membrane $Ca^{+2}$ current in vascular smooth muscle (relaxation), cardiac muscle (reduction in contractility), SA node (decreased pacemaker activity) and AV node (decrease in conduction).

- The $Ca^{+2}$ channels have an activation gate (AG) on its extracellular site and an inactivation gate (IG) on its intracellular site.
- These channels exist in 3 forms :
  1. Resting or closed state with AG closed.
  2. Activated or open state where AG opens and there is inflow of $Ca^{+2}$ and
  3. Inactivated or blocked state as seen with CCBs where occlusion of the channel occurs by IG and $Ca^{+2}$ inflow ceases.
- In skeletal muscles, the $Ca^{+2}$ is intracellular and hence CCBs are ineffective in skeletal muscles.

**Advantages of CCBs on other antihypertensive drugs :**

- No postural hypotension or rebound hypertension.
- Can be safely used in asthma, angina and PVD.
- More beneficial in elderly patients.
- Improve arterial compliance and retard atherogenesis.
- No significant effects on glucose metabolism, lipid profile and uric acid levels.
- They don't impair male sexual activity.
- They do not have significant adverse effects on fetus.

**Pharmacological effects :**

- ***Cardiac depressant effects :*** decreased heart rate, contractility and conduction velocity. These effects are usually seen with Non-DHPs. (Remember **N**on-DHPs-**N**odal depressants).
- Vasodilation of peripheral and pulmonary blood vessels which results in significant reduction of afterload. This effect is usually seen with DHPs. (Remember **D**HPs-**D**ecreased peripheral resistance).
- They also cause coronary vasodilatation.
- All these effects reduce myocardial oxygen demand, reduce BP and cardiac workload. Hence, makes them suitable for treatment of HTN, angina, MI, supraventricular tachycardia.
- Nimodipine is highly lipid soluble and crosses BBB and has higher selectivity for cerebral blood vessels. Hence, used in hemorrhagic stroke.
- Cilnidipine has shown to possess some renoprotective effects also.

**Uses :**

- ***Angina pectoris :*** due to decrease in myocardial oxygen demand, and dilatation of coronary arteries.

- ***Supraventricular arrhythmias :*** because of its depressant action on SA and AV nodes.
- ***Hypertension :*** they control blood pressure by their vasodilatory effect. Previously, short acting DHP group of CCBs like nifedipine (mostly sublingually for emergency management) were used to treat HTN and angina. But, studies have revealed that these drugs have poor outcomes especially in angina because abrupt vasodilation with sympathetic stimulation leads to tachycardia (↑ oxygen demand). This increases the risk of myocardial infarction. Therefore, long acting drugs like amlodipine are preferred nowadays.
- ***Hypertension in pregnancy :*** Though methyldopa and labetolol are used as first line agents, CCBs can also be used as second line agents.
- ***Migraine :*** A special CCB called Flunarizine is used for prophylaxis of migraine but not for acute attack.
- ***Raynaud's phenomenon :*** Due to their peripheral vasodilatory property.
- ***Other uses :*** Hypertrophic cardiomyopathy, premature labor.

**Contraindications :**

- Heart failure, bradycardia, A-V block, hypotension and unstable angina.

**Adverse effects :**

- Hypotension, palpitations, reflex tachycardia, ankle edema, dizziness, constipation, sedation, A-V block, headache, drowsiness and fatigue.

## β-Blockers :

- **Rationale for use :** reduces heart rate and myocardial contractility due to blockade of cardiac β-receptors. This results in decrease in myocardial oxygen demand. Another benefit of them is that they prevent cardiac arrhythmias.
- Cardioselective $\beta_1$-blockers like atenolol and metoprolol are preferred more.
- Non-selective β-blockers (both $\beta_1$ and $\beta_2$ receptor blockers) like propranolol can worsen the prinzmetal angina because of unopposed action of α-receptors which causes coronary vasospasm.
- Celiprolol having an additional vasodilating property is also used.
- Abrupt withdrawal of β-blockers can precipitate angina and MI due to sudden increase in sympathetic tone due to upregulation of β-receptors following prolong blockade by β-blockers.
- More details are covered in chapter on adrenergic antagonists.

## Potassium Channel Opener : Nicorandil :

- **Mechanism of action :**

**Nicorandil**

↓

**Opens $K^+$ channel**

↓

**Efflux of $K^+$**

↓

**Hyperpolarization**

↓

**Smooth muscle relaxation**

- **Effects :** It reduces preload and afterload and also produces coronary vasodilatation. It also exerts nitrates like effect.
- **Adverse effects :** flushing, palpitations, dizziness, headache, nausea etc.

## Cytoprotective Drugs :

### Trimetazidine :

- It is a new calcium channel blocker.
- It is an anti-ischemic drug that has cytoprotective effects on myocardial cells.
- It prevents the degradation of membrane fatty acids by lipid peroxidation and thus reduces myocardial oxygen demand.
- It also inhibits the superoxide cytotoxicity to protect the myocardium from harmful effects of ischemia.
- It is indicated for stable angina, infarction sequelae and ischemia of labyrinths seen in Meniere's disease.

### Ranolazine :

- It is also a cytoprotective drug that has cytoprotective effects on myocardial cells.
- It inhibits inward sodium current during ischemia. As a result, the calcium load in cardiac muscle is reduced indirectly via $Na^+$-$Ca^{+2}$ exchanger.
- The main adverse effect is QTc prolongation.

## Anti-Platelet Drugs :

### Aspirin :

- Aspirin is used in low dose (75-325 mg) for reducing ischemia in patients of coronary artery disease.
- More details are covered in chapter on anti-platelet drugs.

**Clopidogrel, Prasugrel :**

- These are the anti-platelet drugs that does not interfere with prostaglandin synthesis.
- They inhibit the ADP binding to the ADP receptors and thus, prevent platelet aggregation.
- All these drugs are used alone or as an adjuvant in patients of unstable angina and to prevent thrombosis after a coronary intervention.

**Cilostazole :**

- It is phosphodiesterase-3 inhibitor which promotes vasodilation and inhibit platelet aggregation by increasing cAMP in the vessel wall.
- It can be used to treat angina, but it is mainly used to treat intermittent claudication seen in peripheral vascular disease (along with other drugs like pentoxyphylline).

**Dipyridamole :**

- It inhibits adenosine deaminase and phosphodiesterase enzymes.
- This leads to accumulation of adenosine and cAMP respectively.
- Adenosine and cAMP inhibit platelet aggregation and produce coronary vasodilation.
- ***Coronary steal phenomenon :*** Dipyridamole dilates the vessels in the ischemic as well as non-ischemic zones. Dilation of blood vessels in the non-ischemic zones diverts the already reduced blood flow away from the ischaemic zone. This is called as "coronary steal phenomenon" and this can exacerbate the angina. This has lead to therapeutic failure of dipyridamole.

**NOTE :** more details about antiplatelet drugs are covered in the chapter on anticoagulants and antiplatelet drugs.

## Bradycardiac Drugs : *Ivabradine*

- It is a selective If sodium channel blocker in SA node.
- It has no effect on ventricular contractility and has no effect on BP.
- It decreases the myocardial oxygen demand by reducing the heart rate.

## Lipid Lowering Drugs : *Atorvastatin, Rosuvastatin, etc.*

- They are used in prophylaxis and treatment of angina and MI.
- They prevent formation of atheromatous plaques and in higher doses also stabilises the plaque and prevents thromboembolic events.
- Details are covered in the respective chapter.

## Drug Eluting Stents :

- Restenosis of a stent after angioplasty is a common problem. To overcome this, drug eluting medicated stents are being commonly used nowadays. They prevent restenosis and further coronary events.

- Drugs used in drug eluting stents : Sirolimus, Zotarolimus.
- Concurrently antiplatelet therapy has to be continued.

## DRUGS FOR MYOCARDIAL INFARCTION :

### Myocardial infarction :

- It is localised area of ischemic necrosis of myocardium due to sudden occlusion of a branch of coronary artery.

### Pathophysiology :

- There is atherosclerosis in the coronaries. There might be disruption of atherosclerotic plaque and accumulation of platelets & activation of coagulation cascade leading to thrombus formation and occlusion of the coronaries which reduces the cardiac blood supply.

### Risk factors :

- Cigarette smoking, hypertension, dyslipidemia, diabetes mellitus, advanced age, obesity, physical inactivity and stress.

### Clinical features :

- Pain which is deep, visceral, experienced as heavy / squeezing / crushing and which presents in the central portion of chest / epigastrium and radiates to arms, jaws, abdomen, neck.
- Other symptoms : Weakness, sweating, nausea, vomiting, anxiety, sense of impending doom, restlessness, pallor, perspiration & coolness of extremities.

### Diagnosis :

- Clinical diagnosis.
- ***ECG :*** ST segment elevation, T wave inversion and Q waves.
- ***Cardiac biomarkers :*** Troponin-T, CK-MB.
- ***Imaging :*** 2D Echo, Radionuclide imaging techniques, Angiography.

### Treatment :

#### *Prehospital care :*

- Recognition of symptoms by patient or relatives.
- Avoid exertion, activities like walking or climbing stairs.
- Quick transportation of patient to the nearest hospital.
- Admission to ICU or CCU.

#### *Care in emergency department :*

- Confirm the diagnosis by investigations.
- Monitor vitals.
- Aspirin 300 mg and Atorvastatin 80 mg stat. These are given for stabilisation of atherosclerotic plaque and prevent embolism of the thrombus.
- Oxygen support (6-8 liters/min).

- **For anginal pain :** Nitrates (sublingual/ IV), Morphine (IV). Inj. Pentazocine 30 mg IM stat can be given for severe pain and
- **For relieving anxiety :** Inj. Diazepam 10 mg IV.

***Fibrinolysis (Thrombolysis) :***

- Best response is seen if thrombolysed within 3-4 hrs of onset of symptoms.
- **Contraindications :** Surgery within 10 days, serious GI bleeding within 3 months, marked hypertension (>180/110 mm Hg), active internal bleeding, aortic dissection, history of cerebrovascular hemorrhage.
- Inj. Streptokinase 7.5 lakh units in 100 ml NS slow IV infusion to be given over the period of half hour.
- If the patient is sensitive to or has taken streptokinase in the past, give Inj. Urokinase 2.5 lakhs IU IV over 10 min followed by 5 lakhs IU over 1 hr IV.
- More details about fibrinolytics are given in the chapter on fibrinolytics.

***Supportive drugs :***

- **β-blockers :** They reduce the infarct size, prevents re-infarction, reduces duration of ischemia and prevents cardiac arrhythmias and sudden death (Inj. Metoprolol 100 mg IV).
- **Anticoagulants :** Heparin or low molecular weight heparins can be given for prevention of thrombus extension and also in unstable angina.
- **Atropine :** If the patient is having sinus bradycardia.
- **Inotropic agents :** Dopamine or dobutamine are used if the cardiac functions are failing.
- **ACE inhibitors or Angiotensin receptor blockers :** They are used after the patients are stabilised and continued after the discharge of the patient. They prevent remodelling of heart, reduce the chances of CHF and provides long term survival benefits.
- **Antiplatelet drugs :** Aspirin, clopidogrel and other antiplatelet drugs are given on regular basis to prevent future cardiac events.
- **Hypolipidemic drugs :** Drugs like atorvastatin, rosuvastain, fibrates are given for control of hyperlipidemia and prevent further episodes.

***Definitive coronary interventions :***

- PTCA (Percutaneous transluminal coronary angioplasty).
- CABG (Coronary artery bypass grafting).

***Other measures :***

- Control of hypertension, diabetes and other risk factors.
- Lifestyle modifications.
- Quit smoking and regular exercise.

# 50 ANTI-HYPERTENSIVE DRUGS

These are the drugs that are used in the treatment of hypertension.

| BP | Systolic (mm of Hg) | Diastolic (mm of Hg) |
|---|---|---|
| **Normal** | < 120 | < 80 |
| **Pre-hypertension** | 120-139 | 80-89 |
| **Stage I** | 140-159 | 90-99 |
| **Stage II** | > 160 | > 100 |

**Risk factors :**

- ***Primary essential hypertension :*** Advancing age, family history, smoking, stress, dyslipidemia, diabetes, obesity, sedentary lifestyle, excess salt consumption.
- ***Secondary hypertension :*** Pheochromocytoma, renal diseases, Cushing's syndrome.

**Management :**

***Non-Pharmacological Measures :***

- Salt restricted diet, reduce carbohydrates, fats and increase protein intake, daily exercise like brisk walking for 45 min, weight reduction, quit alcohol, smoking and tobacco, stress reduction and control of diabetes.

**ANTI-HYPERTENSIVE DRUG CLASSIFICATION :**

- **α-blockers :** Prazosin, Terazosin, Doxazosin, Phentolamine, Phenoxybenzamine.
- **β-blockers :** Propranolol, Metoprolol, Atenolol, Esmolol, Nebivolol etc.
- **α + β blockers :** Labetalol, Carvedilol.
- **Central sympatholytics :** Clonidine, α-Methyldopa.
- **ACE inhibitors :** Captopril, Enalapril, Lisinopril, Benazapril, Ramipril.
- **Angiotensin receptor blockers :** Losartan, Valsartan, Telmisartan, Olmesartan.
- **Renin inhibitors :** Enalkiren, Remikiren and Aliskiren.
- **Diuretics :** Furosemide, Torasemide, Hydrochlorothiazide, Spironolactone.
- **Vasodilators :** Hydralazine, Minoxidil, Nitrates, Sodium nitroprusside.
- **Calcium channel blockers :** Verapamil, Amlodipine, Nifedipine.

All the drugs are covered in their respective chapters.

## MANAGEMENT OF HYPERTENSIVE EMERGENCIES :

- Hypertensive emergencies include hypertensive encephalopathy, hypertensive nephropathy, intracranial hemorrhage, dissecting aneurysm, pre-eclampsia, unstable angina and myocardial infarction.
- It should be managed quite meticulously because it is associated with high morbidity and mortality.
- Rapid normalisation of BP should be avoided because it leads to cerebral, coronary or renal ischemia.
- The initial goal is to reduce BP by no more than 25% (within few min to 1-2 hrs) and then move towards a level of 160/100 mm of Hg within next 2-6 hrs. Subsequently, the BP can be reduced to normal levels using oral medication over several days or weeks.
- Following drugs are used in management of hypertensive emergencies :
    1. **Sodium nitroprusside :** It is an arteriolar and venous dilator which was used previously but, no longer preferred now. However, along with a beta blocker it is used for treatment of emergency HTN of aortic aneurysm.
    2. **Clevidipine :** It is an ultra-short acting CCB. Infusion of clevidipine is used in severe HTN.
    3. **Nimodipine :** It is again a CCB with higher selectivity for cerebral blood vessels, therefore used in hemorrhagic stroke secondary to HTN.
    4. **Esmolol :** It is a beta blocker used in treatment of supraventricular tachycardia but can also be used for hypertensive emergencies. It can be combined with clevidipine or labetalol. Such a combination is used in HTN associated with aortic dissection and MI.
    5. **Labetalol :** It is a dual alpha and beta blocker which is useful in hypertensive emergencies associated with eclampsia, pre-eclampsia and MI.
    6. **Nitroglycerin :** It is used as IV for management of hypertensive emergencies especially those associated with coronary involvement.
    7. **Fenoldopam :** It is a peripheral $D_1$ receptor agonist which reduces BP without causing tolerance, rebound HTN or deterioration of renal functions. It is used in hypertensive emergencies associated with impaired renal functions.
    8. **Hydralazine :** It is an arteriolar vasodilator which is mainly used in eclampsia and in children but should be avoided in patients with acute coronary disease or dissecting aneurysm. Not preferred nowadays.
    9. **Diuretics :** IV furosemide or bumetanide can be used as adjunct medications in hypertensive emergencies especially if it is associated with pulmonary edema, cerebral edema or acute LVF.
    10. **Phentolamine :** It is a non-selective alpha blocker and is used for hypertensive emergencies of pheochromocytoma.

## HYPERTENSION IN PREGNANCY :

- High BP during pregnancy has implications on both mother and fetus.
- Many drugs are unsafe in pregnancy due to their teratogenic effects on the fetus.
- Antihypertensives that can be used in HTN during pregnancy are :
    1. Methyldopa (Central sympatholytic).
    2. Labetalol (Combined $\alpha$ + $\beta$ blocker).
    3. Nifedipine (Calcium channel blocker).
    4. Hydralazine (vasodilator).
- Antihypertensives that should be avoided during pregnancy are :
    1. ACE inhibitors.
    2. Angiotensin receptor blockers.
    3. Diuretics.
    4. Non-selective beta blockers.
    5. Sodium nitroprusside.

# 51 HYPOLIPIDEMIC DRUGS

Hyperlipidemia or dyslipidemia is one of the leading causes of cardiovascular and cerebrovascular morbidity and mortality. Hypolipidemic drugs lower the levels of lipids and lipoproteins in blood.

## Types of hyperlipidemia :

| Type | Name | Elevation of lipoprotein |
|---|---|---|
| I | Familial Hyperchylomicronemia | Chylomicrons |
| IIa | Familial Hypercholesterolemia | LDL |
| IIb | Familial Combined Hyperlipidemia | VLDL and LDL |
| III | Familial Dysbetalipoproteinemia | Remnants of VLDL and Chylomicrons |
| IV | Familial Hypertriglyceridemia | VLDL |
| V | Familial Combined Hypertriglyceridemia | VLDL and Chylomicrons |

## Non-pharmacological treatment of hyperlipidemia :

- Low fat and high fibre diet, decrease weight, increase physical activity, smoking cessation.

## CLASSIFICATION OF HYPOLIPIDEMIC DRUGS :

- **HMG-CoA Reductase inhibitors (Statins) :** Atorvastatin, Rosuvastatin, Simvastatin, Pravastatin, Pitavastatin.
- **Bile acid binding resins :** Cholestyramine, Colestipol, Colesevelam.
- **Lipoprotein lipase activators (Fibrates) :** Gemfibrozil, Clofibrate, Bezafibrate, Fenofibrate.
- **Inhibitor of intestinal absorption of cholesterol :** Ezetimibe.
- **Inhibitor of lipolysis and triglyceride synthesis :** Nicotinic acid (Niacin).
- **Miscellaneous agents :** Gugulipid and Fish oil derivatives.

## HMG-CoA reductase inhibitors (Statins) :

### Mechanism of action :

- They decrease cholesterol synthesis by competitively inhibiting the enzyme **HMG CoA reductase** (Hydroxy-methyl-glutaryl-co-enzyme-A reductase) which is the rate limiting step in cholesterol synthesis.

## Characteristics :

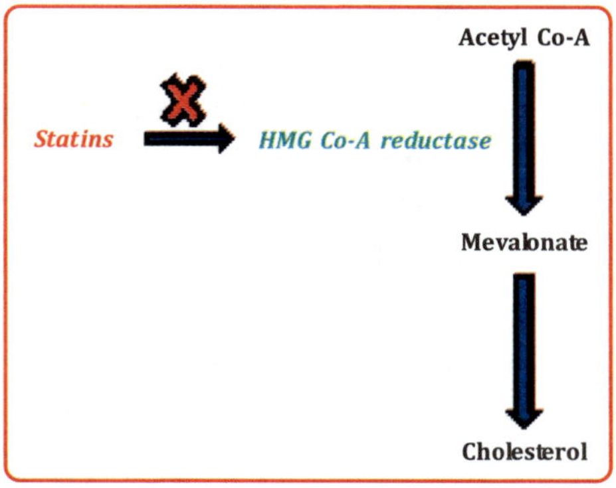


- Statins differ in their potency and max efficacy in reducing LDL cholesterol.
- Dose dependent lowering of LDL cholesterol is seen.
- Triglycerides are reduced by 10-30%.
- Statins also cause rise in HDL by 5-15%.
- HMG-CoA reductase activity is maximum at midnight hence; statins are prefereably administered at bed time. However, Atorvastatin and Rosuvastatin have longer half life and can be administered anytime of the day.
- Statins after prolong use can have reduced effect. This is due to feedback compensatory induction of HMG-CoA reductase.

## Atorvastatin :

- Good LDL cholesterol lowering effect. It has much longer t½ (18-24 hrs). It has additional anti-oxidant property.
- ***Dose :*** 10-40 mg/day (max 80 mg).

## Rosuvastatin :

- The t½ is 18-24 hrs. It raises maximum HDL level compared to other statins.
- ***Dose :*** 5-20 mg/day (max 40 mg/day).

## Simvastatin :

- It also increases HDL significantly.
- The t½ is 2-3 hrs.
- ***Dose :*** 10-40 mg/day.

## Simvastatin :

- It also causes decrease in plasma fibrinogen level.
- ***Dose :*** 20-40 mg/day.

## Simvastatin :

- Most potent statin for reducing LDL.
- ***Dose :*** 1-4 mg/day.

## Use and advantages :

- They are 1st choice in primary and secondary hyper lipidemias mainly type IIa and IIb.
- They decrease CVS mortality by decreasing raised LDL level and also by increasing HDL level.

- They are used in coronary artery diseases, angina, myocardial infarction and prophylactically in high risk cases like diabetes and HTN.
- They also improve coronary compliance and atheromatous plaque stabilisation.
- They also cause improvement in endothelial function and increased NO production.

### Adverse effects :

- Muscle tenderness and rise in CPK levels.
- Myopathy and muscle damage. It is more when given along with nicotinic acid or gemfibrozil or CYP3A4 inhibitors like ketoconazole.
- Headache.
- Sleep disturbances.
- Liver dysfunction.

## Bile acid binding resins (Bile acid sequestrants) :

- Bile acids are synthesised in the liver from Cholesterol and are secreted in the duodenum and helps in dietary fat absorption. They undergo entero-hepatic circulation.

### Mechanism of action :

- Bile acid binding resins are non-absorbable resins that complex with negatively charged bile acids.
- The resin-bile acid complex is non-absorbable and gets excreted through feces, thus preventing bile acids from returning to the liver by entero-hepatic circulation.
- To compensate for absence of bile acids, the biosynthesis of bile acids from cholesterol increases, which leads to partial depletion of hepatic cholesterol pool.
- However, they are unsuitable for long term use because they increase the triglyceride levels and also tend to induce HMG CoA reductase in liver.
- ***Use :*** They are drug of choice for type IIa and type IIb hyperlipidemia along with niacin. Other use is to relieve pruritus in patients with cholestasis.

### Dose :

- Cholestyramine, colestipol granules (16 g daily) with water or juice taken with meals. Palatability is a concern.
- Colesevelam (625 mg tablet) 6 tablets/day. It has better patient compliance.

### Adverse effects :

- Absorption of fat soluble vitamins and folic acid is impaired, constipation, exacerbation of hemorrhoids, GIT distress etc.

## Lipoprotein lipase activators (Fibrates) :

### Mechanism of action :

- They activate lipoprotein lipase which causes increased hydrolyses and removal of VLDL from TGs (Triglycerides), thus lowering circulating TGs level. This effect is exerted through activation of a nuclear receptor called as *peroxisome proliferator activated receptor-α (PPAR-α)*. Its activation enhances lipoprotein lipase activity and synthesis. PPAR-α also enhances LDL receptor expression.
- This class of drugs primarily lower TGs (20-50%). There is 10-15% decrease in LDL and 10-15% increase in HDL.
- ***Use :*** They are drug of choice for hypertriglyceridemia and particularly those which are associated with low HDL levels. They are used in type IV, V and IIb (along with niacin).

### Adverse effects :

- Myopathy (especially when used along with statins), GIT upset, increased aminotransferase levels and increased incidence of gallstones.

## Inhibitor of intestinal absorption of cholesterol : Ezetimibe

### Mechanism of action :

- Inhibit cholesterol absorption by interfering with specific cholesterol transport protein (Neimann pick $C_1$ like $N_1$ protein) in intestinal mucosa. It also inhibits entero-hepatic circulation of cholesterol. The decreased cholesterol in turn increases the uptake of LDL from plasma via LDL receptors in liver.
- There is compensatory increase in cholesterol synthesis due to reduced cholesterol levels. This compensatory increase in cholesterol is blocked by statins and hence, ezetimibe along with statins makes a good combination.
- It reduces LDL by 15-20%, TGs by 8% and increases HDL by 3%.
- ***Use :*** They are used as monotherapy or in combination with statins for type IIa and IIb hyperlipidemia.
- ***Dose :*** 10 mg/day
- ***Adverse effects :*** GIT distress, liver dysfunction etc.

## Inhibitor of Lipolysis and triglyceride synthesis : Nicotinic acid (Niacin)

### Mechanism of action :

- The exact mechanism is still debated. However, it is studied that niacin stimulates a specific receptor on adipose cells which inhibits lipolysis in adipose tissue, reduces levels of circulating free fatty acids and reduces triglyceride synthesis. This results in decreased VLDL and LDL levels.
- It reduces TGs levels by 40%, VLDL by 35%, LDL by 10-15% and increases HDL by 15-25%.

- ***Use :*** It is used for type IIb and IV hyperlipidemia in which both VLDL and LDL are elevated. It is also used for high risk patients with high TGs and low HDL levels.
- ***Dose :*** 1.5-3 g/day.

**Adverse effects :**

- Cutaneous flushing, pruritus which is due to release of prostaglandins. It can be reduced by giving aspirin as premedication or by giving extended release formulations. A new drug called *Laropiprant* can also be used to prevent flushing.
- Cholestasis, hyperuricemia and hepatic dysfunction are sometimes observed.

## Miscellaneous :

**Gugulipid :**

- Developed at Central Drug Research Institute, Lucknow.
- Contains sterones isolated from guggulugum.
- Inhibits cholesterol biosynthesis and enhances its excretion.
- It decreases total cholesterol and LDL, increases HDL and slightly lowers TGs.
- ***Dose :*** 25 mg tablet TDS.
- ***Adverse effects :*** It is usually well tolerated; loose stools are only side effect.

**Fish oil derivatives (Omega-3 fatty acids) :**

- It contains poly unsaturated fatty acids (PUFA); Eicosa-pentanoic and docosa-hexanoic acids.
- It has membrane stabilising and antioxidant action.
- ***Use :*** It is used for prophylaxis in high risk patients of cardiovascular diseases with hyperlipidemia (commonly in combination with Vit. E).

# DRUGS ACTING ON THE KIDNEY

# 52 DIURETICS AND ANTI-DIURETICS

- **Diuretic :** substance that promotes the excretion of urine.
- **Natriuretic :** substance that promotes the renal excretion of sodium.
- **Kaliuretic :** substance which promotes excretion of potassium.
- **Saliuretic :** substance which promotes excretion of sodium and chloride.

**The excretion by kidney is dependent on :**

- Glomerular filtration, Tubular reabsorption and Tubular secretion.

### CLASSIFICATION OF DIURETICS :

- **Loop Diuretics (High ceiling diuretics) :** Furosemide, Bumetanide, Torasemide.
- **Thiazide Diuretics :** Chlorthiazide, Hydrochlorothiazide, Chlorthalidone, Indapamide.
- **Potassium Sparing Diuretics :**
  - **$Na^+$ channel inhibitors :** Triamterene, Ameloride.
  - **Aldosterone receptor antagonist :** Spironolactone, Eplerenone.
- **Carbonic anhydrase inhibitors :** Acetazolamide.
- **Osmotic Diuretics :** Mannitol, Urea, Glycerol.

**Mechanism of action :**

| Diuretics | Site of Action | Mechanism |
|---|---|---|
| Osmotic diuretics | • PCT<br>• Loop of Henle (*Descending limb*)<br>• Collecting duct (CD) | Inhibition of water and $Na^+$ reabsorption. |
| Carbonic Anhydrase Inhibitors | PCT | Inhibition of bicarbonate reabso-rption. |
| Loop diuretics | Loop of Henle (*thick ascending limb*) | Inhibition of $Na^+$, $K^+$, $Cl^-$ cotrans-port. |
| Thiazide diuretics | DCT | Inhibition of $Na^+$, $Cl^-$ cotransport. |
| $K^+$ sparing diuretics | • Late DCT<br>• CD | Inhibition of $Na^+$ reabsorption and $K^+$ secretion. |

## Sites of action of diuretics :

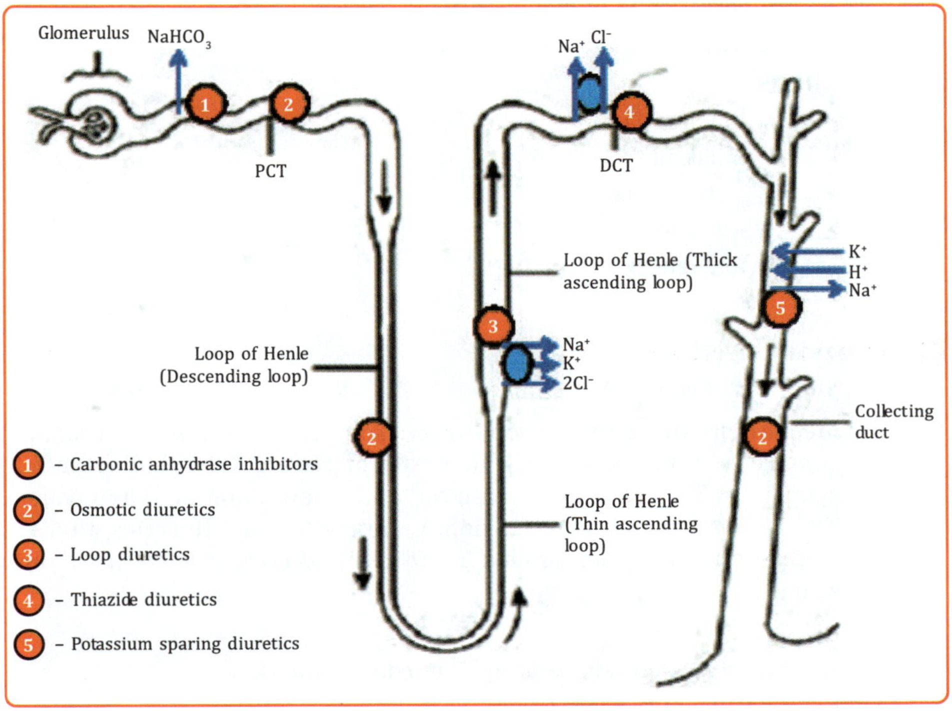


### Loop Diuretics :

- They are also called as *'high ceiling diuretics'* because their dose-response curve is steep and by increasing the dose the sodium excretion can be increased significantly as compared to other diuretics.
- **Site :** Thick ascending limb of loop of Henle.
- **Mechanism of action :** Loop diuretics are secreted into the proximal convoluted tubule and reach their site of action. They **inhibit $Na^+/K^+/2Cl^-$ symporter**. This significantly increases the excretion of $Na^+$, $K^+$ and $Cl^-$. Osmotic gradient for water reabsorption is also decreased leading to increasing water excretion. $Ca^{+2}$ and $Mg^{+2}$ are excreted as well. There is also decreased excretion of uric acid.
- **Drug interactions :** Concomitant use of aminoglycoside or cisplatin increases the risk of nephrotoxicity and ototoxicity. Prostaglandins are important in maintaining Glomerular filtration; NSAIDs reduces the effects of diuretics. They can enhance digitalis toxicity by causing hypokalemia.
- **Uses :**
  - CHF.
  - ***Edema :*** cardiac, pulmonary or renal.
  - Acute pulmonary edema.

- Hypertension.
- Hypercalcemia of malignancy.
- Acute and chronic hyperkalemia.

☞ **Adverse effects :**

- Hyponatremia.
- Hypokalemia.
- Hyperuricemia.
- Hypocalcemia.
- Hypomagnesemia.
- Ototoxicity.

## Thiazide diuretics :

☞ **Site :** Distal convoluted tubule.

☞ **Mechanism of action :** Loop diuretics are secreted into the proximal convoluted tubule and reach their site of action. They inhibit $Na^+/Cl^-$ symporter. This leads to increase $Na^+$ and $Cl^-$ excretion (and also water). There it also favors $K^+$ excretion. Contrary to loop diuretics, there is increased reabsorption of $Ca^{+2}$. There is also decreased excretion of uric acid.

☞ **Uses :**

- Hypertension (single drug or in combination).
- Chronic, mild heart failure.
- Edema (loop diuretic is preferable).
- Nephrogenic Diabetes Insipidus.
- Prevention of $Ca^{+2}$ excretion in osteoporosis and calcium oxalate stones.

☞ **Adverse effects :**

- Hyponatremia.
- Hypokalemia.
- Hyperuricemia.
- Hypercalcemia.
- Hypomagnesemia.
- Hyperglycemia and hypercholesterolemia.
- Sexual dysfunction.

## Potassium Sparing Diuretics :

☞ **Site of action :** $K^+$ sparing diuretics function in DCT and CD.

☞ **Mechanism of action :**

- ***$Na^+$ channel inhibitor (Ameloride, Triamterene) :*** They are secreted at the PCT and act by inhibiting luminal $Na^+$ channels at distal part of DCT and CD. This inhibits $Na^+$ reabsorption and $K^+$ excretion.

- ***Aldosterone antagonist (Spironolactone, Eplerenone) :*** They are competitive antagonist for aldosterone receptors in DCT and CD which prevents aldosterone stimulated increases in $Na^+$ transporter expression. This reduces $Na^+$ reabsorption and $K^+$ secretion.
- Potassium sparing diuretics has a weak diuretic action. They are usually used in combination with other diuretics. The major advantage is that they prevent hypokalemia. Spironolactone is metabolised to its active metabolite, canrenone.

☞ **Uses :**

- Hypertension.
- CHF (with $K^+$ wasting diuretics).
- Hyperaldosteronism (adrenal adenoma, adrenal hyperplasia, Cirrhosis).
- Conditions of hypokalemia.

☞ **Adverse effects :**

- ***Hyperkalemia :*** monitor plasma $K^+$ levels.
- ***Spironolactone :*** gynecomastia.
- GIT Disturbances.

☞ **Contraindications :** Conditions those are prone to cause hyperkalemia like renal failure, drugs like ACE inhibitors, ARBs, NSAIDs, $K^+$ supplementation.

## Osmotic Diuretics :

☞ **Site of action :** PCT, Loop of Henle (descending limb), CD.

☞ **Properties of osmotic diuretics :** They are freely filtrated by glomerulus, have negligible tubular reabsorption, are chemically inert and are usually not metabolised.

☞ **Mechanism of action :** They increase the osmolality in the tubular lumen. Hence, increases excretion of water and electrolytes, increases volume of urine and also rate of urine flow. Mannitol can also reduce brain volume and intracranial pressure by osmotically extracting water from the tissue into the blood. A similar effect occurs in the eye.

☞ **Route of administration :** Mannitol and urea are given IV and glycerol is administered orally.

☞ **Uses :**

- Administered prophylatically for acute renal failure secondary to trauma, cardiovascular disease, surgery or nephrotoxic drugs.
- Glaucoma.
- Raised intracranial pressure; brain bleed, tumors etc.

☞ **Adverse effects :** Transient increased extracellular fluid volume which can worsen cardiac failure and pulmonary edema, if administered orally. It can cause osmotic diarrhea, headache, nausea, vomiting.

## Carbonic Anhydrase Inhibitors :

- **Site of action :** PCT.
- **Mechanism of action :** They inhibit carbonic anhydrase enzyme in renal proximal tubule cells. Carbonic anhydrase catalyses formation of $HCO_3^-$ and $H^+$ from $H_2O$ and $CO_2$. Inhibition of carbonic anhydrase decreases $H^+$ in tubule lumen. As a result, less $H^+$ is available for $Na^+/H^+$ exchange. The net result is increased excretion of $HCO_3^-$, $Na^+$, $K^+$ and water.
- **Uses :**
  - Glaucoma (oral : acetazolamide, topical : dorzolamide, brinzolamide).
  - Acute mountain sickness.
  - Epilepsy (rarely).
  - Metabolic alkalosis.
  - Urinary alkalinisation.
- **Adverse effects :**
  - Tolerance.
  - Metabolic acidosis.
  - Drowsiness, fatigue, Paraesthesias and CNS depression.

## ANTI-DIURETICS :

### Anti-diuretic hormone (ADH, Vasopressin) :

- ***Secretion :*** ADH is secreted by the posterior pituitary in response to rising plasma osmolality of falling blood pressure.
- ***Function :*** It promotes water reabsorption from the collecting ducts. It also constricts blood vessels and can raise BP.
- ***Deficiency :*** Its deficiency results in *Diabetes Insipidus* where there is excretion of large amount of urine, dehydration and thirst. *Diabetes Insipidus* (DI) can be of two types; central DI (Neurogenic cause – head injury, pituitary tumor) and nephrogenic DI (non-function ADH receptors in collecting ducts of kidneys).
- ***Excess secretion :*** Increased ADH secretion can result in SIADH (syndrome of inappropriate secretion of ADH). It is characterised by low plasma osmolality, water retention and dilutional hyponatremia.
- ***ADH receptors :***

| Receptors | Location | Function |
|---|---|---|
| $V_{1a}$ | Vascular and other smooth muscles | Vasoconstriction, visceral smooth muscle contraction |
| $V_{1b}$ | Anterior pituitary | ACTH release |
| $V_2$ | Collecting ducts of kidney | Anti-diuretic action |

## ADH RECEPTOR AGONISTS (Vasopressin analogues) :

- **Drugs : Vasopressin, Desmopressin, Terlipressin, Felypressin, Lypressin.**
- **Uses :**
  - ***Based on $V_1$ action : (Preferred drug is Terlipressin)*** – Bleeding esophageal varices, acute hemorrhagic gastritis, abdominal surgery with portal hypertension and post-operative paralytic ileus.
  - ***Based on $V_2$ action : (Preferred drug is Desmopressin)*** – Diabetes Insipidus (Central DI), nocturnal Enuresis (intranasal/oral), post-lumbar puncture headache, hemophilia and von Willebrand's disease (elevates factor VIII and von Willebrand's factor).
- **Adverse effects :** Facial pallor, abdominal cramps, urge to defecate, precipitation of angina, elevation of BP, fluid retention, hyponatremia.

## ADH RECEPTOR ANTAGONISTS :

- **Drugs : Conivaptan, Tolvaptan, Lixivaptan, Satavaptan.**
- Conivaptan is non-selective in action (acts on both $V_{1a}$ and $V_2$) and has to be given IV. The other vaptans are highly selective ($V_2$) in action and are orally effective.
- **Uses :** SIADH (other drugs; Demeclocycline and Lithium), CHF. Cirrhotic ascites.
- **Adverse effects :** Polydipsia, polyuria, postural hypotension etc.

❑❑❑❑❑

# DRUGS ACTING ON BLOOD AND BLOOD FORMATION

# 53 HEMATINICS (Iron, Vitamin $B_{12}$ and Folic Acid)

**HEMATINICS :**

- These are substances required in the formation of blood, and are used for treatment of anemia.

**Anemia :**

- It is a condition in which there is a deficiency of red cells or of hemoglobin in the blood.

**Types of anemia :**

- Microcytic hypochromic anemia (Iron deficiency).
- Megaloblastic anemia (Vitamin $B_{12}$ and folic acid deficiency).
- Pernicious anemia (It is a type of megaloblastic anemia due to deficiency of intrinsic factor in GIT).
- Hemolytic anemia (Destruction of RBCs).
- Aplastic anemia (Bone marrow depression).
- Sickle cell anemia (sickle cell disease).

**IRON :**

**Total body iron :** 2.5-5.0 gm.

**Distribution :**

- Hemoglobin – 66%
- Iron stores (ferritin and transferrin) – 25%
- Myoglobin – 3%
- Others like enzymes – 6%

**Daily requirement :**

- Adult male – 0.5-1 mg, Adult female – 1-2 mg, Infants – 60 mcg/kg, Children – 25 mcg/kg, Pregnancy – 3-5 mg.

**Dietary sources :**

- Liver, egg yolk, oyster, dry beans, dry fruits, wheat germs, meat, chicken, fish, spinach, banana.

**Factors affecting iron absorption :**

- ***Facilitating :*** Acid - iron reduced to ferric form, reducing substances like ascorbic acid, amino acid having SH group and meat (increases gastric acid).

- ***Decreasing :*** Alkalies - make iron insoluble, phosphates, phytates, tetracyclinas and presence of food in stomach.

### Deficiency : *microcytic hypochromic anemia*

- ***Causes :*** dietary deficiency, faulty absorption and transport, blood loss, excessive demands during pregnancy, lactation and growth.

## ORAL IRON PREPARATIONS :

- **Ferrous sulphate.**
- **Ferrous gluconate.**
- **Ferrous fumarate.**
- **Ferrous lactate.**
- **Ferrous succinate.**
- **Ferrous ascorbate.**
- **Newer oral preparations :**
  - **Iron-polysaccharide complex**
  - **Carbonyl Iron complex**
  - **Ferric hydroxide polymaltose complex**
  - **Ferric citrate**

### Indications :

- Mild to moderate iron deficiency anemia (Microcytic hypochromic anemia).
- Patients who can take orally.

### Dose :

- 200 mg in 3 doses (3-5 mg/kg).
- 3-5 mg / kg in children.
- 30 mg daily for prophylaxis.

### Adverse effects :

- Gastric irritation, abdominal pain, constipation, diarrhea, staining of teeth, metallic taste, bloating etc.

## PARENTERAL IRON PREPARATIONS :

- **Iron dextran.**
- **Iron sorbitol citric acid complex.**
- **Newer Parenteral preparations :**
  - **Iron sucrose complex.**
  - **Iron sodium gluconate complex.**
  - **Ferric carboxymaltose.**
  - **Ferumoxytol.**

### Indications :

- Moderate to severe iron deficiency anemia (Microcytic hypochromic anemia).

- Patients who cannot take orally like in vomiting.
- Oral iron not tolerated.
- Failure of absorption of oral iron *e.g.* Malabsorption.

**Dose :**

- It is calculated by following formula.

**Dose required = 4.4 x Body weight (kg) x Hemoglobin deficit (g/dL)**

**Route :**

- It is better to perform skin sensitivity testing before giving Parenteral Iron to prevent allergic reactions.
- All Parenteral Iron preparations (except Iron sorbitol citric acid complex) can be given IM or IV. Iron sorbitol citric acid complex is given only IM because on IV administration, it binds transferring and saturates its binding site.
- ***Z-technique :*** IM injections are given deeply in the gluteal region by Z track technique (2 ml daily) to avoid staining of skin.
- ***IV :*** 2 ml of iron preparation diluted in 500 ml of dextrose / saline & infused over 6-8 hrs.

**Adverse effects :**

- ***Local :*** pain at the injection site, pigmentation, sterile abscess.
- ***Systemic :*** fever, headache, joint pain, flushing, palpitation, chest pain, dyspnea, lymph node enlargement, metallic taste, anaphylaxis, death.

## ACUTE IRON POISONING :

- It can be accidental or suicidal.
- Mostly seen in children who accidentally swallow iron pills.

**Clinical features :**

- Nausea, vomiting, abdominal pain, hematemesis, diarrhea, lethargy, cyanosis, dehydration, convulsion, shock, death.

**Treatment :**

- *Maintain vitals :* Airway, Breathing, Circulation.
- *Prevent further absorption :* Induce vomiting, gastric lavage with sodium bicarbonate solution.
- *To bind & remove iron already absorbed :* Desferrioxamine (IM), Deferiprone (oral). Calcium edetate can also be used.

## MEGALOBLASTIC ANEMIA :

- It is characterised by retardation of DNA synthesis and cell proliferation in the precursor cells of RBCs.
- **Cause :** Vitamin $B_{12}$ and folic acid deficiency.

## VITAMIN $B_{12}$ :

- It is a water soluble vitamin.
- It is synthesised in nature only by microorganism.

### Daily requirement :

- 1-3 mcg/day. Requirements are increased in pregnancy and lactation.

### Dietary sources :

- The only source available to man is dietary (mostly animal products) : Meat, fish, eggs, liver, kidney, sea fish, milk and milk products.

### Metabolic functions :

- Purine & Pyrimidine synthesis (DNA synthesis).
- Required for synthesis of phospholipid and myelin of nerves.
- Essential for cell growth and multiplication.

### Vitamin $B_{12}$ Absorption :

- Vitamin $B_{12}$ absorption requires Intrinsic Factor.
- Intrinsic Factor - synthesised and secreted by gastric parietal cells.
- Deficiency of Intrinsic Factor results in pernicious anemia.

### Deficiency :

- ***Causes :*** Inadequate dietary intake, intestinal malabsorption, increased requirements like pregnancy & lactation, pernicious anemia (absence of Intrinsic factor), gastric mucosal damage (gastric carcinoma, gastrectomy), drugs that impair vitamin $B_{12}$ absorption (Antiepileptics, phenytoin, alcohol).

### Features of vitamin $B_{12}$ deficiency :

- Megalobalstic anemia.
- Glossitis.
- Neurological : peripheral neuropathy, mental changes due to defective myelin synthesis.

### Preparations :

- Cyanocobalmine.
- Hydroxocobalamine.
- Methylcobalamine.

### Doses :

- Therapeutic : 30-100 mcg/day.
- Prophylactic : 3-10 mcg/day.
- In cases of neuropathy- 500-1500 mcg/day.
- Available as 500, 1000 mcg Tablets / Injections.

### Uses :

- Vit $B_{12}$ deficiency (Iron and Folic acid added).

- Prophylaxis of Vitamin $B_{12}$ deficiency.
- Neuropathy and neurological symptoms.

**Adverse effects :**

- Even larger doses are quite safe.
- Allergic reactions sometimes occur with parenteral preparations.

## FOLIC ACID :

- Humans are incapable to synthesise it so the only source is diet.

**Dietary sources :**

- Liver, green leafy vegetables, egg, meat, milk.

**Daily requirement :**

- 0.2 mg/day, Pregnancy and lactation - 0.8 mg/day.

**Metabolic functions :**

- Converted to folinic acid (active form).
- Purine & Pyrimidine synthesis (DNA synthesis).
- Essential for cell growth and multiplication.

**Deficiency :**

- ***Causes :*** Inadequate dietary intake, intestinal malabsorption (celiac disease, tropical sprue), increased requirement (pregnancy, lactation, growth), drug induced (phenytoin, phenobarbitone).

**Features of Vitamin $B_{12}$ deficiency :**

- Megalobalstic anemia.
- ***Epithelial damage :*** stomatitis, glossitis, enteritis, diarrhea.
- ***Neural tube defects :*** spina bifida (Hence, given prophylactically in pregnancy).
- General debility, weight loss, sterility.

**Preparations :**

- Available as liquid, tablets, injectables.

**Dose :**

- 2-5 mg/day (therapeutic) and 0.5 mg/day (prophylactic).

**Uses :**

- Megaloblastic anemias.
- Supplementation during pregnancy.
- Methotrexate toxicity.

**Adverse effects :**

- Even larger doses are quite safe.

## ERYTHROPOIETIN :

- It is a hormone produced by kidneys and is essential for normal erythropoiesis.
- It stimulates proliferation of colony forming cells of eryhthroid series, induces hemoglobin formation and RBC maturation.

**Preparation : *Epoietin α, β***

- It is made from recombinant DNA technology.
- ***Use :*** anemia due to chronic renal failure, anemia due to cancer chemotherapy, anemia of AIDS, anemia in premature babies.
- ***Dose :*** 25-100 IU/kg SC 3 times a week.

**Darbepoietin :** It is a longer acting analogue which is given once weekly.

❑❑❑❑❑

# 54 ANTI-COAGULANTS, FIBRINOLYTICS, ANTI-FIBRINOLYTICS AND ANTI-PLATELET DRUGS

## HEMOSTASIS :

It refers to control of bleeding to restore normal physiology by 3 mechanisms : Vascular spasm, platelet plug formation and blood coagulation.

### Coagulation factors (clotting factors) :

**Factor I** – Fibrinogen
**Factor II** – Prothrombin
**Factor III** – Tissue Thromboplastin
**Factor IV** – Calcium
**Factor V** – Labile factor
**Factor VII** – Stable factor
**Factor VIII** – Anti-hemophilic factor-A
**Factor IX** – Anti-hemophilic factor-B/christmas factor
**Factor X** – Stuart factor
**Factor XI** – Plasma Thromboplastin antecedent (PTA)
**Factor XII** – Hageman factor
**Factor XIII** – Fibrin stabilising factor

**Vitamin K dependent factors :** Factors II, VII, IX and X.

### Natural anticoagulants :

- Prostacyclin ($PGI_2$), Antithrombin III (Inactivates clotting factors II, IX, X, XI and XII), Protein C, Heparan sulphate.

## ANTICOAGULANTS :

Drugs that prevent coagulation (clotting) of blood are called as anticoagulants.

## CLASSIFICATION :

### Injectable anticoagulants :

- **Heparin.**
- **Low molecular weight heparins (LMWH) :** Enoxaparin, Dalteparin, Ardeparin, Tinzaparin.
- **Synthetic heparins :** Fondaparinux sodium.
- **Direct thrombin inhibitors :** Lepirudin, Bivalirudin, Argatroban.

### Oral anticoagulants :

- **Direct thrombin inhibitors :** Dabigatran.
- **Direct factor Xa inhibitors :** Apixaban, Edoxaban, Rivaroxiban.
- **Vitamin K antagonists :**
  - ☞ ***Coumarin derivatives :*** Warfarin, Dicumarol.
  - ☞ ***Indanedione derivatives :*** Phenindione.

### Injectable Anticoagulants :

**Heparin :**

- ☞ It was first extracted from liver, therefore named heparin.
- ☞ It is also called as UFH (Unfractionised heparin).
- ☞ Molecular weight is 10,000 to 40,000.
- ☞ ***Mechanism of action :*** We know that the natural anticoagulant Antithrombin III exerts its action by inhibiting clotting factors II, IX, X, XI and XII. Heparin activates this Antithrombin III.

**Heparin**

↓

**Activates plasma Antithrombin III**

↓

**Inactivates clotting factors (II, IX, X, XI and XII)**

- ☞ ***Pharmacokinetics :*** Heparin is not absorbed orally. If injected IV, it acts instantaneously. Bioavailability of SC heparin is inconsistent. Half life is short (1-5 hrs) hence, it has to be given in multiple daily dosing. Heparin does not cross blood-brain barrier or placenta *(Hence, it is the anticoagulant of choice during pregnancy).*
- ☞ ***aPTT (Activated partial thromboplastin time)*** is raised by heparin. Therefore, aPTT monitoring is required during therapy.
- ☞ Heparin in higher doses also inhibits platelet aggregation.
- ☞ ***Uses :*** Prophylaxis of deep vein thrombosis (DVT), pulmonary embolism, stroke, myocardial infarction, unstable angina, DVT, to maintain patency of angioplasty stents and to maintain patency of cannulae, rheumatic heart disease; atrial fibrillation, cerebrovascular diseases, vascular surgery, prosthetic heart valves, retinal vessel thrombosis, extracorporeal circulation, hemodialysis.
- ☞ ***Dose :*** 10000-20000 Units every 8-12 hourly.
- ☞ ***Adverse effects :*** Bleeding, thrombocytopenia, transient alopecia, osteoporosis, hypersensitivity reactions.
- ☞ ***Contraindications :*** Bleeding disorders, history of heparin induced thrombocytopenia, severe hypertension, threatened abortion, piles, GI

ulcers, subacute bacterial endocarditis, ocular and neurosurgery, lumbar puncture, chronic alcoholics, cirrhosis, renal failure.

- ***Antidote :*** *Protamine sulphate* (It is used to terminate the action of heparin quickly like in overdose, before cardiac and vascular surgery etc.)

## LMWH (Low Molecular Weight Heparin) :

- *Enoxaparin, Dalteparin, Ardeparin, Tinzaparin.*
- Molecular weight is 3000 to 7000.
- ***Mechanism of action :*** Selectively inhibit factor Xa with little effect on IIa (Thrombin).
- ***Advantages of LMWH over Heparin*** :
  - It can be given subcutaneously.
  - It can be given once daily (longer half life).
  - It does not prolong aPTT. Hence, laboratory monitoring is not needed.
  - Dose is given in 'mg' and not 'U'. Therefore, dose calculation is easy.
- ***Dose :*** Enoxaparin 20-40 mg OD given as SC injections (prefilled syringes).
- ***Uses :*** Same as that of heparin.

## Synthetic heparins :

- *Fondaparinux sodium.*
- It is a synthetic heparin that causes selective inhibition of factor Xa.
- It is administered SC once daily in the dose of 2.5 mg.
- It has lesser antiplatelet action, hence chances of thrombocytopenia is less.
- It is preferred for prophylaxis of DVT in patients undergoing major surgery like hip or knee replacement.
- ***Idraparinux sodium*** is a longer acting congener which is given once weekly.

## Direct thrombin inhibitors :

- ***Parenteral :*** *Lepirudin, Bivalirudin, Argatroban.* ***Oral :*** *Dabigatran.*
- Unlike heparin, these recently developed anticoagulants bind directly to thrombin and inactivate it without the need to combine with and activate Antithrombin III.
- ***Mechanism of action : (See Chart)***
- ***Advantages :*** No laboratory monitoring is required, plasma t½ is 12–14 hours and duration of action is 24 hours.
- ***Use :*** They are being increasingly used in prophylaxis of DVT who have undergone major surgery like hip, knee replacement, prevention of stroke and embolism in patients of atrial fibrillation.

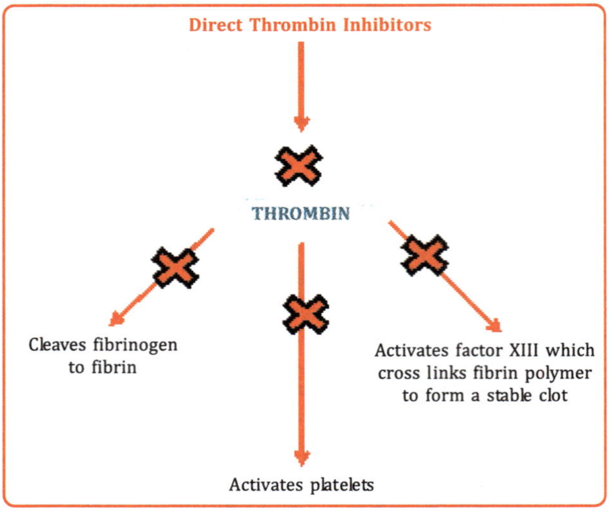


## Oral Anticoagulants :

### Direct thrombin inhibitors :

- *Dabigatran.*
- It is used as Dabigatran etexilate (prodrug of Dabigatran).
- ***Mechanism of action :*** explained above.

### Direct factor Xa inhibitors :

- *Apixaban, Edoxaban, Rivaroxiban.*
- ***Mechanism of action :*** Directly inhibits factor Xa.
- ***Advantages :*** No laboratory monitoring is required, equivalent in safety and efficacy to LMWH.
- ***Use :*** They are being increasingly used in prophylaxis of DVT in Patients who have undergone major surgery like hip, knee replacement, prevention of stroke and embolism in patients of atrial fibrillation.

### Vitamin K antagonists :

- ***Coumarin derivatives :*** *Warfarin, Dicumarol.*
- ***Indanedione derivatives :*** *Phenindione.*
- ***Mechanism of action :*** Act indirectly by interfering with the synthesis of vitamin K dependent clotting factors in liver (II, VII, IX, X). Apparently behave as competitive antagonists of vitamin K and lower the plasma levels of functional clotting factors in a dose dependent manner.
- ***Pharmacokinetics :*** Over 99% of Warfarin is plasma protein bound. Plasma half life is long (36 hrs). Crosses placental barrier *(contraindicated in pregnancy).*
- ***Monitoring :*** Monitoring of therapy is done by *Prothrombin time.*
- ***Contraindication :*** Pregnancy.

- ***Drug interactions :***
  - ***Warfarin activity is enhanced by :*** Enzyme inhibitors, displacement of Warfarin from plasma protein binding sites by drugs like co-trimoxazole, vitamin K deficiency caused by liquid paraffin, and drug that inhibits gut bacterial flora like broad spectrum antibiotics.
  - ***Warfarin activity is reduced by :*** Enzyme inducers, drugs that inhibit its absorption like sucralfate, drugs that increase synthesis of clotting factors like OC pills.
- ***Antidote :*** Vitamin K.

### Uses of Anticoagulants :

- Prophylaxis and treatment of deep vein thrombosis (DVT).
- Pulmonary embolism.
- Stroke.
- Myocardial infarction.
- Unstable angina.
- To maintain patency of angioplasty stents.
- To maintain patency of cannulae.
- Rheumatic heart disease; atrial fibrillation.
- Cerebrovascular diseases.
- Vascular surgery.
- Prosthetic heart valves.
- Retinal vessel thrombosis.
- Extracorporeal circulation; hemodialysis.
- Bedridden patients.
- Major surgeries like knee and hip replacement

## FIBRINOLYTICS AND ANTIFIBRINOLYTICS :

### Fibrinolytics (Thrombolytics) :

- These drugs are used to lyse or dissolve the thrombi or clots in the blood vessels.
- **Drugs available : *Streptokinase, Urokinase, Anistreplase, Alteplase, Reteplase and Tenecteplase. (See Chart)***
- ***Mechanism of action :*** When a clot is formed, an enzyme called plasminogen gets incorporated into the clot. Tissue plasminogen activator activates plasminogen to plasmin. This plasmin digests fibrin leading to lysis of clot (*see* diagram).
- ***Streptokinase :*** It is derived from β-hemolytic streptococci. Being a foreign protein, chances of hypersensitivity are high (therefore cannot be repeated due to formation of anti-streptokinase antibodies). It is least expensive.
- ***Urokinase :*** It was earlier isolated from human urine but now produced from cultured human kidney cells and recombinant DNA technology. It

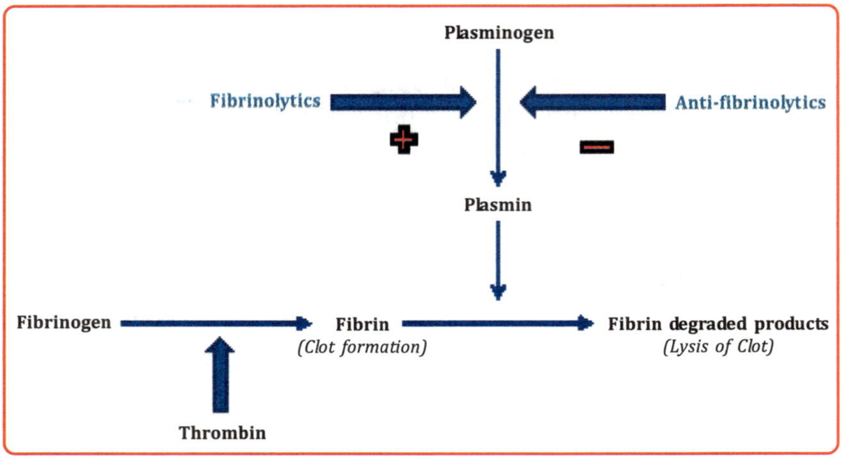


can degrade both fibrin as well as fibrinogen. It is non-allergic, non-pyrogenic. It is used in patients whom streptokinase cannot be repeated. It is less expensive.

- ***Anistreplase :*** It is a complex of plasminogen and streptokinase. This complex is protected by anisoylation. This complex is more fibrin specific than streptokinase. It can also produce hypersensitivity like streptokinase.
- ***Alteplase :*** It was earlier called as tissue plasminogen activator (tPA). It is produced by recombinant DNA technology. It is highly fibrin specific. It has low affinity for circulating plasminogen but has affinity to clot plasminogen. It has shorter half life (5-10 min), thus has higher incidence of reocclusion and therefore should be given along with heparin. It is having no allergenicity, but it is expensive.
- ***Reteplase :*** It is also a recombinant molecule like Alteplase, but it is having longer half life (15-20 min).
- ***Tenecteplase :*** It is also a recombinant molecule and derivative of Alteplase. It has actions similar to Alteplase and Reteplase. The half life is even longer (2 hrs). It is very expensive.
- ***Uses of fibrinolytics :*** Acute myocardial infarction, arterial thrombosis, embolism, for unclotting catheters and shunts.
- ***Adverse effects :*** Allergic reactions, hemorrhage and bleeding.

## Anti-fibrinolytics :

- These drugs decrease the fibrinolytic activity.
- ***Drugs available :*** **Epsilon amino caproic acid (EACA), Tranexemic acid, Ethamsylate, Aprotinin.**
- ***Mechanism of action :*** They inhibit conversion of plasminogen to plasmin (*see* diagram). Ethamsylate has anti-hyaluronidase activity, inhibits $PGI_2$ synthesis and promotes platelet aggregation. Aprotinin inhibits plasmin, Kallikrein and platelets.

☞ ***Uses :*** Overdose of fibrinolytics, abruptio placentae, PPH, menorrhagia, surgical bleeding, surgical procedures in hemophilia patients.

## ANTIPLATELET DRUGS :

- Drugs which interfere with platelet aggregation or adhesion and are useful in prophylaxis of thromboembolic disorders are called antiplatelet drugs. The primary function of platelets is to prevent bleeding by forming a thrombus.
- The various factors that cause platelet aggregation are : binding of Thromboxane $A_2$ ($TXA_2$) to its receptor, binding of ADP to its receptors, binding of fibrinogen to GP IIb/IIIa receptors, binding of thrombin to PAR-1 receptors. cAMP inhibits ADP formation and thus, prevents platelet aggregation but, cAMP is metabolised to inactive 5AMP with the help of enzyme phosphodiesterase 3.
- Balance between $PGI_2$ and $TXA_2$ controls platelet aggregation.

### Classification :

- ***Thromboxane $A_2$ synthesis inhibitor :*** Aspirin.
- ***Phosphodiesterase (PDE) inhibitors :*** Dipyridamole, Cilostazole.
- ***ADP receptor inhibitors :*** Clopidogrel, Prasugrel, Ticlopidine.
- ***Platelet Thrombin Protease activated receptor (PAR-1) inhibitor :*** Vorapraxar.
- ***GP IIb/IIIa receptor inhibitors(antagonists) :*** Abciximab, Eptifibatide, Tirofiban.
- ***Thromboxane $A_2$ receptor inhibitors :*** Terutroban.

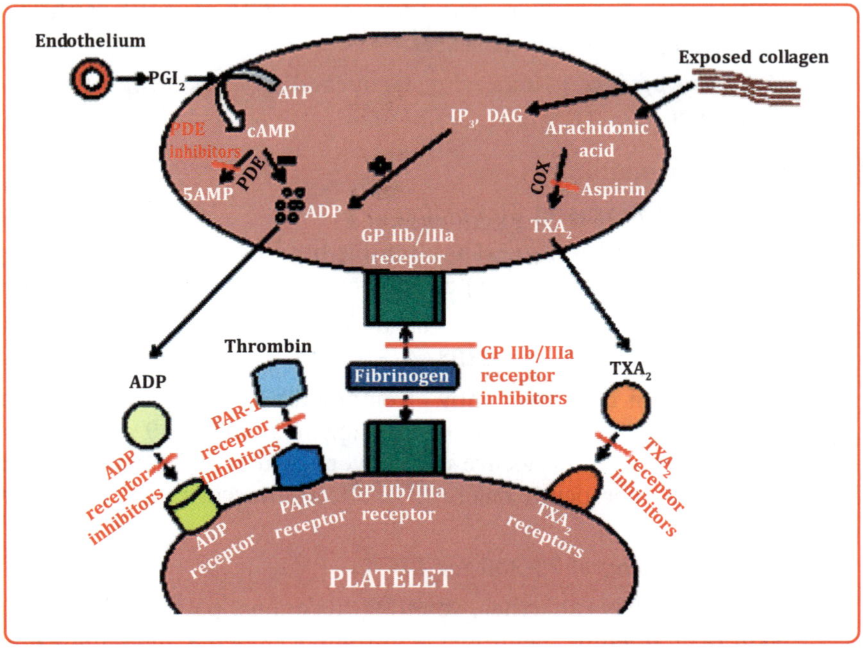

## Aspirin :

- It belongs to NSAIDs class of drugs.
- ***Mechanism of action :*** It inhibits cyclooxygenase *i.e.* COX-1 (it causes irreversible acetylation of COX-1) and thus, inhibits Thromboxane ($TXA_2$) synthesis.
- This inhibition occurs at low doses. At low doses, only $TXA_2$ synthesis is inhibited but, at higher doses both $TXA_2$ and $PGI_2$ synthesis is inhibited (This nullifies the antiplatelet action of $PGI_2$).
- Inhibits platelet aggregation for 7–10 days (lifespan of platelets).
- ***Dose :*** 75–300 mg/day.
- ***Adverse effects :*** Nausea, vomiting, gastritis, peptic ulcer etc.

## Phosphodiesterase inhibitors :

- *Dipyridamole, Cilostazole.*
- ***Mechanism of action :*** Phosphodiesterase enzyme inhibitor increases cAMP concentration. This inhibits platelet aggregation by inhibiting ADP release.
- ***Dipyridamole :*** Is also a powerful coronary vasodilator and is used as anti-anginal drug. It causes a phenomenon called as 'coronary steal phenomenon' in angina pectoris patients in which it diverts the blood from ischemic zones to non-ischemic zones by dilating resistance vessels. This may aggravate angina. Dipyridamole is usually used with Warfarin.
- ***Cilostazole :*** Is usually reserved for treatment of intermittent claudication in peripheral vascular diaseases.
- ***Adverse effects :*** Headache, tachycardia, worsening of angina, GI disturbances.

## ADP receptor inhibitors :

- *Clopidogrel, Prasugrel, Ticlopidine.*
- ***Mechanism of action :*** They inhibit binding of ADP to its receptors (block ADP $P2Y_{12}$ receptor) and thus prevent platelet aggregation.
- All are prodrugs are converted to active metabolite by metabolising enzymes (CYP2C19 and CYP3A4/5).
- If the patient is subsequently given any drug (Omeprazole, Fluconazole) which inhibits these metabolising enzymes (CYP2C19 and CYP3A4/5), these antiplatelet drugs are not converted to active metabolite and this can lead to therapeutic failure (risk of cardiovascular and cerebrovascular events).
- ***Dose :*** Clopidogrel 75-300 mg OD.
- ***Adverse effects :*** Diarrhea, vomiting, abdominal pain, headache, tinnitus, skin rash, bleeding, neutropenia, thrombocytopenia and jaundice.

- ***Ticagrelor and Cangrelor :*** These are newer members of this group. Unlike other drugs of this group, these new drugs are not prodrugs and don't require metabolising enzymes for their activation.

## Platelet Thrombin Protease activated receptor (PAR-1) inhibitor :

- *Vorapraxar.*
- ***Mechanism of action :*** Thrombin facilitates thrombosis by converting fibrinogen to fibrin, stimulating factor XIII and activating PAR-1 receptor on platelets. PAR-1 receptor inhibitors inhibit binding of thrombin on PAR-1 receptors and thus inhibit platelet aggregation.

## GP IIb/IIIa receptor inhibitors (antagonists) :

- *Abciximab, Eptifibatide, Tirofiban.*
- ***Mechanism of action :*** They block the GP IIb/IIIa receptors (inhibit binding of fibrinogen to GP IIb/IIIa receptors) and thus inhibit platelet aggregation.
- Abciximab is a chimeric monoclonal antibody.
- ***Adverse effects :*** Bleeding, thrombocytopenia, constipation.

## Thromboxane $A_2$ receptor inhibitors :

- *Terutroban.*
- ***Mechanism of action :*** It selectively inhibits $TXA_2$ receptors and prevents binding of $TXA_2$ to its receptors.
- Apart from antiplatelet action, it also has vasodilating and anti-atherosclerotic actions.

### Uses of Antiplatelet drugs :

- ***Coronary Artery Disease :***
  - Acute myocardial infarction (AMI).
  - After thrombolytic therapy to prevent re-occlusion.
  - Unstable angina.
  - Primary and secondary prevention of AMI.
- Cerebrovascular disease like transient ischemic attack.
- ***Coronary angioplasty, stents :*** patency of re-canalised artery or implant bypass vessels improved; re-occlusion reduced.
- ***Prosthetic heart valves and arteriovenous shunts :*** reduce formation of microthrombi in heart valves.
- Venous thromboembolism.
- Peripheral vascular disease.

# DRUGS ACTING ON GASTRO-INTESTINAL TRACT (GIT)

# 55 DRUGS FOR ACIDITY, GASTRITIS AND PEPTIC ULCER

Peptic ulcer is mucosal break or defect in the gastrointestinal tract (both, gastric or duodenal). Gastritis is the precursor to Peptic ulcer formation. Peptic ulcer arises when the normal mucosal defense mechanisms like mucus, mucosal blood flow, prostaglandins like $PGE_2$ and bicarbonate ion formation are impaired or inhibited and there is increased gastric acid and pepsin secretion.

### Normal physiology of gastric acid secretion :

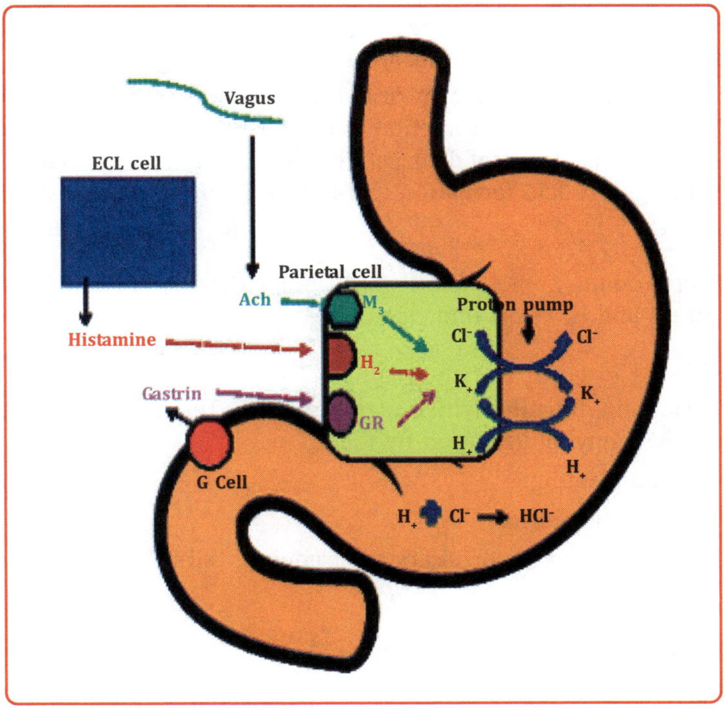


- Gastric acid (HCl) is secreted by the parietal cell in the stomach.
- Main stimulus for gastric acid secretion is : gastrin (from antral G cells), acetylcholine (from vagus) and histamine (from Enterochromaffin cells *i.e.* ECL cells).
- Histamine binds to histaminic $H_2$ receptors on parietal cell, acetylcholine binds to cholinergic muscaranic $M_3$ receptors on parietal cell as well as $M_1$

receptors on ECL cells and gastrin binds to gastrin GR receptors on parietal cell as well as on ECL cells.

- Their primary action is to stimulate the ***$H^+K^+$ATPase pump (Proton pump)*** in the parietal cells.
- First, $Cl^-$ is actively transported into the lumen of stomach accompanied by $K^+$, which is then exchanged for $H^+$ by proton pump. This $H^+$ then combines with $Cl^-$ to form HCl.
- Water and carbondioxide combine and with the help of carbonic anhydrase enzyme (CA) forms carbonic acid ($H_2CO_3$). This $H_2CO_3$ then splits into $HCO3^-$ and $H^+$. $H^+$ ions are used up by the proton pump to form HCl and $HCO3^-$ is exchanged for $Cl^-$ across the parietal cells which are again utilised to form HCl.
- Chief cells in the gastric fundus secrete pepsinogen. When the pH of the gastric acid is below 2, the pepsinogen is cleaved to pepsin. This pepsin erodes the gastric mucosa to form ulcer.
- Prostaglandin ($PGE_2$) inhibits gastric acid secretion. It also enhances mucosal blood flow and stimulates secretion of mucus and bicarbonates which are also protective against mucosal damage. Therefore, $PGE_2$ is a normal physiological protector against acid formation and mucosal damage.

### Risk factors :

- Smoking, Alcohol, Coffee, Tea, Medications (NSAIDs, Corticosteroids), Spicy food, Stress and H. Pylori infection.

### Clinical features :

- Epigastric pain, burning which may radiate to the back. Pain occurs when stomach is empty and relieved by food.
- Belching and bloating.
- Hematemesis or melena.
- NSAID induced gastritis or ulcers are frequently silent in nature.

### Diagnosis :

- Clinical diagnosis.
- ***Investigation :***
  - Complete blood count to evaluate acute or chronic blood loss.
  - *For H. Pylori :*
    - Serologic antibody test for H. Pylori.
    - Fecal antigen test for active H. Pylori.
    - Urea breath test for active H. Pylori.
  - Endoscopy.

### Complications :

- Perforation, peritonitis, bowel obstruction, GI bleeding, gastric carcinoma.

## Treatment :

### *Non-pharmacological treatment :*

- Avoid smoking, alcohol, coffee, tea, medications (NSAIDs, Corticosteroids), spicy food, stress and exercise regularly.

## PHARMACOLOGICAL TREATMENT (DRUGS) :

### Classification :

- ***Acid Neutralising agents (Antacids) :***
  - **Systemic :** Sodium Bicarbonate, Sodium Citrate.
  - **Non-systemic :** Magnesium hydroxide, Magnesium trisilicate, Aluminium hydroxide, Magaldrate, Calcium carbonate.
- ***Drugs that reduce gastric acid secretion :***
  - **$H_2$ receptor antagonists :** Cimetidine, Ranitidine, Famotidine, Nizatidine, Roxatidine.
  - **Proton-Pump Inhibitors :** Omeprazole, Pantoprazole, Rabeprazole, Lansoprazole and Esomeprazole.
  - **Anticholinergics :** Pirenzepine, Telenzepine.
  - **Prostaglandin analogue :** Misoprostol.
- ***Ulcer protectives :***

  Sucralfate, colloidal bismuth subcitrate, bismuth subsalicylate.
- ***Ulcer healing :***

  Carbenoxolone sodium.
- ***Anti-H. pylori Drugs :***

  Amoxycillin, Clarithromycin, Metronidazole, Tinidazole and Tetracycline.

### Antacids :

- **Mechanism of action :** They neutralise the gastric acid. They have no action on gastric acid secretion.
- Non-systemic antacids are poorly absorbed from GIT and do not disturb systemic acid-base balance.
- They are commonly available without prescription over the pharmacy counter.
- Mostly magnesium hydroxide and aluminium hydroxide are combined because :
  - Magnesium hydroxide is fast acting and aluminium hydroxide is slow acting.
  - Magnesium hydroxide has laxative effect and aluminium hydroxide has constipating effect. Thus, their ections get neutralised when used in combination.
- **Uses :** Acidity, gastritis, esophagitis, dyspepsia, GERD.

- ***Adverse effects :***
  - Aluminium antacids – constipation (As they relax gastric smooth muscle & delay gastric emptying), also hypophosphatemia and osteomalacia.
  - Magnesium antacids can cause osmotic diarrhea.
  - In renal failure Aluminium antacids can lead to Aluminium toxicity and Encephalopathy.
  - Systemic antacids have got several limitations like; large doses can cause alkalosis, produces $CO_2$ in stomach leading to distension, belching and risk of ulcer perforation, acid rebound etc.
- ***Drug interactions :*** aluminium, magnesium and calcium containing antacids form complexes and decrease absorption of certain drugs like tetracyclines. Also, by raising the gastric pH, they decrease absorption of certain acidic drugs like barbiturates, phenytoin etc.

## $H_2$ receptor antagonists :

- ***Mechanism of action :*** They are reversible competitive inhibitors of $H_2$ receptor in the parietal cells. This results in reduction in gastric acid secretion.
- They are very effective in inhibiting nocturnal acid secretion.
- ***Preparations :*** Available as tablets, injections.
- ***Uses :*** Acidity, gastritis, esophagitis, dyspepsia, GERD, Peptic ulcer, stress ulcers, NSAIDs induced ulcers, Zollinger-Ellison syndrome (it is a hypersecretory state where there is gastrin secereting tumor). They are also used in chronic urticaria (increases the efficacy of $H_1$ receptor antagonists).
- ***Dose :*** Ranitidine 150 mg BD or Famotidine 20 mg BD. Cimetidine is no longer used due to its adverse effects.
- ***Adverse effects :*** They are extremely safe drugs and well tolerated. Main ADRs are related to Cimetidine : Antiandrogenic effects (gynecomastia, galactorrhea, impotence), Cytochrome P450 inhibition (enzyme inhibitor).

## Proton Pump Inhibitors :

- They are currently most commonly used drugs for these conditions.
- ***Mechanism of action :*** They are inhibitors of *$H^+K^+$ATPase (Proton-Pump)* in the parietal cells. This results in reduction in gastric acid secretion.
- They are given on an empty stomach because food affects their absorption.
- ***Uses :*** Acidity, gastritis, esophagitis, dyspepsia, GERD, Peptic ulcer, stress ulcers, NSAIDs induced ulcers, Zollinger-Ellison syndrome, H. Pylori infections.
- ***Dose :*** Omeprazole 20 mg OD, Lansoprazole 30 mg OD, Pantoprazole 40 mg OD, Rabeprazole 20 mg OD, Esomeprazole 20-40 mg OD.

- ***Adverse effects :*** Nausea, abdominal pain, constipation, flatulence, diarrhea, subacute myopathy, arthralgias, headaches, skin rashes. Prolonged use can cause Gynecomastia, erectile dysfunction, Leucopenia, hepatic dysfunction, Vitamin $B_{12}$ deficiency, achlorhydria which can lead to gastric carcinoma.
- ***Drug Interaction :*** Omeprazole inhibits CYP2C19 which is needed for activation of Antiplatelet drug clopidogrel. Hence, if omeprazole is given along with clopidogrel, it can result in therapeutic failure of clopidogrel.

## Anticholinergics :

- ***Mechanism of action :*** They reduce meal stimulated HCl secretion by reversible blockade of muscarinic receptors on parietal cells and $M_3$ and $M_1$ receptors on the ECL cells.
- They are unpopular as a first choice because of high incidence of anticholinergic side effects.
- Newer anticholinergics like Pirenzepine and Telenzepine have low incidence of anticholinergic side effects.

## Prostaglandin analogues :

- ***Mechanism of action :*** They inhibit histamine stimulated gastric acid secretion. They also stimulate mucus and bicarbonate secretion and increases mucosal blood flow.
- ***Uses :*** They are mostly used in prevention of NSAID induced mucosal injury and ulcers.
- ***Dose :*** Misoprostol 200 mcg 4 times a day.
- ***Adverse effects :*** Diarrhea, abdominal cramps, uterine bleeding, risk of abortion.
- ***Contraindications :*** Pregnancy (may cause abortion).

## Ulcer protectives :

- ***Mechanism of action :*** In acidic environment, it polymerises and forms gel that covers the ulcer and protects it from gastric acid.
- Antacids should not be given along with them; because antacids neutralise gastric acid and the ulcer protectives need acidic pH to get polymerise and perform its action.
- ***Adverse effects :*** Sucralfate can cause hypophosphatemia and adsorbs tetracyclines, phenytoin, fluoroquinolones and inhibit their absorption. Colloidal bismuth can cause blackening of stools and tongue, bismuth toxicity (osteodystrophy and encephalopathy).

## Ulcer healing drugs : *Carbenoxolone sodium.*

- It is outdated and no longer used.
- It has mineralocorticoid like action (sodium and water retention, hypertension)

## Anti- H. Pylori Drugs :

- Helicobacter Pylori is one of the important causes of developing peptic ulcer.
- ***Mechanism of H. Pylori :*** H. pylori secrete urease (which converts urea to ammonia). Ammonia neutralises gastric acid to provide neutral protective environment for H. Pylori. It also produces protease which causes break down of gastric mucosa. This leads to ulcer formation and also causes chronic inflammation.
- There are various drugs used in the treatment of H. Pylori like; Amoxycillin (Penicillin), Clarithromycin (Macrolide), Metronidazole (Anti-amebic), Tinidazole (Anti-amebic) and Tetracycline (Broad spectrum antibiotic).
- Their mechanism and pharmacology are discussed in their respective chapters :
    - The most commonly used regimes for H. Pylori are : Triple therapy, Quadruple therapy and Sequential therapy.
- In place of Omeprazole, we can also use Lansoprazole 30 mg BD.
- After the therapy, Proton-Pump inhibitors are continued for additional 4-6 weeks.

**TRIPLE THERAPY**

| | | |
|---|---|---|
| Omeprazole 20 mg BD | | Omeprazole 20 mg BD |
| Clarithromycin 500 mg BD | OR | Clarithromycin 500 mg BD |
| Amoxycillin 1000 mg BD | | Metronidazole 500 mg BD |

**For 2 Weeks**

**QUADRUPLE THERAPY**

Omeprazole 20 mg BD
Bismuth subsalicylate 525 mg QID
Tetracycline 500 mg QID
Metronidazole 500 mg BD

**For 2 Weeks**

**SEQUENTIAL THERAPY**

| For 1st 5 days | For next 5 days |
|---|---|
| Omeprazole 20 mg BD | Omeprazole 20 mg BD |
| Amoxycillin 1000 mg BD | Clarithromycin 500 mgBD |
| | Tinidazole 500 mg BD |

For 10 days

# 56 ANTI-EMETICS, PROKINETICS AND DRUGS FOR GASTRO-ESOPHAGEAL REFLUX DISEASE

- **Emesis :** vomiting
- **Anti-emetics :** drugs that reduce or control vomiting

## ANTIEMETIC DRUGS :

### Pathophysiology of emesis :

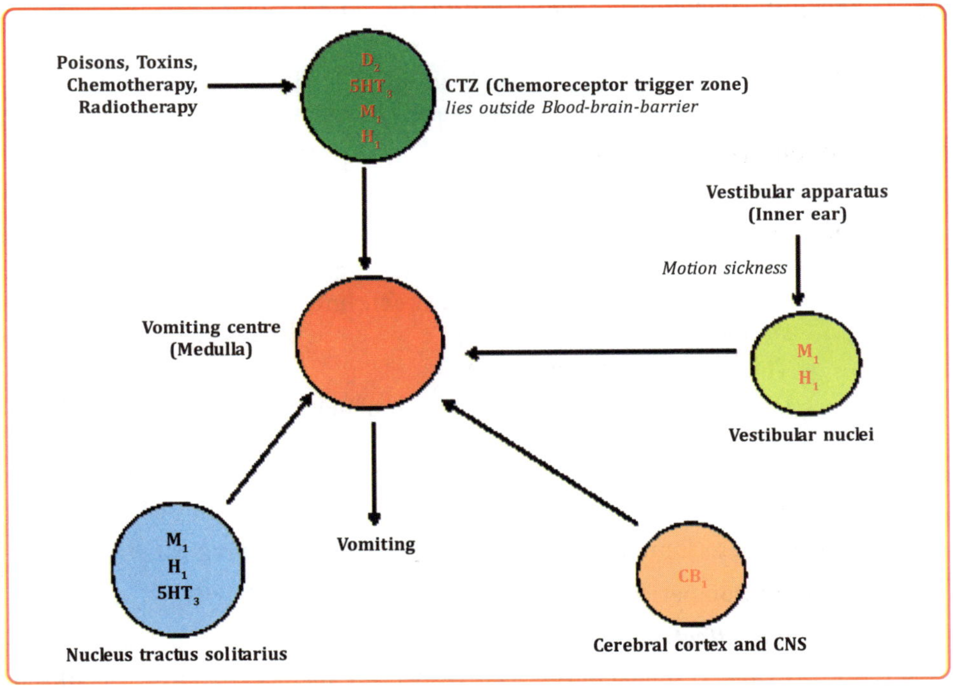


- *The main inputs to the vomiting centre in the medulla are from :* CTZ which lies outside blood brain barrier, from vestibular apparatus of inner ear via vestibular nuclei, from nucleus tractus solitarius and from cerebral cortex.
- *The main receptors that regulate vomiting are :* Dopaminergic ($D_2$), Serotonergic ($5HT_3$), Muscaranic ($M_1$), Histaminic ($H_1$) and Cannabinoid ($CB_1$) receptors.

## CLASSIFICATION OF ANTIEMETIC DRUGS :

- **$D_2$ receptor antagonists :** Metoclopramide, Domperidone.

- **$5HT_3$ receptor antagonists :** Ondansetron, Granisetron, Dolasetron, Palanosetron.
- **$H_1$ receptor antagonists (Antihistaminics) :** Promethazine, Doxylamine, Meclizine.
- **$M_1$ receptor antagonists (Anticholinergics) :** Hyoscine (Scopalamine).
- **Neurolepts :** Chlorpromazine, Haloperidol.
- **Others :**
  - **Glucocorticoids :** Dexamethasone.
  - **Cannabinoid receptor agonists :** Dronabinol, Nabilone.

## $D_2$ receptor antagonists : *Metoclopramide, Domperidone*

- Both drugs are also prokinetic agents due to their 5 $HT_4$ agonist activity.
- Metoclopramide crosses Blood-brain-barrier but domperidone does not. Therefore, metoclopramide can cause extrapyramidal side effects.
- ***Mechanism of action :*** They are antagonists of dopaminergic $D_2$ receptors in CTZ.
- ***Uses :***
  - As an antiemetic in vomiting due to gastroenteritis, post surgery, pre-operatively (as pre-anethetic medication), drug induced vomiting.
  - They are also used in GERD.
  - One of the important uses is as a prokinetic agent *i.e.* they accelerate gastric emptying and increase the tone of lower esophageal sphincter, which is required in emergency surgeries to prevent aspiration of gastric contents in the lungs (metoclopramide).
- ***Dose :*** Metoclopramide 2.5 mg BD, Domperidone 10 mg BD.
- ***Route :*** Domperidone – oral; Metoclopramide – oral or IV.
- ***Adverse effects :***
  - Extra-Pyramidal Side Effects (especially metoclopramide) : Akathisia, dystonia, tardive dyskinesia, parkinsonism, restlessness and prolonged muscle contraction.
  - Dry mouth, headache, galactorrhea (due to $D_2$ block).

## $5HT_3$ receptor antagonists : *Ondansetron, Granisetron, Dolasetron, Palanosetron*

- They are potent antiemetics. Have high first pass metabolism. Excreted by liver & kidney. No dose reduction in renal insufficiency is required but needed in hepatic insufficiency. Given once or twice daily – orally or intravenously.
- ***Mechanism of action :*** They are antagonists of $5HT_3$ receptors in CTZ and nucleus tractus solitaries.

- ***Uses :*** They are drug of choice for cancer chemotherapy induced nausea & vomiting (given 30 minutes before chemotherapy). They are also used for postoperative & postradiation nausea & vomiting.
- ***Dose :*** Ondansetron; 4-8 mg BD.
- ***Adverse effects :*** They have got excellent safety profile. Headache & constipation are seen sometimes. Prolongation of QT interval is seen with dolasetron.

## $H_1$ receptor antagonists (Antihistaminics) : Promethazine, Doxylamine, Meclizine

- Along with anticholinergics, they are most potent drugs for motion sickness.
- ***Mechanism of action :*** They are antagonists of histaminic $H_1$ receptors in vestibular nuclei, CTZ and nucleus tractus solitaries.
- ***Uses :***
    - Motion sickness (Promethazine / Meclizine) – 1 hour before journey. Once motion sickness starts, there is no use of these drugs.
    - Sea sickness (Meclizine).
    - Morning sickness in pregnancy / hyperemesis gravidarum – Doxylamine (Vitamin $B_6$ *i.e.* pyridoxine also offer some benefit).
- ***Adverse effects :*** Sedation, dryness of mouth etc.

## $M_1$ receptor antagonists (Anticholinergics) : *Hyoscine (Scopalamine)*

- ***Mechanism of action :*** They are antagonists of cholinergic muscaranic $M_1$ receptors in vestibular nuclei, CTZ and nucleus tractus solitaries.
- ***Use :*** Hyoscine is used as oral (0.4 mg) or transdermal patch (1.5 mg) behind the ear for motion sickness; 30-60 minutes before journey.
- ***Adverse effects :*** anticholinergic side effects like blurring of vision, constipation, urinary retention etc.

## Neurolepts : *Chlorpromazine, Haloperidol*

- These are antipsychotic drugs with potent antiemetic property.
- ***Mechanism of action :*** They are antagonists of $D_2$ receptors.
- They are less frequently used due to availability of better drugs.
- ***Uses :*** drug induced vomiting, post chemotherapy and radiotherapy induced vomiting and post anesthesia vomiting.
- ***Adverse effects :*** sedation, acute muscle dystonia etc.

## Glucocorticoids : *Dexamethasone*

- They can alleviate nausea and vomiting especially in cancer chemotherapy.
- They are less frequently used for this purpose, due to availability of better drugs like $5HT_3$ antagonists.

### Cannabinoid receptor agonists : *Dronabinol, Nabilone*

- Tetrahydrocannabinol is the active principle of *cannabis Indica.*
- It posseses anti-emetic activity.
- The actions are mediated by cannabinoid $CB_1$ receptors in CNS.
- Dronabinol and Nabilone are agonists of this $CB_1$ receptors and causes anti-emetic effect.
- They are used for cancer chemotherapy induced nausea & vomiting.

## MOTION SICKNESS :

- Nausea and vomiting while travelling in a car, bus or any other modes of transport.
- **Treatment :**
    - Tab. Hyoscine (Scopalamine) 0.2-0.4 mg orally or 1.5 mg transdermal patch behind the ear 30-60 minutes before journey. Or
    - Tab. Promethazine 25 mg 1 hour before travel.

## CANCER CHEMOTHERAPY INDUCED NAUSEA AND VOMITING :

**Treatment :**

- ***$D_2$ receptor antagonists :***
    - Metoclopramide, Domperidone.
    - They are not used commonly nowadays due to availability of more efficacious and safe drugs like $5HT_3$ receptor antagonists.
- ***$5HT_3$ receptor antagonists :***
    - Ondansetron, Granisetron, Dolasetron, Palanosetron.
    - They are the most commonly used drugs for this purpose.
- ***Neurolepts :***
    - Chlorpromazine, Haloperidol.
    - They are sometimes used in cases not responding to other drugs.
- ***Glucocorticoids :***
    - Dexamethasone.
    - They are used in cases not responding to other drugs.
- ***Cannabinoid receptor agonists :***
    - Dronabinol, Nabilone.
    - They are upcoming drugs used where $5HT_3$ antagonists fail to control nausea and vomiting in cancer chemotherapy patients.
- ***Benzodiazepines :***
    - Diazepam.
    - They increase the effect of inhibitory transmitter GABA on the CTZ.

- ***NK-1 receptor antagonists :***
  - Aprepitant, Fosaprepitant.
  - These are newer drugs being used in Cancer chemotherapy induced nausea and vomiting. They inhibit a new receptor which is identified in vomiting centre *i.e.* Neurokinin-1 receptor (NK-1).

## PROKINETIC DRUGS :

- These are the drugs that increase motility of GIT and enhance gastric emptying.
- It includes the following drugs.

### $D_2$ antagonist : *Metoclopramide, Domperidone.*

- They are also antiemetic drugs.
- ***Mechanism of action :*** They accelerate gastric emptying and increase the tone of lower esophageal sphincter.
- ***Uses :***
  - As an antiemetic
  - GERD
  - As a prokinetic agent (which is required in emergency surgeries to prevent aspiration of gastric contents in the lungs).

### 5-$HT_4$ agonists : *Cisapride, Mosapride, Itopride, Renzapride, Zacopride*

- ***Mechanism of action :*** They are devoid of any $D_2$ blocking property (no antiemetic action). The main action is mediated by $5HT_4$ agonism which promotes Acetylcholine release from the myenteric plexus. This increases gut motility and promotes gastric emptying.
- ***Uses :***
  - GERD
  - Non-ulcer dyspepsia.
- ***Adverse effects :*** Abdominal cramps, diarrhea. Cisapride causes QT prolongation and predisposes to ventricular arrhythmias (therefore withdrawn from market). Newer congeners like Mosapride, Itopride, Renzapride, Zacopride does not cause this problem.

### Macrolide antibiotics : *Erythromycin, Azithromycin*

- They stimulate *motilin* receptors in the GIT.
- This increases GI motility.
- Lower esophageal sphincter tone is increased and intestinal contractility is increased.
- They can be used in patients with diabetic gastroparesis.

## DRUGS FOR GERD :

- GERD is gastro-esophageal reflux disease. It is the condition in which the contents of the stomach especially gastric acid is going in the esophagus.

- **Causes :** Obesity, hiatus hernia, lower esophageal sphincter problems, pregnancy.
- **Clinical features :** Retrosternal burning (especially after a large meal or on lying down), dry cough, belching, chest pain.
- **Diagnosis :** Clinical diagnosis, endoscopy, esophageal pH monitoring.
- **Treatment :**
  - ***Non-pharmacological treatment :*** Avoid spicy food, weight reduction, early and light dinner, head end elevation of bed.
  - ***Drugs for GERD :***
    - **Proton pump inhibitors :** Omeprazole, Lansoprazole, Esomeprazole etc.
    - **$H_2$ receptor antagonists :** Ranitidine, Famotidine etc
    - **Antacids :** Magnesium hydroxide, Aluminium hydroxide etc.
    - **Prokinetic agents :** Metoclopramide, Domperidone, Cisapride, Mosapride, Itopride, macrolides etc.

*These drugs are already covered in this chapter and chapter on drugs for acidity, gastritis and peptic ulcer.*

❑❑❑❑❑

# 57 DRUGS FOR CONSTIPATION, DIARRHEA AND INFLAMMATORY BOWEL DISEASE

## DRUGS FOR CONSTIPATION :

### Constipation :

- Infrequent passage of stool (Less than 3 per week with or without straining) that may be due to decreased motility in colon or due to difficulty in evacuation.

### Some common terms :

- ***Laxatives :*** Elimination of soft but formed stools.
- ***Purgatives :*** Stronger action and more watery stools.
- ***Cathartics :*** Makes you defecate sooner.

### Causes of constipation :

- Decrease intake of water and fibre in diet, local painful conditions like anal fissures and piles, lack of exercise, certain drugs like anticholinergics, calcium channel blockers and antidepressants, diseases like hypothyroidism and diabetes.

### Uses of laxatives / purgatives :

- Constipation, pre and post surgery, hernia, piles, fissures, pregnancy, hepatic coma, preoperatively in bowel surgery, colonoscopy, aneurysms (to avoid straining), myocardial infarction, abdominal X-ray, poisonings.

### Treatment of constipation :

***Non-pharmacological treatment :***

- High fibre diet, avoid refined and junk foods, adequate water intake, regular exercises, avoid drugs that cause constipation, treatment of associated diseases that cause constipation.

## DRUGS FOR CONSTIPATION :

- **Bulk forming laxatives :**
  - ***Dietary fibres :*** Vegetables, Fruits, Grains, Bran, Pectin.
  - ***Natural plant products :*** Psyllium husk, Isaphghula husk.
  - ***Semi synthetic :*** Methyl cellulose.
- **Osmotic purgatives :**
  - ***Sugars :*** Lactulose, Sorbitol.

- ***Saline purgatives :*** Magnesium hydroxide (milk of magnesia), magnesium sulphate.
- ***Electrolyte osmotic purgative :*** PEG (Polyethylene glycol).

- **Stimulant Purgatives (cathartics) :**
  - Bisacodyl, Castor oil, Senna.

- **Fecal Softeners (Lubricants) :**
  - Liquid paraffin, Glycerin, Docusate sodium (surfactant purgative).

## Bulk forming laxative :

- ***Mechanism of Action :*** They are non absorbable dietary fibres which increase the bulk of intestinal contents by water absorption. This increases the mechanical pressure on the walls of intestine and causes stimulation of stretch receptors and thus stimulates peristalsis leading to bowel evacuation.
- Adequate amount of water should be taken with bulk forming laxatives.
- Effect occurs within 1-3 days.
- ***Adverse effects :*** They are not absorbed and are quite safe. However, there are certain drawbacks like delayed onset of action (1-3 days), intestinal obstruction (should be taken with enough water), malabsorption syndrome, abdominal distension, interfere with absorption of iron, calcium, and cardiac glycosides.

## Osmotic purgatives :

- ***Mechanism of Action :*** They are water Soluble but non absorbable compounds that increase water content in large intestine.

***Lactulose :***

- It is metabolised by gut bacteria into fructose and galactose. These sugars are fermented into lactic acid and acetic acid that function as osmotic laxatives.
- ***Dose :*** 10 gm BD or TDS (10 gm/15 ml).
- ***Adverse Effects :*** Delayed onset of action (2-3 days), abdominal cramps, flatulence and electrolyte disturbance.
- ***Lactulose in hepatic encephalopathy :*** In hepatic encephalopathy, there is accumulation of ammonia in the blood leading to encephalopathy. Lactulose reduces this ammonia production. Therefore, it is used in hepatic encephalopathy (20 gm TDS).

***Saline Purgatives (Milk of magnesia) :***

- ***Mechanism of Action :*** They are poorly absorbed salts. They remain in the bowel and retain water by osmosis thereby increasing the volume of feces. This increases peristalsis and causes evacuation of watery stool.
- ***Adverse effects :*** Intravascular volume depletion, electrolyte fluctuations.

***PEG :***

- It is an electrolyte osmotic purgative.
- It is used in a form of balanced isotonic solution prepared by adding sodium chloride, sodium sulphate, sodium bicarbonate and potassium chloride.
- The advantage of Polyethylene glycol solution is that no electrolyte shift occurs across the intestinal wall. Therefore, it is safe.

## Stimulant Purgatives (Cathartics) :

- ***Mechanism of Action :*** They act by direct stimulation of enteric nervous system which increases peristalsis and causes purgation.

***Bisacodyl :***

- It acts on the large intestine.
- Onset time 6-10 hours, usually taken at night.
- Also available as suppository for emergency evacuation of bowel.

***Castor Oil :***

- ***Mechanism :*** It is degraded by lipase in small intestine to ricinoleic acid and glycerin. This ricinoleic acid irritates intestinal mucosa and causes evacuation of bowel.
- Onset of action is only 2-3 hours. Therefore, it is taken in the early morning.
- ***Dose :*** 5-20 ml on empty stomach.

***Senna :***

- ***Mechanism :*** In colon, it is hydrolysed by bacteria into emodin. Emodin has direct stimulant action on myenteric plexus and increases smooth muscle contraction leading to defecation.
- Bowel movements occur in 12 hours. It is taken orally and at night.
- Brown pigmentation of the colon (melanosis coli) can occur.
- ***Adverse effects of Stimulant Purgative :***
    - Abdominal cramps may occur.
    - Prolonged use can lead to dependence & destruction of myenteric plexus and atonic colon, leading to chronic constipation.
- ***Contraindications :***
    - Senna in lactation.
    - Castor oil in pregnancy (may cause reflex contraction of uterus leading to abortion).

## Fecal Softeners (Lubricants) :

- ***Mechanism of action :*** They are non-absorbable drugs that soften the feces thus promoting defecation.

***Docusate sodium (Surfactants) :***

- ***Mechanism :*** They decrease the surface tension of fluids in the bowel. This makes the stool soft.
- It is given orally or as enema.
- Is commonly prescribed in hospitalised patients to minimise straining.

***Glycerin :***

- It is commonly used as Suppository.
- Quite commonly used in constipation after Surgery.

***Liquid paraffin :***

- It is inert mineral oil and inhibits water absorption from the stool and softens the stool.
- ***Dose :*** 15-30 ml / day at bedtime. Takes 1-3 days for effect.
- ***Adverse effects :*** Not palatable, impairs absorption of fat soluble vitamins, anal leaking, aspiration lipoid pneumonia.

## DRUGS FOR DIARRHEA (Anti-diarrhoeal drugs) :

### Diarrhea :

- Diarrhea is defined by the WHO as having 3 or more loose or liquid stools per day, or as having more stools than is normal for that person.

### Types of diarrhea :

- ***Acute Diarrhea :*** Food poisoning, typhoid (Salmonella), bacillary dysentery (Shigella), traveller's diarrhea (E.coli), cholera (vibrio cholerae), amebic (E. Histolytica), viral *e.g.* rotavirus.
- ***Chronic Diarrhea :*** Malabsorption, chron's disease and ulcerative colitis, diabetic diarrhea.
- ***Drug induced :*** Penicillins, cephalosporins etc

### Clinical features :

- Loose motions, nausea, vomiting, abdominal pain, dehydration, hypotension, fever, tachycardia, shock and death, if severe dehydration.

### Treatment :

***Goals :***

- Rehydration.
- Drug Therapy :
  - i. Nonspecific anti-diarrheal drugs.
  - ii. Specific antimicrobial drugs (bacterial diarrhea).
- Maintenance of Nutrition.

***Rehydration :***

**IV Fluids :**

- If fluid loss more than 10% of body weight.

- Fluids used :
  - Normal saline (NS).
  - Ringer lactate (RL).
  - Dextrose normal saline (DNS).

***ORS (Oral rehydration solution) :***

- It is an orally given salt which replenishes the electrolytes which are lost in diarrhea. It is constituted in water and given orally.
- ***Composition :***

| ORS (ORAL REHYDRATION SALT) | |
|---|---|
| Sodium chloride | 3.5 g |
| Potassium chloride | 1.5 g |
| Sodium citrate | 2.9 g |
| Glucose | 20.0 g |
| Water | 1 litre |

- WHO has given new formula ORS in the year 2002 :

| ORS (ORAL REHYDRATION SALT) New | |
|---|---|
| Sodium chloride | 2.6 g |
| Potassium chloride | 1.5 g |
| Sodium citrate | 2.9 g |
| Glucose | 13.5 g |
| Water | 1 litre |

- ***Super-ORS :*** It is the ORS which also contains amino acids. This is especially useful in malnourished children.
- ***Zinc :*** Recent studies have shown that zinc along with ORS reduces severity and duration of acute diarrhea.

## CLASSIFICATION OF ANTI-DIARRHEAL DRUGS :

- **Anti Motility and antisecretory agents :**
  - ***Opioid derivatives :*** Diphenoxylate, Loperamide.
  - ***Anticholinergics :*** Atropine, Dicyclomine, Hyoscine.
  - ***Others :*** Racecadotril.
- **Adsorbents :**
  - Kaolin, Pectin, Charcoal, Bismuth subsalicylate.
- **Agents that modify fluid & electrolyte transport :**
  - Bile salt binding resins, Octreotide, Clonidine.
- **Antimicrobial Agents :**
  - Ciprofloxacin, Ofloxacin. Tetracyclines.

- **Antiamebic agents :**
  - Metronidazole, Tinidazole.
- **Probiotics :**
  - Lactobacillus sp, Bifidobacterium, Saccharomyces boulardi.

## Diphenoxylate, Loperamide :

- ***Mechanism of action :*** They are opioid agonists that decrease propulsive activity of large intestine. This is mediated by μ opioid receptors, thus lead to increase colonic transit time, decreases secretions.
- These should not be used in bacterial diarrheas because, suppression of motions will lead to decrease clearance of pathogens from the body and can lead to systemic invasion of these pathogens and aggravate the patient's condition.

## Loperamide :

- It does not cross blood brain barrier, have no analgesic property and does not cause addiction.
- ***Dose :*** 4 mg followed by 2 mg after each motion.

## Diphenoxylate :

- It does not have morphine like activity in the CNS but higher doses produce typical opioid effects.
- Commercial preparations contains 2.5 mg Diphenoxylate with 0.025 mg Atropine *(Lomotil)* The presence of atropine prevents abuse because, though atropine present in the combination is in very less concentration, if such tablets are taken in more quantity in abuse, then the uncomfortable anticholinergic effects of atropine kicks in.
- ***Dose :*** 2 tablets TDS.

## Anticholinergics :

- They are used as antimotility and antisecretory agents and also in combination with diphenoxylate (as mentioned above).
- They can also be used to treat symptoms of abdominal colic associated with gastroenteritis.

## Racecadotril :

- It is the inhibitor of enzyme enkephalinase. This increases the concentration of enkephalins in intestinal mucosa then stimulates μ and δ opioid receptors like loperamide to produce antidiarrheal effect.
- ***Dose :*** 100-300 mg TDS.

## Adsorbents :

- ***Kaolin :*** Naturally occurring hydrated Magnesium-Aluminium-Silicate.
- ***Pectin :*** Indigestible carbohydrate derived from apples.

- Both act as adsorbents of bacteria, toxins and fluids and decreases stool liquidity and number.
- They are used in acute but not in chronic diarrhea.
- ***Dose :*** 1.2-1.5 g after each loose stool.
- ***Adverse effects :*** Kaolin / pectin preparations not absorbed, so no significant adverse effects are seen except constipation & binding with medicines.

### Bile salt binding resins : *Cholestyramine, Colestipol & Colesevelam*

- Conjugated bile salts are normally absorbed in the terminal ileum. Diseases of terminal ileum like Crohn's disease or surgical resection leads to malabsorption of bile salts which leads to colonic secretory diarrhea.
- These bile salt binding resins bind to the bile acids in the intestinal lumen and prevent excess fecal loss of bile acids.
- ***Dose :*** 4–5 gm, 1-3 times / day before meals.

### Octreotide :

- Refer chapter of anterior pituitary hormones.

### Clonidine :

- It is an $\alpha_2$ agonist. It enhances salt & water absorption from the intestine.
- ***Use :*** diabetic diarrhea.

### Antimicrobial agents and antiamebic agents :

- They are used in bacterial and amebic diarrhea respectively.
- They have no role in viral diarrhea and chronic diarrhea.
- For details, refer to respective chapters in chemotherapy system.

### Probiotics :

- The presence of normal bacterial flora of the gut is disturbed in diarrhea.
- It can also be disturbed after taking antibiotics.
- In order to maintain the balance and to replenish the healthy bacterial flora of the intestine, Probiotics are used.

## DRUGS FOR INFLAMMATORY BOWEL DISEASE :

It includes :

- Ulcerative colitis.
- Crohn's disease.

### Drugs :

- ***Corticosteroids :*** Prednisolone, Budesonide.
- ***Antidiarrheal agents :*** Loperamide, Diphenoxylate, Anticholinergics.
- ***Aminosalicylates :*** Sulphasalazine, Mesalazine, Olsalazine, Balsalazine.

- *Immunosuppressants :* Azathioprine, Methotrexate, Cyclosporine.
- *TNF-α inhibitors :* Infliximab.

## Corticosteroids :

- Prednisone, Prednisolone are for oral use.
- Budesonide enemas, foam or suppositories are used.
- For mechanism of action and adverse effects, refer chapter on corticosteroids.

## Antidiarrheal agents :

- Patients of inflammatory bowel diseases can get diarrhea. To treat this symptom, antidiarrheals are used.
- Mechanism is explained in detail above.

## Aminosalicylates :

***Sulphasalazine :***

- Sulphasalazine is poorly absorbed from the intestine and gets converted in the GIT to 5-aminosalicylic acid (5-ASA) and sulphapyridine.
- This 5-ASA exerts local anti-inflammatory response in the GIT. It inhibits production of cytokines, PAF, TNF-α, prostaglandins and leukotrienes. Migration of inflammatory cells is interfered and mucosal secretion is reduced. Sulphapyridine is absorbed systemically and exerts its effects which are used in the treatment of rheumatoid arthritis.
- ***Dose :*** 3-4 g/day.
- ***Uses :*** Ulcerative colitis, Crohn's disease and Rheumatoid arthritis.

***Mesalazine :***

- It is the official name of 5-ASA.
- As, 5-ASA is the active moiety, it is used.
- It is available as coated polymer.
- 5-ASA is also available as enema.

***Osalazine :***

- It consists of 2 molecules of 5-ASA joined by azo bond.
- Osalazine is poorly absorbed in the ileum, the azo bond is split in the colon providing 5-ASA locally.

## Immunosuppressants : (Details are covered under immunosuppressant drugs chapter)

***Azathioprine :***

- It has immunosuppressive properties. It is important agent for maintenance of remission of ulcerative colitis and Crohn's disease.

***Methotrexate :***

- It has effect in number of anti-inflammatory diseases including Crohn's disease and rheumatoid arthritis. It can be given orally, SC or IM.

***Cyclosporine :***

- It is inhibitor of calcineurin preventing clonal expansion of T-cells. Indicated in severe ulcerative colitis. No value in Crohn's disease.

## Infliximab :

- ***Mechanism :*** anti-TNF-α monoclonal antibody.
- Indicated active and fistulating Crohn's disease, in severe Crohn's disease refractory or intolerant to steroids & immunosuppressants, for whom surgery is inappropriate. Also has potent anti-inflammatory action.

❑❑❑❑❑

# ANTI-MICROBIAL DRUGS

# 58 INTRODUCTION TO CHEMOTHERAPY

**Chemotherapy :** It deals with the treatment of various infections and malignancies with drugs.

**Antibiotics :** Substances produced by microorganisms, which selectively suppress the growth of or kill other microorganisms.

**Antimicrobials :** Any substance of natural, synthetic or semisynthetic origin which selectively suppresses the growth of or kill other microorganisms.

**Bacteriostatic and bactericidal :** Bacteriostatic drugs arrest the growth and development of bacteria whereas, bactericidal drugs kill the bacteria.

## MECHANISM OF ACTION OF ANTIBIOTICS :

### 1. Inhibition of folic acid synthesis :

T – Trimethoprim
P – Pyrimethamine
S – Sulphonamides
D – Dapsone

### 2. Inhibition of protein synthesis :

| 50 S Ribosomal | 30 S Ribosomal |
|---|---|
| C – Chloramphenicol | A – Aminoglycosides |
| M – Macrolides | T – Tetracyclines |
| L – Lincosamides (clindamycin, lincomycin) | G – Glycylcyclines |
| O – Oxazolidinones (Linezolid) | |
| K – Ketolids (Telthromycin) | |
| S – Streptogramins | |

***Steps in bacterial protein synthesis :***

The protein synthesis of bacteria takes place in ribosomes (50 S and 30 S units). It occurs in following steps :

1. Messenger RNA (m-RNA) gets attached to the 30 S subunit of ribosome and then the 50 S ribosome unit binds to 30 S subunit. This complete unit moves along the m-RNA. The codons of m-RNA pass from the acceptor site ('A' site) to the peptidyl site ('P' site). This stage is known as the formation of **'Initiation complex'**. A transfer RNA (t-RNA) with its

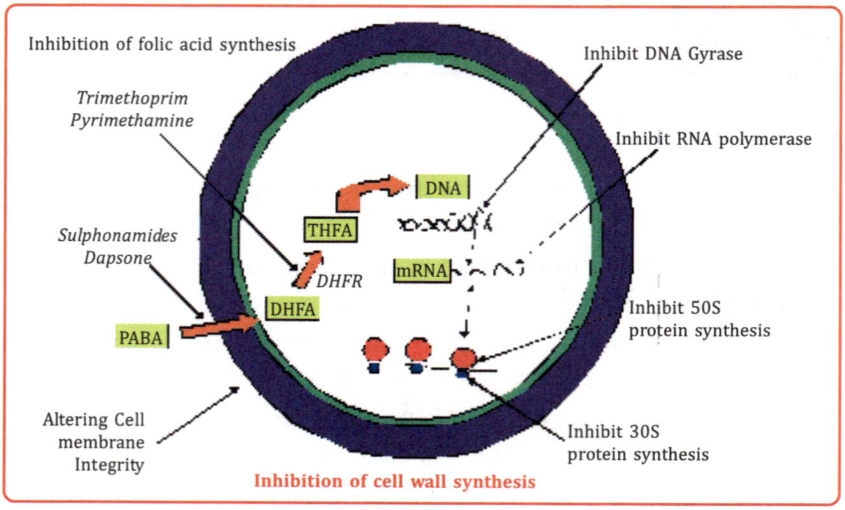


amino acids is already attached to the 'P' site. The incoming t-RNA carries another amino acid to be added to the peptide chain.

2. The incoming t-RNA with a new amino acid attaches to the acceptor site ('A' site).
3. The peptide chain on the t-RNA attached to the 'P' site is then transferred

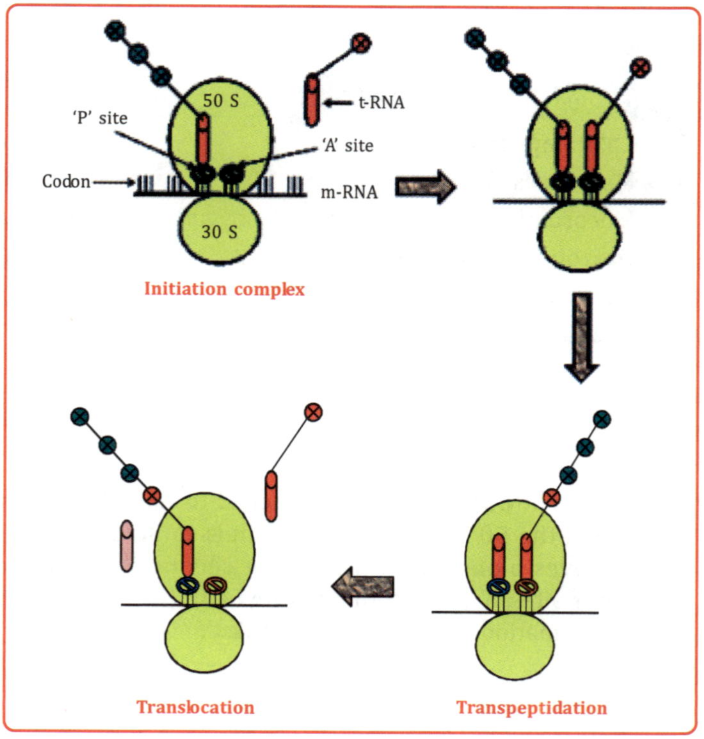

to the t-RNA attached to the 'A' site. This process is called as **'transpeptidation'**.

4. The t-RNA which has lost its peptide chain is then ejected out from the 'P' site and t-RNA at the 'A' site along with attached 4 amino acids is translocated to the 'P' site. This process is called as **'translocation'**. Now, the 'A' site is ready to accept new t-RNA with new amino acid. This is how a peptide chain is formed and protein synthesis occurs.

### 3. Inhibition of cell wall synthesis :

| β-Lactam antibiotics | Anti-TB Drugs |
|---|---|
| Penicillins | Isoniazid |
| Cephalosporins | Ethambutol |
| Carbapenems | Pyrizinamide |
| Monobactams | |
| Glycopeptides (Vancomycin) | |

### 4. Inhibits DNA gyrase / Topoisomerase :

Fluoroquinolones.

### 5. Inhibit DNA dependent RNA polymerase :

Rifampicin.

### 6. Alteration of cell wall integrity :

P – Polymyxins

A – Amphotericin-B

A – Azole antifungals

C – Chlorhexidine

## DEVELOPMENT OF RESISTANCE TO ANTIBIOTICS IN BACTERIA :

Due to widespread and indiscriminate use of antibiotics, there is emergence of a potentially serious challenge in front of medical fraternity of antibiotic resistance. Resistance refers to unresponsiveness of bacteria to a given antibiotic to which it was responding previously. Antibiotic resistance could be intrinsic (natural) or acquired due to irrational antibiotic use. Acquired antibiotic resistance develops due to genetic or biochemical methods.

### Genetic methods of antibiotic resistance :

1. Chromosomal mutations.
2. Plasmid mediated.
3. Methods of transfer of resistant genes (r-gene) from one bacteria to another by :
   - ☞ ***Conjugation*** : plasmids that contain r-genes, makes connecting tube between two bacteria through which the plasmids can pass.

- ☞ ***Transduction*** : plasmid DNA enclosed in a bacterial virus (bacteriophage) is transferred to another bacterium.
- ☞ ***Transformation*** : it's the ability of certain bacteria to pick up free DNA from the environment.

4. **Transposons :** Transfer of r-genes between plasmids within the bacteria with the help of transposons.

**Biochemical methods of antibiotic resistance :**

1. By producing antibiotic inactivating enzymes. *E.g.* production of β-lactamase enzyme by staphylococcus against β-lactam antibiotics like penicillins.
2. Preventing influx of drug inside the bacteria.
3. Promoting efflux of drug from the bacteria.
4. Modification of target sites.
5. Using alternate pathway by bacteria for its growth and metabolic requirements.

❑❑❑❑❑

# 59 SULPHONAMIDES

- Sulphonamides are structural analogues of PABA (Para amino benzoic acid).

## CLASSIFICATION :

- ***Short acting (6-9 hours) :***
  Sulphadiazine and Sulphisoxazole.
- ***Intermediate acting (10-12 hours) :***
  Sulphamethaxazole and Sulphamoxole.
- ***Long acting (7-8 days) :***
  Sulphadoxine.
- ***Special purpose sulphonamides :***
  Sulphasalazine, Silver sulphadiazine, Sulphacetamide and Mafenide.

## SPECTRUM :

- Sulphonamides are bacteriostatic. They are mainly active against gram negative bacteria like E. coli, Salmonella, Shigella, H. Influenzae, Vibrio cholera and proteus but not pseudomonas. They are also having activity against Meningitidis, N. gonorrheae, Nocardia, toxoplasma gondii, Chlamydia.

## MECHANISM OF ACTION :

- Folic acid is synthesised from PABA and Pteridine.

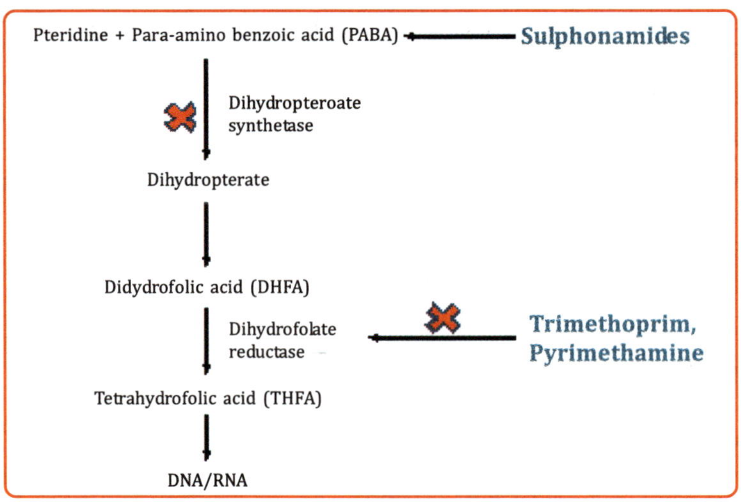

- All sulphonamides are analogue of PABA. Because of their structural similarity to PABA, they compete with this substrate for the bacterial enzyme, dihydropteroate synthetase. They thus inhibit the synthesis of bacterial folic acid, which is essential for synthesis of DNA.
- *Trimethoprim* is another drug which is structural analogue of Pteridine, but unlike sulphonamides it blocks the conversion of dihydrofolic acid to tetrahydrofolic acid (active form) by inhibiting enzyme dihydrofolate reductase.
- *Pyrimethamine* like trimethoprim also blocks the conversion of dihydrofolic acid to tetrahydrofolic acid (active form) by inhibiting enzyme dihydrofolate reductase, but has greater affinity for protozoal dihydrofolate reductase.

## COMBINATIONS OF SULPHONAMIDES :

### Co-trimoxazole (Trimethoprim + sulphamethoxazole) :

- Sulphonamides are rarely used as single agents. They are usually used in fixed dose combination. The most common combination is that of Trimethoprim + sulphamethoxazole which is also called as **"Co-trimoxazole'.**
- ***Justification for combination :*** Sulphamethoxazole is analogue of PABA. Because of its structural similarity to PABA, it competes with PABA for the bacterial enzyme dihydropteroate synthetase, while trimethoprim blocks enzyme dihydrofolate reductase. Both these drugs produce sequential blockade of synthesis of tetrahydrofolic acid (active form of folic acid) from PABA. This mechanism is known as wood field's theory.
- ***Advantages of combination :*** Individually, there are bacteriostatic, but the combination makes them bactericidal. This is also a synergistic combination. Both drugs have same half life of 10 hr.
- ***Dose :*** The dose of co-trimoxazole is trimethoprim 80 mg + sulphamethaxozole 400 mg, *i.e.* in the ratio of 1:5. The double strength tablet contains dose of trimethoprim 160 mg + sulphamethaxozole 800 mg.

### Sulphadoxine + Pyrimethamine :

- It is also a synergistic fixed dose combination and provides sequential blockage of folic acid synthesis like co-trimoxazole (*see* above).
- ***Dose :*** sulphadoxine 500 mg + pyrimethamine 25 mg or sulphadoxine 1500 mg + pyrimethamine 75 mg *i.e.* in the ratio of 20 :1.

## USES :

### Co-trimoxazole :

- UTI (Urinary tract infections).
- Prostatitis.
- Respiratory tract infections.
- Typhoid.
- Bacterial diarrheas and dysentery.
- Pneumocystis carinii pneumonia.

- Sexually transmitted diseases.
- Cholera.
- Nocardiasis.

**Special purpose sulphonamides :**

- ***Sulphasalazine :*** It is not absorbed from GIT. Therefore high concentration is reached in GIT. Intestinal flora splits sulphasalazine into sulphapyridine and 5-aminosalicylic acid (5-ASA). This 5-ASA exerts the anti-inflammatory effect in the intestines. This property is used for treatment of chronic inflammatory bowel disease (*e.g.* Crohn's disease and ulcerative colitis). The sulphapyridine component of sulphasalazine is absorbed in the body and is used in the treatment of rheumatoid arthritis.
- ***Silver sulphadiazine :*** It is topically used in burns. It is active against gram negative bacteria including pseudomonas. It slowly releases silver ions which also provide additional antimicrobial action.
- ***Sulphacetamide :*** Usually used as eye drops or eye ointment for treatment of trachoma and bacterial conjunctivitis.
- ***Mafenide :*** It is topically used. The advantage is that it is active even in the presence of pus and is also effective against pseudomonas and clostridia.

**Sulphadoxine + Pyrimethamine :**

- Chloroquine resistant falciparum malaria.
- Toxoplasmosis.

## ADVERSE EFFECTS :

- **Blood :** Hemolytic and aplastic anemia especially in G6PD deficiency patients, Thrombocytopenia.
- *Hypersensitivity :* Photosensitivity, Exfoliative dermatitis, Stevens Johnson's syndrome, Drug fever and Eosinophilia.
- **Crystalluria and renal toxicity :** It can be prevented by Adequate intake of water and by making urine alkaline.
- **Kernicterus in neonates :** Sulphonamides displace bilirubin from protein binding sites. Free bilirubin crosses the blood brain barrier and gets deposited in basal ganglia leading to toxic encephalopathy. Therefore, should be avoided in neonates & pregnancy (last trimester).
- **GI :** Nausea, vomiting, diarrhea, pancreatitis.

□□□□□

# 60 FLUOROQUINOLONES

- They are synthetic antimicrobial agents.
- Before fluoroquinolones, *Nalidixic acid* which is a quinolone derivative was used to treat gram negative infections of urinary tract, but not for systemic infections because it is highly protein bound.

## CLASSIFICATION :

- ***1$^{st}$ generation :*** Norfloxacin, Ciprofloxacin, Ofloxacin and Pefloxacin.
- ***2$^{nd}$ generation :*** Levofloxacin and Prulifloxacin.
- ***3$^{rd}$ generation :*** Sparfloxacin and gatifloxacin.
- ***4$^{th}$ generation :*** Moxifloxacin, Trovafloxacin and Finafloxacin.

## Spectrum :

| Generation | Spectrum |
|---|---|
| 1$^{st}$ | Gram negative bacteria, bacillus anthracis, Mycobacterium tuberculosis |
| 2$^{nd}$ | Similar to 1$^{st}$ generation plus better activity against gram positive cocci. |
| 3$^{rd}$ | Similar to 2$^{nd}$ generation plus enhanced activity against gram positive cocci. |
| 4$^{th}$ | Similar to 3$^{rd}$ generation plus enhanced activity against anaerobes. |

## Mechanism of action :

- The fluoroquinolones (FQs) work by inhibiting one or more of a group of enzymes called as topoisomerase, enzymes needed for supercoiling, replication and separation of circular bacterial DNA. FQs **inhibit** both **topisomerase II (DNA gyrase)**, especially in gram negative bacteria and **topisomerase IV**, especially in gram positive bacteria.
- ***Topoisomerase II (DNA Gyrase) :*** catalyzes the negative supercoiling of the circular DNA found in bacteria.
- ***Topoisomerase IV :*** is involved in the relaxation of the supercoiled circular DNA, enabling the separation of the interlinked daughter chromosomes at the end of bacterial DNA replication.

## Drug interactions :

- FQs increases the plasma concentration of drugs like theophylline, Warfarin due to inhibition of metabolism. Thus, can result in toxicity of these drugs.
- Antacids, sucralfate and iron salts decreases absorption of FQs.
- NSAIDs can increase CNS toxicity of FQs.

**Uses :**

- ***Urinary tract infections :*** Usually ciprofloxacin 500 mg BD or Norfloxacin 400 mg BD or ofloxacin 400 mg BD are used. Norfloxacin has got poor bioavailability, hence not used to treat systemic infections.
- ***Typhoid :*** Ciprofloxacin 500 mg BD for 10 days or ofloxacin 400 mg BD for 10 days are used. Ceftriaxone (cephalosporin antibiotic) is being increasingly used drug of choice nowadays.
- ***Bacterial diarrheas :*** Acute bacterial diarrheas like traveller's diarrhea are treated with norfloxacin 400 mg BD or ciprofloxacin 500 mg BD or ofloxacin 400 mg BD.
- ***Skin and soft tissue infections :*** Ciprofloxacin 500 mg BD or ofloxacin 400 mg BD for 7 days or pefloxacin 400 mg BD for 7 days are used. FQs are also used to treat diabetic foot and other gram negative infections. For complicated infections moxifloxacin 400 mg OD can be used.
- ***Respiratory infections :*** FQs are used to treat bronchitis, sinusitis and pneumonia. Levofloxacin 500 mg OD or prulifloxacin 600 mg OD can be used.
- ***Sexually transmitted diseases :*** Gonorrhea, chancroid are treated with FQs. Ciprofloxacin 500 mg BD or ofloxacin 400 mg BD can be used.
- ***Anthrax :*** Ciprofloxacin 500 mg BD for 60 days is used. For severe infection, Ciprofloxacin 400 mg IV 12 hrly along with ampicillin and clarithromycin is used for 60 days.
- ***Tuberculosis :*** Ciprofloxacin and ofloxacin are used for treatment of MDR-TB.
- ***Eye infections :*** Ciprofloxacin or moxifloxacin eye drops are used for treatment of bacterial conjunctivitis or other eye infections.
- ***Intra-abdominal infections :*** Severe intra-abdominal infections are treated with trovafloxacin or finafloxacin.
- ***Bone & Joint infections :*** Ciprofloxacin 750 mg BD for 6 wks for chronic osteomyelitis is used.

**Adverse effects :**

- Tendonitis and Tendon rupture.
- ***Articular cartilage damage :*** FQs can cause arthropathy including articular cartilage damage, arthralgias, and joint swelling. Contraindicated in pediatric patients and pregnant or breast feeding women.
- ***Cardiac :*** Prolongation of QTc interval (sparfloxacin, gatifloxacin).
- ***CNS :*** Headache, agitation, insomnia, dizziness, rarely, hallucinations and seizures (elderly).
- ***Hepatotoxicity :*** LFT elevation (trovafloxacin).
- ***Phototoxicity :*** More common with older FQs.
- ***Gastrointestinal :*** Nausea, vomiting, diarrhea, dyspepsia.

□□□□□

# 61 β-LACTAM ANTIBIOTICS

All of the drugs in this group contain a β-*lactam ring* in their structure. They share similar features of chemistry, mechanism of action, pharmacologic effects and clinical effects. They have short elimination half-life and are primarily excreted through kidneys. They show cross-allergenicity. They can be degraded by β-Lactamase enzyme produced by bacteria, which can result in resistance to the antibiotic.

### β-lactam Antibiotics include :

- Penicillins.
- Cephalosporins.
- Monobactams.
- Carbapenems.

## PENICILLINS :

### Classification :

- ***Natural Penicillins :*** Penicillin G (Benzyl penicillin).
- ***Semisynthetic penicillins :***
  - **Acid-stable penicillins :** Penicillin V.
  - **Penicillinase (β-lactamase) resistant penicillins :** Nafcillin, Oxacillin, Methicillin, Cloxacillin.
- ***Extended-spectrum penicillins :***
  - **Aminopenicillins :** Ampicillin, Amoxycillin.
  - **Carboxypenicillins :** Carbencillin, Ticarcillin.
  - **Ureidopenicillin :** Piperacillin, Azlocillin.

### Mechanisms of Action :

- Inhibit bacterial cell wall synthesis. They bind to penicillin binding protein (PBPs) on cell wall and specifically inhibits the cross linking of peptides chains (cross-bridging / Transpeptidation). If cell walls are improperly made cell walls allow water to flow into the cell causing it to burst and killing the bacteria.

### Natural Penicillins (Penicillin G / Benzyl penicillin) :

- It is extracted from penicillium notatum. Prototype is penicillin G (Benzyl penicillin). It is pH sensitive, therefore not given orally. Only given parenterally.

- It is effective against Gram-positive microorganisms and is susceptible to penicillinase (β-lactamase) enzyme produced by the bacteria.

- ***Spectrum :***
  - ***Gram-positive :*** S. aureus, S. pneumonia, streptococci, viridans streptococci and Enterococcus.
  - ***Gram negative :*** Neiserria sp.
  - ***Anaerobes :*** Clostridium sp.
  - ***Others :*** Treponema pallidum (syphilis).

- ***Parenteral preparations of penicillin G :*** The two parenteral preparations of penicillin G are :
  - *Procaine penicillin G*
  - *Benzathine penicillin G*

  Such agents release penicillin G slowly from the area in which they are injected and produce relatively low but persistent concentrations of antibiotic in the blood.

- ***Uses of penicillin G :***
  - *Pneumococcal Infections* (Pneumococcal Meningitis and Pneumonia).
  - *Streptococcal Infections* (Streptococcal Pharyngitis including Scarlet Fever, Streptococcal Pneumonia, Arthritis, Meningitis, and Endocarditis).
  - *Enterococcal endocarditis* (along with an aminoglycoside like gentamicin).
  - *Staphylococcal Infections.*
  - *Meningococcal Infections.*
  - *Gonococcal Infections.*
  - *Diphtheria* (along with diphtheria antitoxin).
  - *Anthrax.*
  - *Clostridial Infections like Tetanus* (along with Tetanus antitoxin).
  - *Syphilis.* Procaine penicillin G in the dose of 1.2 MU daily for 10 days.
  - *Prophylactic use :* Surgical Procedures like dental extraction, tonsillectomy in Patients with Valvular Heart Disease. For Rheumatic fever, benzathine penicillin G 1.2 MU every 4 weekly till 18 years of age or 5 years after the attack.
  - *Actinomycosis.*
  - *Rat-Bite Fever.*
  - *Lyme Disease.*

- ***Adverse effects :***
  - ***Hypersensitivity :*** Skin rashes, fever, eosinophilia, angio-edema, serum sickness and *anaphylactic shock.* Cross-reactivity exists among

all penicillins and even other β-lactams. The most serious hypersensitivity reaction is anaphylactic shock. Prompt treatment with adrenaline is necessary to relieve angio-edema and bronchospasm.

- ***Local pain and irritation at injection site.***
- ***Jarisch-Herxheimer reaction :*** Seen with treatment of syphilis with penicillins. Features include shivering, fever, myalgia and vascular collapse. This is due to sudden release of degradation products of treponema pallidum. It can get relieved by aspirin.
- ***Superinfections :*** Results from alterations in intestinal flora. A higher incidence occurs with broad-spectrum penicillins.

**Acid-stable Penicillins (Penicillin V) :**

- This Penicillin is given orally.
- Indicated only in minor infections because of their relatively poor bioavailability, weaker antimicrobial activity, the need for dosing many times.
- Has narrow antimicrobial spectrum.

**Penicillinase (β-lactamase) resistant penicillins :** ***Nafcillin, Oxacillin, Methicillin, Cloxacillin***

- They were developed to overcome the penicillinase enzyme of *S. aureus* which inactivated natural penicillins.
- Active against gram-positive bacteria like methicillin susceptible *S. aureus*, group streptococci and viridans streptococci.

**Aminopenicillin :** ***Ampicillin, Amoxycillin***

- Developed to increase activity against gram negative aerobes.
- ***Spectrum :***
  - ***Gram positive :*** S. aureus, Group streptococci, viridans streptococci, Enterococcus sp, Listeria monocytogenes.
  - ***Gram negative :*** Proteus mirabilis, Salmonella, Shigella, E. coli, H. influenzae.
- ***Uses :***
  - *Urinary tract infections.*
  - *Respiratory tract infections.*
  - *Gonorrhea.*
  - *Meningitis.*
  - *Bacillary dysentery.*
  - *H. pylori gastritis.*
  - *Subacute bacterial endocarditis* : Ampicillin along with gentamicin is used.
  - *Skin and soft tissue infections.*

- ***Adverse effects :***
  - ***Diarrhea :*** the most common adverse effects seen especially with oral ampicillin and amoxycillin is diarrhea due to suppression of bacterial flora.
  - ***Hypersensitivity reactions.***

### Carboxypenicillin (carbenicillin, ticarcillin) :

- Developed to increase activity against resistant gram negative organisms like Proteus mirabilis, Salmonella, Shigella, some E. coli, H. influenza, Enterobacter sp and Pseudomonas aeruginosa.

### Antipseudomonal Penicillins :

- These are the penicillins which are active against pseudomonas aeruginosa, indole positive proteus and enterobacter. They include :
  - ***Carboxypenicillins :*** Carbencillin, Ticarcillin.
  - ***Ureidopenicillin :*** Piperacillin, Azlocillin.
- Mechanism of action, uses (+ also used for pseudomonas infections) and adverse effects are similar to all conventional penicillins.
- Piperacillin is usually given with a β-lactamase inhibitor like tazobactum.

### Beta-Lactamase inhibitors :

- ***Drugs :*** **Clavulanic acid, Sulbactam and Tazobactam.**
- ***Mechanism :*** They bind irreversibly to and inactivate bacterial beta-lactamase enzyme (can protect penicillins from inactivation by the enzyme) and are used to enhance the antibacterial actions of beta-lactam antibiotics. They are also called as *'suicide inhibitors'.*
- They only have weak antibacterial action.
- Only clavulanic acid is orally absorbed, others are given parenterally.
- They are available in fixed combinations.

  *E.g. :*
  - Tablet Amoxycillin 500 mg + Tablet Clavulanic acid 125 mg.
  - Injection Ampicillin 1 gm + Injection Sulbactum 0.5 gm.
  - Injection Piperacillin 4 gm + Injection Tazobactum 0.5 gm.

## CEPHALOSPORINS :

- They are also beta lactam antibiotics.
- Except 1st generation drugs, rest are more resistant to β-lactamase enzyme, therefore are having broader spectrum.

### Mechanisms of Action :

- Inhibit bacterial cell wall synthesis. They bind to penicillin binding protein (PBPs) on cell wall and specifically inhibits the cross linking of peptides chains (cross-bridging / Transpeptidation). If cell walls are improperly made cell walls allow water to flow into the cell causing it to burst and killing the bacteria.

## Classification :

- ***1st generation :***
  ***Oral :*** Cephalexin, Cefadroxil.
  ***Parenteral :*** Cefazolin, Cefalothin.
- ***2nd generation :***
  ***Oral :*** Cefuroxime axetil, cefaclor.
  ***Parenteral :*** Cefuroxime, cefoxitine, cefotetan.
- ***3rd generation :***
  ***Oral :*** Cefixime, cefpodoxime, cefdinir.
  ***Parenteral :*** Ceftriaxone, cefotaxime, ceftazidime, cefoperazone, ceftizoxime.
- ***4th generation :***
  ***Parenteral :*** Cefepime, cefpirome.
- ***5th generation :***
  ***Parenteral :*** Ceftaroline, ceftobiprole.

## 1st generation cephalosporins :

- **Spectrum :**
  - ***Gram positive cocci :*** Streptococci, Staphylococci.
  - ***Gram negative :*** Moraxella catarrhalis, E. coli, K. pneumonia, P. mirabilis.
  - Penicillin susceptible anaerobes in oral cavity except B. fragilis.
  - ***Exception :*** Enterococci, MRSA, Penicillin resistant Streptococci, S. epidermidis, pseudomonas, salmonella.
- **Uses :** Due to emergence of resistance, they are less frequently used nowadays. The primary uses are :
  - Skin & Soft tissue infections.
  - Prophylaxis before surgery (especially cefazolin).
  - Upper respiratory tract infections.
- Except for cefadroxil which is given 12 hrly, rests are given 6-8 hrly.

## 2nd generation cephalosporins :

- **Spectrum :**
  - ***Gram negative aerobes :*** H. influenza, M. catarrhalis, P. mirabilis, E. coli, Klebsiella, Neisseria gonorrhea.
  - ***Gram positive cocci :*** less active.
  - ***Anaerobes :*** B. fragilis.
  - No efficacy against Pseudomonas, Enterococci.
- **Uses :**
  - Respiratory tract infections.
  - Acute sinusitis.

- Otitis media.
- Uncomplicated UTI.
- Skin & soft tissues.
- Intra abdominal and Gynecological infections.
- Gonorrhea.
- Community acquired pneumonia.

## 3rd generation cephalosporins :

- **Spectrum :**
  - Less active than 1st generation against Gram positive organisms.
  - More active against gram negative organisms like E. coli, N. meningitides, H. influenza, Klebsilla Pneumoniae and proteus.
  - Ceftriaxone and cefoperazone : Salmonella typhi.
  - ***Ceftazidime :*** Pseudomonas aeruginosa.
  - Adequate therapeutic levels are achieved in CSF.
- **Uses :**
  - ***With or without aminoglycosides :*** infections by Klebsiella, Enterobacter, Proteus, Haemophilus sp, Providencia.
  - ***Ceftriaxone :*** all forms of gonorrhea; severe Lyme disease, *Drug of choice for Typhoid* (1 gm IV 12 hrly).
  - ***Cefotaxime & Ceftriaxone :*** initial treatment of meningitis.
  - ***Ceftazidime + aminoglycoside :*** Pseudomonas infections.
  - Community acquired Pneumonia.
  - Uncomplicated gonorrhea (cefixime 400 mg single dose).
  - Upper respiratory infections (cefixime 200 mg BD).

## 4th generation cephalosporins :

- **Spectrum :**
  - Active against Gram positive, Enterobacteriaceae, Pseudomonas.
  - ***No activity :*** penicillin-resistant S. pneumonia, MRSA, MRSE, Staphylococci, Enterococcus, L. monocytogenes, Legionella, C. difficile, Campylobacter.
- **Uses :**
  - Hospital acquired infections.
  - Septicemia.
  - Bacteremia.
  - UTIs.
  - RTIs.

## 5th generation cephalosporins :

- **Spectrum :**
  - ***Gram positive cocci :*** MRSA, MRSE, Penicillin Resistant Streptococcus, Enterococcus fecalis.
  - ***Gram negative :*** E. coli, Pseudomonas.

- **Uses :**
  - Skin and soft tissue Infections.
  - Community acquired pneumonia.
  - Diabetic foot.

**Adverse effects :**

- Hypersensitivity reactions :
  - ***Immediate :*** anaphylaxis, bronchospasm, urticaria.
  - ***Late :*** Maculopapular rash with/without fever, eosinophilia.
  - Cross reactivity
- Nephrotoxicity.
- Antibiotic induced colitis, diarrhea.
- Intolerance to alcohol (disulfiram like reaction with cefoperazone).
- Thrombocytopenia/ platelet dysfunction.
- Rarely, bone marrow depression, granulocytopenia.

## MONOBACTAMS :

- **Drugs : *Aztreonam, Tigemonam and Carumonam.***
- **Mechanism of action :** Inhibit bacterial cell wall synthesis.
- **Spectrum :** spectrum resembles that of aminoglycosides and include mostly gram negative bacteria like enterobacteriacae, pseudomonas, klebsiella, proteus, haemophilus, salmonella, shigella, neisseria etc.
- Oral bioavailability is poor, therefore is given IM or IV in the dose of 1 gm 8 hrly.
- **Use :** infections caused by gram negative bacteria as an alternative to aminoglycoside. Recently an inhalational formulation of aztreonam is approved for treatment of cystic fibrosis due to pseudomonas.

## CARBEPENEMS :

- **Drugs : *Imipenem, Meropenem, Ertapenem, Faropenem, Doripenem, Razupenem.***
- **Mechanism of action :** Inhibit bacterial cell wall synthesis.
- **Spectrum :** their spectrum is wide and includes gram negative bacteria, gram positive bacteria and anerobes. They are resistant to many β-lactamases.
- **Imipenem + Cilastatin :** Imipenem is hydrolysed by renal dehydropeptidase present in renal brush border resulting in lower urinary concentration. It is therefore administered with Cilastatin which inhibits this enzyme and prevents its degradation.
- Meropenem, Ertapenem and Doripenem are not degraded by renal dehydropeptidase.
- Faropenem is given orally.

# 62 TETRACYCLINES AND CHLORAMPHENICOL (Broad Spectrum Antibiotics)

## TETRACYCLINES :

- They are broad spectrum antibiotic.
- It is commonly used to treat common bacterial infections.

### Classification :

- ***Short acting (6-10 hrs) :*** Tetracycline, Chlortetracycline and Oxytetracycline.
- ***Intermediate acting (12-13 hrs) :*** Demeclocycline and Methacycline.
- ***Long acting (18-20 hrs) :*** Doxycycline and Minocycline.

### Antimicrobial Spectrum :

They are active against the following microorganisms :

- gram-positive and gram-negative bacteria, spirochetes, rickettsiae, candida, mycoplasma pneumonia, vibrio, streptococcus pneumonia, neisseria gonorrheae.

### Mechanism of action :

- They bind to 30S ribosomal unit. Blocks the binding of t-RNA to the 'A' site on mRNA. Ultimately, they inhibit protein synthesis of the microorganism.

### Dosing :

- ***Tetracycline :*** 250-500 mg QID or TDS.
- ***Doxycycline :*** 100 mg 12 hourly on 1$^{st}$ day then 100 mg OD.

### Uses :

#### *Primary uses :*

- Peptic ulcers caused by *H. pylori.*
- Atypical Pneumonia (*M. pneumoniae).*
- Pneumonia (Chlamydia).
- Typhus fever (Rickettsia).
- Cholera.
- Rocky mountain spotted fever.
- Brucellosis.
- Granuloma inguinale.

### *Secondary uses :*

- Alternative drug for syphilis.
- Plague.
- Psittacosis.
- Leptospirosis.
- Treatment of acne.
- SIADH (Demeclocycline).
- Leprosy (minocycline).

### Adverse effects :

1. ***GI disturbances :*** nausea, vomiting, gastritis.
2. ***Bony structures and teeth :***
    - **Fetal exposure :**
        - Tooth enamel dysplasia.
        - Irregularities in bone growth.
    - **Younger children (under age 8) :**
        - Enamel dysplasia and crown deformation when permanent teeth appears.
        - Bind with calcium and deposit in newly formed bones (impaired long bone formation) and teeth (discoloration of teeth).

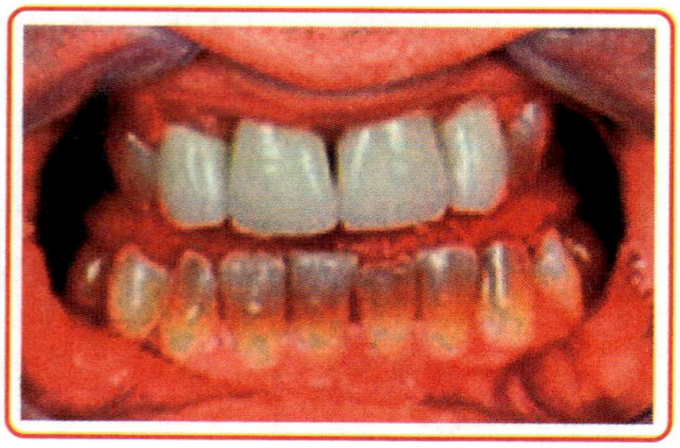

3. Hepatotoxicity.
4. Bacterial superinfection.
5. Renal toxicity (*Fanconi's syndrome)* :
    - Renal tubular damage.
    - Due to toxic metabolites (epitetracycline and epianhydrotetracycline).
    - Seen with use of expired tetracycline.
6. Photosensitivity (Demeclocycline).
7. Vestibular toxicity (Doxycycline and minocycline) : Dizziness and Vertigo.

### Drug Interactions :

- Aluminium, calcium and iron containing preparations like antacids, milk and iron supplements should not be given with tetracyclines because they decrease absorption of tetracyclines by chelation.
- Tetracyclines inhibit intestinal flora that produces vitamin K and therefore may potentiate anticoagulant effect of warfarin.

## GLYCYLCYCLINES :

- **Drug : Tigelcycline.**
- It is a minocycline (tetracycline) analogue.
- **Mechanism of action :** They bind to 30S ribosomal unit. Blocks the binding of t-RNA to the 'A' site on mRNA. Ultimately, they inhibit protein synthesis of the microorganism.
- **Spectrum :** It has broad spectrum activity against tetracycline resistant strains as well as multiple drug resistant strains of gram positive bacteria including MRSA, vancomycin resistant enterococci and S. pneumonia.
- **Uses :** Complicated intra-abdominal infections, skin and soft tissue infections, septicemia.
- **Adverse effects :** Nausea, vomiting, allergic reaction.

## CHLORAMPHENICOL :

- Chloramphenicol was initially obtained from streptomyces venezuelae in 1947.
- It is bacteriostatic but in higher concentration exerts bactericidal effect.

### Antimicrobial Spectrum :

- Effective against wide range of gram negative bacteria (*E.g.* S. Typhi, H. Influenzae and N. meningitidis), gram positive (*E.g.* S. Pneumoniae) and anaerobes as well.

### Mechanism of action :

- They bind to 50S ribosomal unit. Blocks the binding of t-RNA to the 'A' site on mRNA. Ultimately, they inhibit protein synthesis of the microorganism.

### Uses :

- Meningitis (H.Influenzae, N. Meningitidis and S. Pneumoniae).
- Typhoid fever – 500 mg QID (Its use declined due to resistance, adverse effects and emergence of new drugs like fluoroquinolones and ceftriaxone).
- Anaerobic infections (clindamycin and metronidazole are preferred nowadays).
- Urinary tract infection.
- Topically (conjunctivitis, ear infections).
- Complicated skin, soft tissues and intra-abdominal infections.

### Adverse effects :

1. ***GI disturbances :*** Due to direct irritation and due to superinfection.
2. ***Bone marrow depression :*** Leads to anemia, leucopenia and thrombocytopenia. Usually seen when dose > 3-4 gm/day for 1-2 weeks. Periodic blood counts advised.

3. ***Aplastic anemia :*** Idiosyncratic, Irreversible and may be fatal. Non-dose related.

4. ***Grey baby syndrome :*** Neonates cannot adequately metabolised Chloramphenicol due to immature liver. They also have slow kidney functions. This leads to higher levels of free Chloramphenicol in the body leading to toxicity. It is characterised by abdominal distension, progressive cyanosis (grey baby), hypothermia, vomiting, decreased intake, cardiovascular collapse and death.

# 63 AMINOGLYCOSIDE ANTI-BIOTICS

## DRUGS :

- **Tobramycin, Amikacin, Netilmicin, Gentamicin, Kanamycin, Streptomycin, Paromomycin, Neomycin, Framycetin.**

### How to remember the drugs ?

(**T**-Tobramycin, **A**-Amikacin, **N**-Netilmicin, **G**-Gentamicin, **KA**-Kanamycin, **SHARBAT**-Streptomycin, **PIYO**-Paromomycin, **NEW**-Neomycin, **FRIEND**-Framycetin).

***'Tang Ka Sharbat Piyo New Friend'***

## CHARACTERISTICS :

- All derived from streptomyces, micromonospora or are semisynthetic derivatives. Consists of two or more amino sugars linked to an aminocyclitol ring by glycosidic bonds, therefore the name aminoglycoside. They are polar compounds which are polycationic, water soluble, and incapable of crossing lipid containing cell membranes. They are bactericidal.

## MECHANISM OF ACTION :

- **Inhibition of protein synthesis** by binding to **30S** ribosomal unit and prevents the formation of **initiation complex**.
- They must first diffuse through outer membrane and cytoplasmic membrane to bind to ribosome. On the other hand β-lactam antibiotics inhibit cell wall synthesis, which facilitates entry of aminoglycoside in the bacteria. Thus, aminoglycosides and β-lactam antibiotics are having synergistic action.

## POST-ANTIBIOTIC EFFECT :

- Aminoglycosides exhibit **concentration dependent killing** (increased concentration kills more bacteria and at faster rate) and they also exhibit **post-antibiotic effect** which means that they continue to kill bacteria for several hours even when their plasma concentration falls below minimum inhibitory concentration. Due to this post-antibiotic effect, they are usually given as single daily dose despite their short half life.

## SPECTRUM :

- **Mainly : Gram -ve aerobes :** E. coli, Klebsiella, Shigella, Proteus, Enterobacter, Pseudomonas aeruginosa, Yersinia, Brucella, Vibrio cholerae.
- **Gram +ve aerobes :** S. aureus, viridans streptococci, Enterococcus.
- **Mycobacteria :** M. Tuberculosis, atypical mycobacteria.

## PHARMACOKINETICS :

- **Absorption :** They are poorly absorbed from GIT. Therefore, they are given parenterally or applied topically.
- **Distribution :** Primarily in extracellular fluid volume; are widely distributed into body fluids but not the CSF.
- **Elimination :** Eliminated unchanged by the kidney via glomerular filtration.

## DRUG INTERACTIONS AND PRECAUTIONS :

- Aminoglycosides should be avoided in pregnancy as it causes Teratogenicity.
- Do not mix aminoglycoside with any other drug in the same syringe.
- Should not be used with other nephrotoxic drugs like amphotericin-B or ototoxic drugs like furosemide.

## USES :

### Streptomycin (1 gm/day IM) :

- Tuberculosis.
- Plague, tularemia and brucellosis in combination with tetracycline.
- Subacute bacterial endocarditis along with penicillin (Gentamicin is more preferred).

### Gentamicin (3-5 mg/kg/day IM or IV) :

- Severe gram-negative infections.
- Burns, UTI, pneumonia, lung abscess, osteomyelitis, middle ear infection, conjunctivitis, septicemia etc.
- Pseudomonas aeruginosa infections : in combination with anti-pseudomonal penicillin or a 3rd generation cephalosporin.
- Severe gram negative meningitis, SABE, for preventing and treating serious respiratory tract infections in critically ill and immunocompromised patients.

### Kanamycin :

- Topical administration only.
- Oral administration in preparation for elective bowel surgery.
- Most ototoxic amongst all hence largely replaced by other aminoglycosides.
- Recently found place in management of MDR-TB.

### Amikacin (7.5-15 mg/kg/day IM or IV in 2 divided doses) :

- Has the most wide antibacterial spectrum amongst aminoglycosides.
- Resistant to many enzyme that inactivate gentamicin and tobramycin.
- Should be used as reserved alternative to Gentamicin.
- It is the synthetic derivative of Kanamycin.
- Uses same as Gentamicin.

### Netilmicin :

- Resistant to many enzymes that inactivate gentamicin and tobramycin.

- Lowest toxicity among aminoglycosides.
- It can be used as an alternative to gentamicin.

**Tobramycin :**
- Similar antibacterial spectrum with gentamicin.
- More active against P. aeruginosa.
- Should be used as reserved alternative to Gentamicin.
- Not useful in enterococcal endocarditis.
- It is mainly used to treat infections caused by P. aeruginosa that are resistant to gentamicin.
- Used topically in eye and ear infections as eye drops.

**Neomycin :**
- It is too toxic for parenteral use.
- Used only topically as drops, ointment and creams.
- It is also used for preparation for elective bowel surgery.
- Neomycin in the dose of 1 g TDS is useful in hepatic coma as it suppresses ammonia producing bacteria and thus prevents encephalopathy.

**Paromomycin :**
- It is mainly used to treat intestinal amebiasis.
- Also used in cryptosporidiosis in AIDS patients.

**Framycetin :**
- Similar to neomycin.
- Too toxic for systemic use.
- Used topically.
- Brand : soframycin.

## ADVERSE EFFECTS :

**Nephrotoxicity :**
- Neomycin, Gentamicin, Amikacin and Tobramycin are more nephrotoxic than others.
- Proximal tubule damage, increase in blood urea nitrogen and serum creatinine, low GFR, albuminuria.
- Reversible if caught early.
- Risk factors : long term use, higher doses, elderly and children, renal insufficiency, concurrent use with loop diuretics or other nephrotoxic drugs like Amphotericin-B.

**Ototoxicity :**
- ***$8^{th}$ cranial nerve damage :*** vestibular and auditory toxicity which is usually irreversible.
- ***Vestibular damage :*** dizziness, vertigo, ataxia (more with Streptomycin and Gentamicin).

- ***Cochlear damage :*** tinnitus decreased hearing (more with Amikacin and Neomycin).

**Neuromuscular blockade :**

- They block postsynaptic $N_M$ receptors and also inhibit $Ca^{+2}$ mediated release of Ach.

**Allergic reactions :**

- Same like that with other drugs.

**ARBEKACIN :**

- Newer Aminoglycoside antibiotic.
- Approved in 2017 in India.

❑❑❑❑❑

# 64 MACROLIDES AND RELATED ANTI-BIOTICS

## MACROLIDES :

### Drugs :

- **Erythromycin (prototype).**
- **Clarithromycin.**
- **Roxithromycin.**
- **Azithromycin.**
- **Spiramycin.**

## ERYTHROMYCIN :

- Derived from *Streptomyces erythreus.*
- Problems - acid labile, narrow spectrum, poor GI intolerance, short half-life.

### Structural derivatives like clarithromycin and azithromycin :

- Broader spectrum of activity.
- Improved Pharmacokinetics – better bioavailability, better tissue penetration, prolonged half-lives.
- Improved tolerability.

### Mechanism of Action :

- Inhibits protein synthesis by reversibly binding to the 50S ribosomal subunit (Inhibition of translocation of mRNA).

### Spectrum of Activity :

- ***Gram-Positive Aerobes :*** Methicillin susceptible Staphylococcus aureus, streptococcus pneumonia, streptococcus pyogenes, bacillus sp, corynebacterium (erythromycin and clarithromycin display the best activity).
- ***Gram-Negative Aerobes :*** H. influenza, M. catarrhalis, Neisseria sp. (Azithro> Clarithro>Erythro). Dont have activity against any Enterobacteriaceae
- ***Anaerobes :*** Activity against upper airway anaerobes.
- ***Atypical Bacteria :*** Excellent activity against atypical bacteria like : Legionella pneumophila – Drug of choice, Chlamydia, Mycoplasma, Ureaplasma.
- ***Other Bacteria :*** Mycobacterium avium complex, Treponema pallidum, Campylobacter, Borrelia, Bordetella, Brucella, Pasteurella.

### Pharmacokinetics :

- ***Erythromycin*** – variable absorption; food may decrease the absorption :
  - ☞ Destroyed by gastric acid that's why used as enteric coated tablet.
  - ☞ Esters (stearate) and ester salts (estolate) are more acid stable.
- ***Roxithromycin*** – long acting (half life – 12 hours. Therefore twice daily dosing), acid stable, food does not interfere with absorption.
- ***Clarithromycin*** – acid stable and well-absorbed regardless of presence of food. Half life – 6 to 7 hours, twice daily dosing.
- ***Azithromycin*** – More acid stable, food decreases absorption, half life is 68 hrs which permits OD dosing and shortening the duration of treatment (3 days).
- ***Erythromycin and Clarithromycin***– are *inhibitors* of cytochrome p450 system in the liver (enzyme inducers).

### Adverse Effects :

- ***Gastrointestinal :*** Nausea, vomiting, diarrhea, dyspepsia. Most common with erythromycin; less with new agents.
- ***Cholestatic hepatitis :*** Rare
- ***Thrombophlebitis :*** With IV Erythromycin and Azithromycin.
- ***Other :*** Ototoxicity (high dose erythromycin), QTc prolongation, allergy

### Drug Interactions :

- Erythromycin and Clarithromycin – are *inhibitors* of cytochrome p450 system in the liver (enzyme inducers); may increase concentrations of : Theophylline, Digoxin, Disopyramide, Carbamazepine, Valproic acid, Cyclosporin, Terfenadine, Astemizole, Phenytoin, Cisapride and Warfarin.

### Uses :

#### Erythromycin :

- ☞ Mycoplasma pneumoniae infections.
- ☞ Legionnaires Disease.
- ☞ Diphtheria.
- ☞ Whooping cough caused by B. Pertussis.
- ☞ Chlamydial infections.
- ☞ Anti-inflammatory property of erythromycin – asthma, rheumatoid arthritis and cystic fibrosis.
- ☞ Erythromycin is also motilin receptor agonist in GIT and improves gastric emptying and thus it is used in diabetic gastroparesis.

#### Roxithromycin :

- ☞ Uses are similar to erythromycin but are more preferred for upper respiratory tract infections like sinusitis, otitis media and pneumonia.
- ☞ **Dose :** 150 mg orally 12 hourly.

## Clarithromycin :

- Uses are similar to erythromycin. Certain additional uses of clarithromycin are :
  - MAC (mycobacterium avium complex) infection in AIDS.
  - H.pylori gastritis / peptic ulcer.
  - Ususal dose used is clarithromycin 500 mg BD.

## Azithromycin :

- Uses are similar to clarithromycin.
- Strep/Staph Infections; alternatives in patients allergic to Penicillin.
- It is highly effective against Chlamydia. A single dose of 1 gram is used in chlamydial cervicitis and urethritis.
- Mycobacterium avium complex infection in AIDS - alternative to clarithromycin.
- Community acquired pneumonia. **Dose :** 500 mg loading dose followed by 250 mg once daily for next 4 days.
- Skin and soft tissue infections.
- Respiratory tract infections.
- Acne vulgaris.

## Spiramycin :

- Its use is limited for treatment of toxoplasma gondii infection in pregnancy.

## KETOLIDES :

- **Drugs : Telithromycin and Cethromycin.**
- Telithromycin is a semisynthetic derivative of erythromycin with a keto group which makes it sensitive to macrolide resistant bacteria.
- **Mechanism of action :** is similar to macrolides.
- **Uses :** Macrolide resistant community acquired pneumonia, sinusitis, acute exacerbations of chronic bronchitis and streptococcal pharyngitis.
- **Adverse effects :** Nausea, vomiting, diarrhea, enzyme induction (increases levels of theophylline, terfenadine), prolongs QT interval.
- Cethromycin is more potent.

## LINCOSAMIDES :

- **Drugs : clindamycin, lincomycin.**
- **Mechanism of action :** is similar to macrolides.
- **Activity :** similar to macrolides.
- **Uses :** Severe anaerobic infection, Aerobic Gram positive cocci infection (but not MRSA) like liver abscess, staphylococcal bone and joint infections, topically for acne. Combination with pyrimethamine for AIDS related toxoplasmosis. Combination with primaquine for AIDS-related *pneumocystis carinii* pneumonia.

- **Dose :** The usual adult dose is 150-300 mg QID.
- **Adverse effects :** Antibiotic associated diarrhea (pseudomembranous colitis), Allergic reaction, Impaired liver function.

## GLYCOPEPTIDES :

- **Drugs : Vancomycin and Teicoplanin.**
- **Antibacterial activity :** Bactericidal for Gram positive bacteria (especially Gram positive cocci, including MRSA).
- **Mechanism of action :** Inhibit bacterial cell wall synthesis.
- **Uses :** Severe infection caused by MRSA, alternative for β-lactam antibiotics, enterococcal or staphylococcal endocarditis (combination with gentamicin), Pseudomembranous colitis.
- **Dose :** 1 gm IV given BD.
- **Adverse effects :** Hypersensitive reaction – it releases histamine (*e.g.* red man syndrome), ototoxicity, nephrotoxicity, nausea and gastritis.

## OXAZOLIDINONES :

- **Drugs : Linezolid, torzolid, radezolid.**
- **Mechanism of action :** is similar to macrolides.
- **Spectrum :** multidrug resistance Gram positive bacteria like MRSA (methicilin resistant staph aureus) and VRSA (vancomycin resistant staph aureus).
- **Dose :** Linezolid 600 mg BD (oral/iv).
- **Uses :** MRSA and VRSA infections, Skin infections, diabetic foot.
- **Adverse effects :** myelosuppression, neutropenia, thrombocytopenia (These adverse effects are less with second generation drugs like torzolid and radezolid).

## STREPTOGRAMINS (PRISTINAMYCIN) :

- It is a synergistic combination of Streptogramin-B (Quinupristin) and Streptogramin-A (Dalfopristin).
- **Mechanism of action :** They bind to 50 S ribosomal unit and prevent extrusion of newly synthesised peptide chain from the ribosome, leading to death of bacteria.
- **Spectrum :** Its spectrum closely resembles vancomycin and linezolid.
- **Uses :** vancomycin resistant enterococcus faecium, MRSA and VRSA infections, Skin infections.
- **Adverse effects :** injection site pain, thrombophlebitis, arthralgia.

## POLYMYXIN-B AND COLISTIN (POLYMYXIN-E) :

- Both are peptide antibiotics. Both are rarely used because of their toxicity.
- Colistin is used as colistin sulphate for oral and colistimethate sodium for parenteral use.
- **Mechanism of action :** Both, Polymyxin-B and colistin disrupt the integrity of bacterial cell membrane leading to leakage of intracellular constituents.

- **Spectrum :** They are effective mostly against gram negative bacteria except proteus, serratia and B. fragilis.
- **Uses :** Polymyxin-B is used topically mostly in combination for skin, ear and eye infections, colistin sulphate is given orally in GIT infections, colistimethate is used as inhalation for pulmonary infections like in cystic fibrosis, injectable for eye and bladder infection.
- **Adverse effects :** nephrotoxicity, flushing and bronchoconstriction due to histamine release, ataxia, paraesthesia.

**MUPIROCIN :**

- It is rapidly inactivated after absorption in the body, therefore, not used systemically and only used topically.
- **Mechanism of action :** inhibits bacterial protein synthesis.
- **Uses :** staphylococcal and streptoccal infections of skin like boils, furuncle, impetigo, ulcers, burns.

**FUSIDIC ACID :**

- Used topically.
- **Mechanism of action :** inhibits bacterial protein synthesis.
- **Uses :** staphylococcal and streptococcal infections of skin like boils, furuncle, impetigo, ulcers, burns.

❑❑❑❑❑

# 65 URINARY ANTI-SEPTICS AND TREATMENT OF URINARY TRACT INFECTION (UTI)

## URINARY TRACT INFECTION :

### Etiology :

- ***Acute uncomplicated UTI :*** Escherichia coli (80%), Klebsiella, Proteus, Streptococcus faecalis and Staphylococcus saprophyticus.
- ***Complicated UTI :*** Pseudomonas aeruginosa, Enterobacter & Serratia, Viruses - Rubella, Mumps and HIV, Fungi - Candida, Protozoa - Trichomonas vaginalis.

### Risk factors :

- Diabetes mellitus, urine retention, calculi, impaired immunity, shorter urethra, sexual intercourse, contraceptive devices, incomplete bladder emptying, prostatic hypertrophy, advanced age.

### Clinical features :

- Dysuria / burning micturition, increased frequency, hematuria, fever with chills, nausea and vomiting (pyelonephritis), flank pain (pyelonephritis).

### Treatment :

- ***Non-specific therapy :*** More water and fluid intake, removal of indwelling catheter, send urine for culture and sensitivity, start empiric therapy till the reports come, and change over to specific antibiotic after urine culture and sensitivity report comes.
- ***Antibiotic therapy :*** following regimes can be used :

  **Single dose therapy :**

  - Any of the following drugs is used :
    1. Trimethoprim 160 mg + sulphamethaxole 800 mg (*co-trimoxazole-DS).*
    2. Amoxycillin 500 mg + clavulanic acid 125 mg.
    3. Amoxycillin 3 gm.
    4. Ciprofloxacin 500 mg.
    5. Norfloxacin 400 mg.
  - Single dose therapy is for uncomplicated UTI. Not used for patients with past history of complicated UTI, antibiotic resistance and relapse with single dose.
  - ***Advantages :*** compliance, cost, less side effects, less resistance.
  - ***Disadvantages :*** increased recurrence or relapse.

**3 day therapy :**

- Efficacy same as 7 day therapy with less adverse effects.
- Drugs used include :
  1. Fluoroquinolones (*e.g.* ciprofloxacin 250-500 mg 12 hrly, ofloxacin 200-400 mg 12 hrly).
  2. TMP-SMZ (960 mg 12 hrly).
  3. Beta-lactam antibiotics (penicillins like Amoxycillin + clavulanic acid 625 mg 8 hrly, cephalosporins like cefixime 200 mg BD).
  4. ***Gentamicin :*** 80-120 mg i.v. 12 hrly.

**7 day therapy :**

- ***Useful in :*** recurrent cases, pregnancy, UTI with other risk factors. Same drugs used as mentioned above.

**14 day therapy :**

- For upper UTI (Pyelonephritis), for complicated UTI. Same drugs used as mentioned above but for 2 weeks.

**Catheter associated UTI :**

- Catheter removal before treatment is beneficial. Usually, infection is by pseudomonas aeruginosa. Treatment is by anti-pseudomonal penicillin combination (Piperacillin + tazobactum 4.5 gm 8 hrly).

## NITROFURANTOIN :

- It's a *urinary antiseptic.*
- Bacteriostatic but cidal at higher concentration.
- Reduced to reactive forms by bacterial nitroreductase - damage DNA, ribosomes. Damages bacterial DNA.
- **Adverse effects :** Hypersensitivity pneumonitis, GI upset, hemolytic anemia.
- Contraindications : Renal failure, neonates, pregnancy.
- **Dose :** 100 mg TDS for 10 days.

## PHENAZOPYRIDINE :

- *Urinary analgesic.*
- Orange color dye.
- Offers symptomatic relief from burning sensation, dysuria and urgency.
- It does not have antibacterial property.
- **Dose :** 200-400 mg TDS.

## ROLE OF URINARY PH IN UTI :

- Certain antimicrobials work better in acidic pH whereas some work better in alkaline pH.
- But, changing pH is seldom required because most of the antimicrobials used for UTI are well concentrated in urine and changing pH would not alter the outcomes much.

- Urine can be made acidic by vitamin C or cranberry juice and can be made alkaline by urinary alkaliser like disodium hydrogen citrate.
- The antimicrobials which work better in acidic pH are : Nitrofurantoin, tetracyclines and cloxacillin.
- The antimicrobials which work better in alkaline pH are : Fluoroquinolones, cephalosporins, Aminoglycosides and co-trimoxazole.

# 66 ANTI-TUBERCULAR DRUGS

Tuberculosis (TB) is a chronic infection caused by Mycobacterium tuberculosis. It can affect the lungs (pulmonary tuberculosis) or bones, joints, meninges, intestine etc. (extrapulmonary tuberculosis). It is more commonly seen in developing countries like India because of overcrowding, poor financial conditions, bad hygiene, lack of education and awareness and irrational use of antibiotics. Irrational use of antibiotics had lead to emergence of more dangerous variants of TB like MDR-TB (multiple drug resistant tuberculosis) and XDR-TB (Extensive drug resistant tuberculosis) which are difficult to treat.

## CLASSIFICATION OF ANTI-TB DRUGS :

### First line drugs :

- Isoniazid (H), Rifampicin (R), Ethambutol (E), Streptomycin (S), Pyrazinamide (Z).

### Second line drugs :

- Fluoroquinolones (ciprofloxacin, ofloxacin etc), Ethionamide, Prothionamide, Para amino salicylic acid (PAS), Cycloserine, Thiacetazone, Rifabutin and Rifapentin, Capreomycin, Aminoglycosides (Kanamycin / Amikacin).

### Newer drugs :

- Clarithromycin, Amoxycillin + clavulanic acid (Amoxiclav), Linezolid, Clofazimine, Bedaquiline, Pretomanid, Delamanid.

## FIRST LINE DRUGS :

### Isoniazid (H / INH) :

- Isonicotinic acid hydrazide. It's a prodrug.
- Bactericidal to actively growing mycobacteria / Bacteriostatic to dormant mycobacteria.
- ***Mechanism of action :*** Inhibits biosynthesis of mycolic acids which are important components of mycobacterial cell wall.
- Metabolism of INH is by acetylation. Two types of genetic variation is seen in acetylation. The first group is *rapid acetylators* (Japanese, Eskimos, 30-40% Indians) while the second group is of *slow acetylators* (Mediterranian jews, Egyptians and 60-70% Indians). The acetylator status of an individual decides the nature of INH toxicity.
- ***Adverse effects :***
  - ***Peripheral neuritis :*** It is more common in slow acetylators

because INH causes increased excretion of pyridoxine (vit. $B_6$) from urine and INH also inhibits conversion of pyridoxine to its active form pyridoxal phosphate. This neuropathy can be prevented by giving prophylactic vitamin $B_6$ *i.e.* pyridoxine in the dose of 10-40 mg per day.

- ***Hepatotoxicity :*** It is more common in fast acetylators because fast metabolism produces increased quantities of metabolised products like acetylisoniazid and acetylhydrazine which are hepatotoxic.
- ***Nausea, vomiting, gastritis, drug rash, allergic reaction.***

### Rifampicin (R) :

- Bactericidal, broad spectrum anti TB drug.
- Active against *Neisseria meningitides, Haemophilus influenzae, M.Leprae and S. aureus* also.
- It's a potent microsomal enzyme inducer.
- Usually given before breakfast.
- ***Mechanism of action :*** *Inhibit DNA dependent* RNA polymerase of bacteria.
- ***Uses :*** Tuberculosis, leprosy, H. influenza meningitis, prophylaxis of meningococcal meningitis, brucellosis.
- ***Adverse effects :***
  - *Secretions of body like tears, saliva, urine turns orange red in color.* This can make the patient frightened as it is perceived as blood and the patient can stop the treatment.
  - *Flu like syndrome* (fever, chills, myalgia).
  - *Hepatitis.*
  - *GI upset.*

### Ethambutol (E) :

- Bacteriostatic agent. All strain of *M. tuberculosis* sensitive including *M. avium.*
- ***Mechanism of action :*** Inhibits arabinosyl transferase which prevents polymerisation of arabinoglycans which are essential constituents of mycobacterial cell wall.
- ***Adverse effect :***
  - ***Optic neuritis*** : This leads to impairment of vision and also impairs red-green color discrimination. It should therefore be avoided in children less than 5 years of age where these problems can go unnoticed.
  - ***Hyperuricemia*** (This can precipitate gouty arthritis).
  - ***GI upset.***

### Streptomycin (S) :

- Bactericidal agent. Belongs to aminoglycoside group of antibiotics.

- Poorly absorbed from gut, therefore given as injection.
- ***Mechanism of action :*** Inhibits 30 S ribosomal protein synthesis of mycobacteria.
- ***Adverse effects :***
  - *Ototoxicity*
  - *Nephrotoxicity*

**Pyrazinamide (Z) :**

- Bactericidal agent.
- ***Mechanism of action :*** Inhibits Mycobacterial fatty acid synthase I enzyme and disrupts mycolic acid synthesis.
- ***Adverse effect :***
  - *Hepatotoxicity.*
  - *Hyperuricemia.*

**Doses of first line drugs :**

| Drug | Dose |
|---|---|
| Isoniazid (H) | 5 mg/kg (300 mg) |
| Rifampicin (R) | 10 mg/kg (600 mg) |
| Ethambutol (E) | 15 mg/kg (1000 mg) |
| Streptomycin (S) | 15 mg/kg (1000 mg) |
| Pyrazinamide (Z) | 25 mg/kg (1500 mg) |

## SECOND LINE DRUGS :

**Fluoroquinolones :**

- Already covered in fluoroquinolones chapter.

**Ethionamide :**

- It's a Tuberculostatic drug.
- It acts by inhibiting the synthesis of mycolic acid.
- The drug is not used commonly nowadays because the dose used is 1 gram per day which causes severe gastritis and neurological symptoms.
- It also causes Hepatotoxicity.

**Prothionamide :**

- It is a congener of ethionamide having similar pharmacology.
- The advantage is that it is better tolerated than ethionamide.
- ***Used*** for drug resistant TB.

**PAS (Para-aminosalicylic acid) :**

- It is structural analogue of PABA.
- It inhibits folic acid synthesis of mycobacteria.

- It causes severe GI disturbances which lead to poor compliance by patients.
- ***Dose :*** 8-12 gm/day in 3 divided doses.

**Cycloserine :**

- It is bacteriostatic.
- It acts by inhibiting bacterial wall synthesis.
- It is excreted unchanged in urine, therefore it is an excellent drug for renal tuberculosis. It is also used for MDR-TB.
- ***Dose*** is 500 mg BD.
- ***Adverse effects*** are peripheral neuropathy (prevented by prophylactic vit. $B_6$), dizziness, GI disturbances.

**Thiocetazone :**

- It is rarely used nowadays.
- Causes ototoxicity, hepatitis, neutropenia and thrombocytopenia.

**Rifabutin and Rifapentin :**

- Are structural analogues of rifampicin.
- Advantages are that they are less potent enzyme inducers, have longer plasma half lives and are having better activity against MAC (mycobacterium avium complex) infection as compared to rifampicin.

**Capreomycin :**

- It's a polypeptide antibiotic. Poorly absorbed from gut; given as injection.
- Usual dose is 1 g/day.
- ***Adverse effects*** are Ototoxicity and Nephrotoxicity.

**Aminoglycosides (kanamycin, amikacin) :**

- Already covered under aminoglycosides chapter.

## NEWER DRUGS :

- **Clarithromycin, Amoxycillin + clavulanic acid (Amoxiclav), Linezolid and Clofazimine.**
- These drugs are already covered under respective chapters.

**Bedaquiline :**

- It has a resemblance with fluoroquinolones chemically.
- It acts by inhibiting the enzyme ATP synthase of mycobacterium. Without this enzyme, the mycobacterium cannot generate energy.
- It is given orally as 400 mg OD for 2 weeks, then 200 mg thrice a week for next 22 weeks.
- It is reserved for MDR-TB.
- ***Adverse effects*** are Hepatotoxicity and Prolongation of QTc interval.

### Delamanid :

- It is new drug for treatment of drug resistant TB (MDR and XDR).
- It acts by inhibiting mycolic acid synthesis of mycobacterium.
- ***Dose*** is 100 mg OD.
- It is metabolised by CYP3A4.
- It can cause prolongation of QTc interval.

### Pretomanid :

- It is also a newer drug for drug resistant TB (MDR and XDR).
- It acts by dual mechanism. It acts by inhibiting mycolic acid synthesis of mycobacterium. It also acts as a respiratory poison like cyanide.
- ***Dose*** is 100 mg OD.
- It is relatively safe.
- No CYP3A4 drug interactions seen.

## REVISED NATIONAL TUBERCULOSIS CONTROL PROGRAMME 2017 :

The RNTCP had recommended DOTS (directly observed treatment short course) where the anti-TB drugs are given under direct supervision. Previously DOTS was given three days a week. But, this leads to high incidences of relapse, failure and emergence of resistance. Now, the anti-TB drugs are given on a daily basis. The anti-TB drugs are given in 2 phases : the intensive phase followed by continuation phase. The following regimes are recommended under RNTCP :

### Drug sensitive TB :

Here, the patients are divided into 2 categories : category I and II. Category I consists of all new patients and category II patients are those who were treated previously but had failure of treatment, relapse of TB or defaulted the treatment. In category I, drugs given are Isoniazid (H), Rifampicin (R), Pyrazinamide (Z) and Ethambutol (E) for 2 months in tensive phase followed by Isoniazid (H), Rifampicin (R) and Ethambutol (E) for 4 months. Total duration of treatment is 6 months.

| TB category | Intensive phase | Continuation phase | Total duration |
|---|---|---|---|
| **Category I** (New cases) | 2 HRZE | 4 HRE | 6 Months (2+4) |
| **Category II**<br>(Previously treated cases)<br>• Relapse<br>• Failure<br>• Default | 2 HRZES +<br>1 HRZE | 5 HRE | 8 Months<br>(2+1+5) |

In category II, the drugs given in intensive phase are Isoniazid (H), Rifampicin (R), Pyrazinamide (Z), Ethambutol (E) and Streptomycin (S) for 2 months followed by Isoniazid (H), Rifampicin (R), Pyrazinamide (Z) and Ethambutol (E) for 1 month and then followed by continuation phase with drugs Isoniazid (H), Rifampicin (R) and Ethambutol (E) for 5 months. Total duration of category II treatment is 8 months.

## MDR-TB (Multiple drug resistant TB) :

It is resistance to isoniazid and rifampicin with or without resistance to other drugs. The intensive phase consists of K-Kanamycin, L-levofloxacin, Eto-Ethionamide, C-cycloserine, Z-Pyrazinamide, E-Ethambutol for 6 months duration. After 6 months, patient will be reviewed based on the reports of sputum LC and DST (Liquid culture and drug susceptibility testing) and treatment is change to continuation phase if LC report is negative. If the 6th or 7th month LC report comes out to be positive, the intensive phase is extended for one month. Maximum extension upto 3 months can be done (Intensive phase 6-9 months). This is followed by continuation phase in which kanamycin is stopped and rest of the intensive phase drugs are continued upto 18 months. Pyridoxine 100 mg is given to prevent cycloserine neurotoxicity.

| TB category | Intensive phase | Continuation phase | Total duration |
|---|---|---|---|
| MDR-TB | K<br>L<br>Eto<br>C<br>Z<br>E<br>(6-9 Months) | L<br>Eto<br>C<br>Z<br>E<br>(18 Months) | 24-27 Months |

K-Kanamycin, L-levofloxacin, Eto-Ethionamide, C-Cycloserine, Z-Pyrazinamide, E-Ethambutol. **(Remember KLECZE and LECZE).**

## XDR-TB (Extensive drug resistant TB) :

It is type of MDR-TB where the mycobacteria are additionally resistant to fluoroquinolones and a second line injectable anti-TB drug like amikacin, kanamycin and or capreomycin. Here, the intensive phase consist of Capreomycin, Moxifloxacin, PAS, High dose Isoniazid, Clofazimine, Linezolid and Amoxiclav for 6 months followed by LC and DST testing, if negative then continuation phase started. If LC is positive, intensive phase is extended by 1 month and again LC and DST testing is done. Intensive phase can be extended by 1 month each for maximum of 6 months (Intensive phase 6-12 months). This is followed by continuation phase where injection capreomycin is stopped and rest of the drugs is continued for 18 months. The total duration of treatment is 24-30 months.

| TB category | Intensive phase | Continuation phase | Total duration |
|---|---|---|---|
| XDR-TB | C<br>M<br>P<br>HH<br>Cfz<br>L<br>A<br>(6-12 Months) | M<br>P<br>HH<br>Cfz<br>L<br>A<br>(18 Months) | 24-30 Months |

C-Capreomycin, M-Moxifloxacin, P-PAS, HH-High dose Isoniazid, Cfz-Clofazimine, L-Linezolid, A-Amoxiclav. **(Remember CMPHHCLA and MPHHCLA)**

### Chemoprophylaxis of TB :

It is indicated in :

1. All household contacts under 6 years of age.
2. Neonate of tubercular mother.
3. Children with positive mantoux test.
4. Patients of HIV, Diabetes, leukaemia who are showing positive mantoux test.

***Drug used :*** Isoniazid 10 mg/kg for 6 months.

### Role of corticosteroids in TB :

Corticosteroids should not be used normally in TB patients because it will worsen the infection. However, in certain scenarios we can use corticosteroids. They are :

- In meningeal, renal and pericardial TB, to reduce the exudation.
- In seriously ill patients, to reduce the inflammatory changes.
- In allergic reactions to anti-TB drugs.
- In HIV patients with severe manifestations.

# 67 ANTI-LEPROTIC DRUGS

Leprosy is also known as **'Hansen's Disease'**. It is a chronic granulomatous infection caused by Mycobacterium Leprae which is an Acid fast bacillus. It is called as Kustharoga in India. It is usually seen in Low socio-economic strata of society. Transmission is usually from person to person when the bacilli are shed from nose and skin lesions.

### Clinical features :

- Skin lesions, typically hypoaesthetic.
- Thickened peripheral nerves.
- Leonine faces.

### Classification of leprosy (Ridley-Jopling classification) :

- Lepromatous leprosy.
- Borderline lepromatous leprosy.
- Borderline leprosy.
- Tuberculoid leprosy.
- Borderline Tuberculoid leprosy.

For the purpose of categorising the patients for treatment, leprosy is classified into paucibacillary and multibacillary leprosy.

| Paucibacillary Leprosy | Multibacillary Leprosy |
|---|---|
| Tuberculoid | Lepromatous |
| Non-infectious | Infectious |
| Cell mediated immunity is normal | Cell mediated immunity is decreased |
| < 5 hypoasthetic lesions | > 5 hypoaesthetic lesions |
| Lepromin test +ve | Lepromin test –ve |
| Bacilli not seen on biopsy | Bacilli seen on biopsy |

## CLASSIFICATION OF ANTILEPROTIC DRUGS :

- **Sulphones :** Dapsone.
- **Phenazine derivative :** Clofazimine.
- **Antitubercular drugs :** Rifampicin, Ethionamide.
- **Other antibiotics :** Ofloxacin, Minocycline, Clarithromycin.

### Dapsone :

- Simplest, oldest, cheapest, most active & most commonly used drug.

- It is leprostatic drug.
- It is related to sulphonamides.
- Converted in body to DDS (diamino diphenyl sulphone).
- ***Mechanism of action :*** It inhibits bacterial folic acid synthesis.
- ***Dose :*** 100 mg/day orally.
- ***Uses :*** Paucibacillary leprosy, multibacillary leprosy, pneumocystis carinii pneumonia in AIDS patient, Nodulocystic acne, Pustular psoriasis, Madura foot, Actinomycosis.
- ***Adverse effects :*** Nonhemolytic anemia and methemoglobinemia in G6PD deficiency patients, nausea, vomiting, neuropathy, rash and Hepatotoxicity. During treatment with dapsone, some reactions occur which are called as lepra reaction.
- ***Type 1 lepra reaction :*** They are delayed hypersensitivity (type 4 allergic reaction) reactions to M. leprae antigens. It is characterised by cutaneous ulceration and various nerve involvements. Treatment is usually with Glucocorticoids like prednisolone.
- ***Type 2 lepra reaction (erythema nodosum leprosum) :*** They are humoral antibody response (type 3 allergic reaction) to dead leprae bacteria. It is acute onset, the lesions become enlarged, become red, inflamed and painful. Treatment is with clofazimine, Glucocorticoids and thalidomide.

## Clofazimine :

- It's a Phenazine dye.
- One of the primary antileprotic drugs along with dapsone.
- It has a potent anti-inflammatory action as well.
- It is bacteriostatic.
- ***Mechanism of action :*** Clofazimine binds to mycobacterial DNA to inhibit its templete function. Ultimately it inhibits mycobacterial growth.
- ***Dose :*** Usual dose is 50 mg/day orally.
- ***Uses :*** Leprosy and Chronic skin ulcers (Buruli ulcer) produced by *Mycobacterium ulcerans.*
- ***Adverse effects :*** Reddish black discoloration of skin, especially in fair complexion people, discoloration of hair & body secretions may also occur, phototoxicity, enteritis with intermittent loose stools, abdominal pain, diarrhea, nausea & vomiting, weight loss with higher doses.

## Rifampicin :

- Details covered under anti-tubercular drugs.

## Ofloxacin :

- Details covered under fluoroquinolone antibiotics.

### Minocycline :

- Details covered under tetracyclines (broad spectrum antibiotics).

## WHO REGIME FOR TREATMENT OF LEPROSY :

| For paucibacillary leprosy | For multiibacillary leprosy |
|---|---|
| • Dapsone 100 mg daily<br>• Rifampicin 600 mg once a month | • Dapsone 100 mg daily<br>• Rifampicin 600 mg once a month<br>• Clofazimine 50 mg daily for 29 days and 300 mg on 30$^{th}$ day |
| **Duration :** 6 months | **Duration :** 12 months |

❑❑❑❑❑

# 68 ANTI-FUNGAL DRUGS

**Most common fungal pathogens :**

- ***Dermatophytes*** – Microsporum, Epidermophyton and Trichophyton, Candida albicans, Aspergillus, Mucormycosis, Cryptococcus, Rhizopus.

**Superficial fungal infections :**

- ***Dermatophytes (ring worms) :*** Athlete's foot or tinea pedis, tinea cruris, tinea capitis etc. Candida : oral thrush, vaginitis and diaper candidiasis etc.

**Deep fungal infections :**

- ***Candidiasis :*** Mucocutaneous candidiasis, systemic candidiasis etc, Aspergillosis : broncho-pulmonary aspergillosis, Coccidiondomycosis : pulmonary and disseminated, Histoplasmosis : (common in HIV).

**CLASSIFICATION OF ANTIFUNGALS :**

- **Drugs that increase cell membrane permeability (Polyenes) :**
  Amphotericin B and Nystatin.
- **Drugs that inhibit Ergosterol synthesis (Azole antifungals) :**
  Clotrimazole, Miconazole, Ketoconazole, Fluconazole, Itraconazole and Voriconazole.
- **Drugs that inhibit protein synthesis :**
  5-Flucytosine.
- **Drugs that inhibit Ergosterol+lanosterol synthesis :**
  Terbinafine.
- **Drugs that inhibit fungal cell wall synthesis (Echinocandins) :**
  Capsofungin, Micafungin.
- **Drugs that cause disruption of mitotic spindle :**
  Griseofulvin.
- **Miscellaneous topical agents :**
  Ciclopirox, Tolnaftate, Nystatin, Topical azoles.

**Polyenes :**

**Amphotericin B :**

- ***Mechanism of action :*** It binds to the ergosterol in the fungal cell

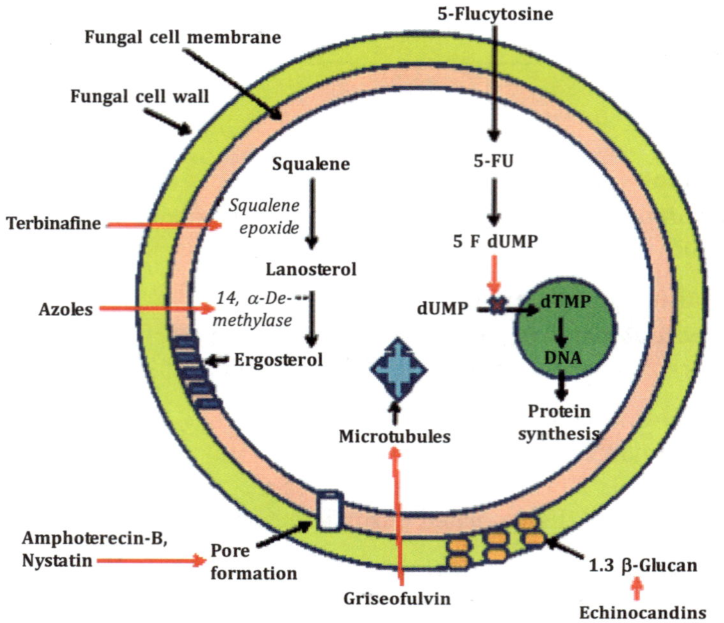

*Mechanism of action of all antifungals*

membrane (high affinity for ergosterol present in fungal cell membrane, affinity is less for host cell membrane) and forms pores. Cell contents and nutrients leak out from these pores leading to fungal cell death.

- ***Uses :*** It is a broad spectrum antifungal useful for :
  1. Oral, vaginal and cutaneous candidiasis.
  2. Cryptococcal meningitis
  3. Histoplasmosis
  4. Invasive Aspergillosis
  5. Mucormycosis
  6. Blastomycosis
  7. Leishmaniasis (Reserve drug for resistant cases of Kala Azar)

- ***Dose :*** 0.5-0.6 mg/kg/day as slow IV infusion in 5% glucose.

- ***Adverse effects :*** It is the most toxic antifungal agent :
  - Nephrotoxicity.
  - Acute reactions - Chills, Nausea, Vomiting, Pain, Fever, Aches, Dyspnea.
  - Thrombophlebitis.
  - Bone marrow depression.
  - On intrathecal injection – Headache, Vomiting, Nerve paralysis.
  - **Newer Amphotericin B preparations.**

- *They are developed to overcome :*
    1. Side effects of amphotericin-B.
    2. To improve tolerability.
    3. To get the drug at site of action.
    4. To reduce the toxicity *i.e.* less nephrotoxic (they deliver amphotericin-B selectively to ergosterol of fungi).
- *Formulations are :*
    1. Amphotericin B lipid complex.
    2. Amphotericin B colloidal dispersion.
    3. Liposomal Amphotericin B.

    (Only drawback of these formulations is that they are costly)

☞ ***Drug Interactions of Amphotericin B :***

- With Flucytosine - synergistic action.
- With Vancomycin and Aminoglycoside – Both increase risk of nephrotoxicity.

## Nystatin :

☞ Similar to Amphotericin B but more toxic than Amphotericin B.

☞ Used only topically for superficial candidiasis of Skin, Mouth, Vagina, Intestine.

☞ As ointment, oral tablets & suppositories.

☞ Available as tablets and ointments (1 to 5 lacs U) – also vaginal tablets.

## Azole antifungals :

☞ **Clotrimazole, Miconazole, Ketoconazole, Fluconazole, Itraconazole, Voriconazole and Posaconazole.**

☞ ***Mechanism of action :*** Azoles bind to 14$\alpha$-demethylase and inhibiting the production of ergosterol which is important component of fungal cell membrane.

## Ketoconazole :

☞ ***Spectrum :*** Generally used in mucosal infections only (dermatophytosis)

☞ ***Pharmacokinetics :*** Variable oral absorption, dependent on pH (often given with cola or fruit juice). T½ = 7-10 hours. Topical shampoos available.

☞ ***Adverse effects :*** Nausea and vomiting, Hepatotoxicity, Gynecomastia, oligospermia, decreased libido, microsomal enzyme inhibitor.

## Fluconazole :

☞ Water soluble having wider range of activity than Ketoconazole.

☞ Good activity against C. albicans and Cryptococcus neoformans.

- ***Dosing :***
  - **Mucosal candidiasis :** 100-200 mg/day (150 mg tablet vulvovaginal candidiasis).
  - **Systemic fungal infections :** 400-800 mg q24h.

**Itraconazole :**

- Orally active triazole. Broader spectrun than Ketoconazole and Fluconazole – includes moulds like aspergillus.
- Lacks adverse effects of Ketoconazole.

**Voriconazole :**

- It is a newer azole antifungal which has good CSF penetration and its absorption is not dependent on gastric pH.
- ***Uses :*** invasive aspergillosis, esophageal candidiasis.
- ***Dose :*** 200 mg 12 hourly.

**Topical azoles :**

- Popular local azoles are – Clotrimazole, Miconazole (For Tinea, Ring worm, Athlete's foot, otomycosis, oral, cutaneous & vaginal candidiasis).
- Mechanism of action is same as that of Ketoconazole *i.e.* ergosterol inhibition.
- Clotrimazole is *favored in vaginitis* because of long lasting residual effect and once daily dosing.
- Available as lotion, cream, powder, vaginal tablet etc.

## 5-Flucytosine :

- Fluorinated pyrimidine related to anticancer drug 5-fluorouracil (5FU).
- **Kinetics :** Orally absorbed, widely distributed even in CSF, converted in fungal cell to 5-FU which is antimetabolite.
- Mammalian cells remain unaffected except few bone marrow cells.
- **Mechanism of action :** Inhibits fungal DNA / Protein synthesis.
- **Uses :** It is used in combination with Amphotericin-B because there is increased uptake of 5-FC in the fungal cell when given with Amphotericin-B (synergistic effect). This combination is used for Candidiasis, Cryptococcal meningitis.
- **Adverse effects :** Bone marrow depression, loss of hair, nausea.

## Terbinafine :

- Belongs to a newer allylamine class of antifungals. Given both orally & locally.
- Fungicidal in contrast to azoles (fungistatic).
- **Mechanism of action :** Acts by non-competitive inhibition of "squalene epoxidase" (early step enzyme in ergosterol synthesis) – accumulation of squalene in fungal cells – cidal effect

- **Use :** Used for fungal infections of nails, tinea, athlete foot, pityriasis versicolor & candida infection.
- **Adverse effects :** With oral : GIT upset, Hepatic dysfunction, Rash, Taste disturbance (No interaction with CYP450). On local application - dryness, Erythema, Rash, itching etc.
- **Preparations and doses :** 1% cream, 125/250 mg tablets, Tinea pedis : 250 mg OD for 2-6 weeks, Onychomycosis : 250 mg OD 3-12 months.

## Echinocandins :

- Capsofungin, micafungin.
- **Mechanism :** Inhibit fungal cell wall synthesis by inhibiting 1,3 β glucan synthesis.
- **Uses :** Invasive aspergillosis, esophageal candidiasis.
- Not absorbed orally therefore given as slow IV infusion.
- **Adverse effects :** Thrombophlebitis, abnormal liver functions, flushing, rash.

## Griseofulvin :

- Used for superficial fungal infections caused by dermatophytes.
- Derived from Penicillium griseofulvum.
- Effective against most dermatophytes, but not against candida causing deep mycosis.
- Dermatophytes actively concentrate it – accounts for selective toxicity against them. It is taken up by newly formed keratin.
- **Mechanism of action :** causes disruption of fungal mitotic spindle.
- **Pharmacokinetics :** Given orally and fats improve absorption. Absorption depends on the particle size. Microsomal enzyme inducer.
- Duration of treatment depends upon tissue turn over (3-6 weeks for skin & hair and 3-6 months for nails). Should continue till whole infected tissue is shed off.
- **Uses and dose :** Used orally only for dermatophytosis (125 to 250 mg 4 times daily) but depends on site of infection.
- **Adverse effects :** GIT upset, CNS symptoms, Hepatotoxicity, Leucopenia, Photo-sensitivity, Allergy etc.

## Topical antifungals :

### Ciclopirox :

- Used as 1% cream and lotion for topical management of superficial fungal infections like candidiasis and tenia versicolor. It acts by inhibiting membrane uptake of amino acids by fungus.

### Tolnaftate :

- It is also used for topical treatment of fungal infections.
- It acts by distorting hyphae of fungi.
- Relapses are common.

# 69 ANTI-VIRAL DRUGS (Non-retroviral)

### STRUCTURE OF A VIRUS :

A virus consists of a core genome (DNA or RNA) surrounded by protein shell (Capsid) and which is surrounded by a membrane (envelope).

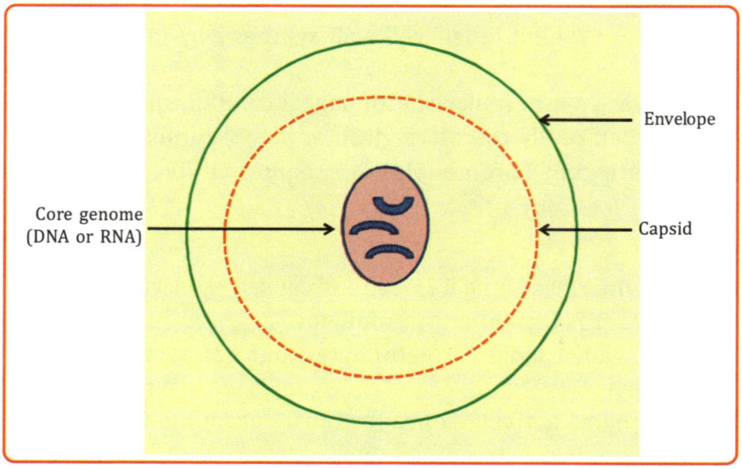


### TYPES OF VIRUSES :

#### DNA viruses :

- ***Adenovirus*** (Respiratory tract infections).
- ***Hepadna virus*** (Hepatitis-B).
- ***Herpes virus*** (*Herpes simplex type 1* : herpes labialis, oral herpes, ocular herpes), (*Herpes simplex type 2* : genital herpes), (*Varicella zoster virus* : chickenpox, herpes zoster or shingles), (*Cytomegalovirus* : CMV retinitis in AIDS) and (*Epstein Barr virus* : infectious mononucleosis, B cell lymphoma).
- ***Poxvirus*** (smallpox).
- ***Papilloma virus*** (warts or papillomas).

#### RNA viruses :

- ***Orthomyxovirus*** (*Influenza virus* which causes Influenza, $H_1N_1$ *virus* which cause swine flu).
- ***Rotavirus*** (diarrhea in children).
- ***Picorna virus*** (*Poliovirus* – polio, *Hepatovirus* – Hepatitis-A).

- ***Paramyxovirus*** (*Respiratory syncitial virus* – respiratory tract infections, *Morbillivirus* – Measles, *Rubulavirus* – mumps).
- ***Rhabdovirus*** (Rabies).
- ***Arbovirus*** (chickengunya, dengue, yellow fever, encephalitis).
- ***Retrovirus*** (HIV virus, human T-cell leukaemia virus).

## STEPS OF VIRAL REPLICATION :

### DNA virus :

- ***Step 1*** : Attachment of DNA virus to host cell.
- ***Step 2*** : Penetrates the host cell by endocytosis.
- ***Step 3*** : Capsid is removed and genome containing DNA is released.
- ***Step 4*** : After the entry of viral genome in the nucleus, its DNA is transcribed into viral m-RNA by host's RNA polymerase.
- ***Step 5*** : Host cell's ribosomes utilise this viral m-RNA for synthesising viral enzymes and proteins.
- ***Step 6*** : Replication of viral DNA by DNA polymerase.
- ***Step 7*** : Assembly of virus components to form a fully matured virus (Virion).
- ***Step 8*** : Release of virion by budding.

### RNA virus :

- ***Step 1*** : Attachment of DNA virus to host cell.
- ***Step 2*** : Penetrates the host cell by endocytosis.
- ***Step 3*** : The $M_2$ protein (ion channels) of the virus then allow an influx of $H^+$ ions in the virion.
- ***Step 4*** : RNA virus is released in the cytoplasm of host cell.
- ***Step 5*** : There is synthesis of viral m-RNA from viral genomic RNA with the help of RNA polymerase enzyme.
- ***Step 6*** : Host cell's ribosomes utilise this viral m-RNA for synthesising viral enzymes and proteins.
- ***Step 7*** : Viral RNA replication can also take place via cRNA using RNA polymerase.
- ***Step 8*** : Assembly of virus components to form a fully matured virus (Virion).
- ***Step 9*** : Release of virion by budding. Neuraminidase which is an important enzyme present in virions plays an important role in release of virions.

## CLASSIFICATION OF ANTIVIRAL DRUGS :

- **Anti-herpes virus agents :**

  Acyclovir, Valacyclovir, Ganciclovir, Valganciclovir, Penciclovir, Famciclovir, Cidofovir, Foscarnet, Vidarabine, Idoxuridine, Trifluridine.

- **Anti-influenza agents :**
  Amantadine, Rimantadine, Ribavirin, Oseltamivir, Zanamivir, Peramivir.

- **Anti-hepatitis-B virus agents :**
  Entecavir, Telbivudine, Adefovir dipivoxil, Tenofovir, Interferons, Lamivudine (anti-HIV drug).

- **Anti-hepatitis-C virus agents :**
  Ribavirin, Interferons, Boceprevir, Sofosbovir, Daclatasvir, Ledipasvir.

- **Anti-respiratory syncitial (RSV) virus agents :**
  Ribavirin, Palivizumab.

- **Anti-papilloma virus agents :**
  Imiquimod.

## Anti-herpes virus agents :

### Acyclovir and valacyclovir :

- ***Mechanism of action :*** Acyclovir is first converted to its active metabolite acyclovir triphosphate which then inhibits viral DNA polymerase and prevents its replication by terminating the elongation of viral DNA chain. Valacyclovir is a prodrug which is converted to acyclovir and has advantage that its bioavailability is more and requires less frequent dosing.
- ***Effective against the following :*** Herpes simplex virus type 1 (HSV-1), Herpes simplex virus type 2 (HASV-2), Varicella zoster virus (VZV), Epstein-barr virus (EBV), Cytomegalovirus (CMV).
- ***Uses :***
  - Herpes labialis.
  - Herpes esophagitis, herpes keratitis.
  - Ocular herpes, genital herpes, chickenpox and shingles (VZV).
- ***Formulations :*** Oral tablets, parenteral and ointment.
- ***Dose :*** Orally 400 mg TDS or 200 mg 4-5 times a day.
- ***Adverse effects :*** **Local** : stinging and burning sensation on application, **Oral** : headache, nausea, malaise, **IV** : rash, sweating, emesis, hypotension, neurologic toxicity (*e.g.* tremors, delirium, seizures, disorientation, hallucinations and coma).

### Ganciclovir and valganciclovir :

- They are analogue of acyclovir having similar mechanism of action. Valganciclovir is a prodrug of ganciclovir.
- ***Uses :*** They are used for treatment of serious and vision threatening CMV retinitis in AIDS patient. They are also used for acyclovir resistant HSV infections.
- ***Adverse effects :*** Myelosuppression, fever, phlebitis, pain.

**Penciclovir and Famciclovir :**

- Penciclovir is structurally related to acyclovir with similar mechanism of action. It is used mainly for acyclovir resistant HSV strains.
- Famciclovir is a prodrug which is converted to penciclovir. The bioavailability of the resultant penciclovir is more. Topical penciclovir is used for herpes labialis, acute localized varicella zoster infections.

**Cidofovir :**

- Effective against HSV resistant to acyclovir and CMV resistant to ganciclovir.
- Gets converted to cidofovir diphosphate.
- ***Uses :*** AIDS patients with CMV retinitis especially in ganciclovir failed cases; and also in acyclovir resistant mucocutaneous herpes simplex in immunocompromised.
- ***Adverse effects :*** Nephrotoxicity and hypersensitivity reactions.

**Foscarnet :**

- ***Mechanism of action :*** Inhibits viral DNA polymerase and reverse transcriptase.
- ***Spectrum :*** Effective against HSV (resistant to acyclovir), CMV (ganciclovir resistant), other herpes viruses and HIV.
- ***Drawback :*** Low viral selectivity, toxicity high, kidney damage, anemia, phlebitis, tremor, convulsion.
- ***Uses :*** CMV retinitis and other CMV infections in AIDS, acyclovir resistant mucocutaneous herpes simplex type 2 and VZV infection in AIDS.

**Vidarabine :**

- ***Mechanism of action :*** Inhibits viral DNA polymerase.
- Because of its poor GIT absorption, poor lipid solubility, it is used only topically.
- ***Uses :*** HSV keratoconjunctivitis not responding to idoxuridine.

**Idoxuridine and trifluridine :**

- It is iodinated derivative of deoxyuridine.
- ***Mechanism of action :*** Inhibits viral DNA polymerase.
- ***Uses :*** It is used only topically for HSV keratoconjunctivitis.
- ***Adverse effects :*** Irritation in the eye, corneal blurring, lacrimation and photophobia.
- ***Trifluridine :*** It is a derivative of idoxuridine which is used topically in patients unresponsive to topical idoxuridine or vidarabine.

## Anti-influenza agents :

**Amantadine and Rimantadine :**

- Tricyclic amine unrelated to any nucleic acid precursor. to treat Influenza A (not Influenza B), resistant to $H_5N_1$ (avian) and $H_1N_1$ (swine).

- ***Mechanism of action :*** It inhibits the uncoating of the viral genome and also viral assembly in late step, specifically targets a protein called $M_2$ (an ion channel) but inactive against Influenza B, which lacks $M_2$ protein.
- ***Uses :*** Prophylaxis of Influenza A (epidemic or seasonal); treatment of influenza and parkinsonism.
- ***Dose :*** 100 mg BD or 200 mg OD.
- ***Adverse effects :*** Nausea, anorexia, insomnia and some CNS side effects (nightmares and scary hallucinations).
- ***Rimantadine*** – methyl derivative of amantadine with similar actions and uses.

**Ribavirin :**

- ***Mechanism of action :*** It inhibits the synthesis of viral mRNA.
- Its oral absorption is rapid and its bioavailability increases with fatty foods. It can also be given as aerosol.
- ***Uses :*** *As aerosol* : Treatment of Influenza and Respiratory syncitial virus infections. *As oral tablets* : (800-1200 mg / day) along with injectable interferon $\alpha_{2b}$ is used to treat chronic hepatitis C infection.
- ***Adverse effects :*** Worsening of COPD, can be teratogenic or mutagenic in nature.

**Oseltamivir (TAMIFLU) :**

- ***Broad spectrum :*** Against Influenza A and B, $H_5N_1$ (bird flu) and $H_1N_1$ (swine flu).
- ***Mechanism of action :*** Neuraminidase inhibitor (important for viral progeny release).
- ***Pharmacokinetics :*** Oseltamivir is a prodrug that is activated in the GIT and liver to oseltamivir carboxylate. well absorbed orally (bioavailability - 80%), excreted by kidney. Plasma half life is 6-10 hrs.
- ***Uses :*** Prophylaxis and treatment of Influenza A and B, $H_5N_1$ and $H_1N_1$. (Reduces the severity, duration and complications).
- ***Dose :*** 75 mg bd for 5 days.
- ***Adverse effects :*** Gastric irritation like nausea and vomiting, headache, weakness, seizures, cough and insomnia.

**Zanamivir :**

- ***Mechanism of action :*** Neuraminidase inhibitor (important for viral progeny release).
- Oral bioavailability of zanamivir is very less; therefore it is used as disc inhaler.
- ***Uses :*** Prophylaxis and treatment of Influenza A and B, $H_5N_1$ and $H_1N_1$. (Reduces the severity, duration and complications).
- ***Dose :*** 10 mg bd inhalation for treatment and od for prevention.
- ***Adverse effects :*** Nasal irritation and bronchosecretions.

### Peramivir :

- It is a newer drug belonging to same league of oseltamivir and zanamivir.
- ***Mechanism of action :*** Neuraminidase inhibitor (important for viral progeny release).
- Oral bioavailability is low therefore used as IV.
- ***Uses :*** It is used for emergency treatment of hospitalised patients of $H_1N_1$ (swine flu) infection especially those who are resistant to oseltamivir and zanamivir.

## Anti-hepatitis-B virus agents :

### Entecavir :

- ***Mechanism of action :*** Inhibits viral DNA polymerase and thus inhibits its replication.
- ***Uses :*** It is used in patients with chronic Hepatitis-B infections in adults with HIV or without HIV especially lamivudine resistant cases.
- ***Dose :*** 0.5-1 mg od orally.
- ***Adverse effects :*** Headache, nausea, dizziness.

### Telbivudine :

- ***Mechanism of action :*** Inhibits viral DNA polymerase and thus inhibits its replication.
- ***Uses :*** It is used in patients with chronic Hepatitis-B infections.
- ***Adverse effects :*** Headache, nausea, elevated creatinine phosphokinase.

### Adefovir dipivoxil :

- It is effective against hepatitis B virus and other DNA viruses.
- ***Mechanism of action :*** After entering cell, it is phosphorylated to diphosphate which has high affinity for hepatitis B virus DNA polymerase and not to host DNA polymerase. Adevofir gets incorporated in DNA and terminates DNA chain.
- ***Uses :*** Chronic hepatitis B, lamivudine resistant cases and hepatitis B with concurrent HIV infection.
- ***Doses :*** 10 mg/day.
- ***Adverse effects :*** Headache, sore throat, flu syndrome, nephrotoxicity.

### Tenofovir :

- It is an anti-retroviral drug but also effective against Hepatitis-B.
- It has low oral absorption, therefore administered as prodrug (tenofovir disoproxil).
- ***Mechanism of action :*** Inhibits Hepatitis-B viral DNA polymerase and also HIV reverse transcriptase (low affinity for host DNA polymerase).
- ***Uses :*** 300 mg daily in Hepatitis-B virus infection (including lamivudine resistant cases).

**Interferons :**

- Interferons are cytokines produced by host cells in response to viral infections; they are body's defence against viral infection.
- ***Mechanism of action :*** They bind to cell surface receptors and act on multiple steps of viral replication like viral penetration, viral synthesis of mRNA, assembly, and release of virions.
- ***Types of interferons :*** α, β, γ. But, only *Interferon α-2a and Interferon α-2b* are available for use as IM and SC preparations. Pegylated forms are available for SC use (peg IFN$\alpha_{2a}$ longer duration than peg IFN$\alpha_{2b}$).
- ***Uses :*** Chronic hepatitis-B infection, AIDS related Kaposi's sarcoma, chronic hepatitis-C, hairy cell leukaemia, anogenital warts.
- ***Dose :*** 3 mU three times weekly SC or IM.

**Lamivudine :**

- It is an antiretroviral drug used for HIV-AIDS belonging to class Nucleoside reverse transcriptase inhibitors (NRTI).
- ***Mechanism of action :*** It gets incorporated in viral (hepatitis-B) DNA by DNA polymerase and terminates DNA chain elongation. It also inhibits DNA polymerase.
- ***Uses :*** HIV, Hepatitis-B.

## Anti-hepatitis-C virus agents :

**Ribavirin :**

- Already covered under anti-influenza agents.

**Interferons :**

- Already covered under anti-Hepatitis-B agents.

**Boceprevir :**

- It is an oral drug for hepatitis-C infection.
- ***Mechanism of action :*** It inhibits non-structural proteins of hepatitis-C virus namely NS 3/4 A.
- It is mainly used along with pegylated interferons $\alpha_{2a}$ and $\alpha_{2b}$.

**Sofosbuvir :**

- It is an orally effective nucleotide analogue.
- ***Mechanism of action :*** Inhibits RNA dependent RNA polymerase of Hepatitis-C virus.
- It is used along with pegylated interferons $\alpha_{2a}$ and $\alpha_{2b}$ and ribavirin.
- ***Adverse effects :*** Headache, nausea, vomiting, joint pain.

**Daclatasvir and Ledipasvir :**

- ***Mechanism of action :*** They inhibit non-structural proteins of hepatitis-C virus namely NS 5 A.

- They are usually given in a combination along with sofosbuvir.
- ***Adverse effects :*** Headache, nausea, vomiting, joint pain.

## Anti-respiratory syncitial (RSV) virus agents :

**Ribavirin :**

- Already covered under anti-influenza agents.

**Palivizumab :**

- It is a monoclonal antibody against RSV (Respiratory syncitial virus).
- ***Mechanism of action :*** It neutralises RSV and inhibits its fusion with host cell membrane.
- ***Use :*** Used to prevent RSV infection in high risk patients especially infants and neonates with bronchopulmonary dysplasia.
- ***Dose :*** 15 mg/kg IM once a month for 5 months.
- ***Adverse effects :*** Pain at the injection site, elevated serum aminotransferases.

## Anti-papilloma virus agents :

**Imiquimod :**

- It is a topical antiviral preparation.
- ***Mechanism of action :*** It acts as immunomodulator and causes production of cytokines such as interferons.
- ***Use :*** For management of warts on external genitalia and perineal warts/ condyloma acuminate caused by human papilloma virus.
- ***Preparation :*** 5% cream.
- ***Adverse effects :*** Local burning, irritation and itching.

# 70 ANTI-RETROVIRAL DRUGS (Anti-HIV Drugs)

- AIDS (Acquired immunodeficiency syndrome) caused by HIV (Human immunodeficiency virus) is one of the most dreadful infections in the world. HIV attaches to cells with $CD_4$ receptors ($T_4$ cells and macrophages).
- The 3 important enzymes necessary for growth and survival of HIV virus are :
  - ☞ **Reverse transcriptase, Integrase and Protease.**

## HIV LIFE CYCLE :

- ***Step 1*** : Attachment of virus at the $CD_4$ receptor and chemokine co-receptors $CXCR_4$ or $CCR_5$.
- ***Step 2*** : Viral fusion and uncoating.
- ***Step 3*** : Reverse transcriptase makes a single DNA copy of the viral RNA and then makes another to form a double stranded viral DNA.
- ***Step 4*** : Migration to nucleus.
- ***Step 5*** : Integration of the viral DNA into cellular DNA by the enzyme integrase.
- ***Step 6*** : Transcription and RNA processing.
- ***Step 7*** : Protein synthesis.
- ***Step 8*** : Protease cleaves polypeptides into functional HIV proteins and the virion (newly formed virus) assembles.
- ***Step 9*** : Virion budding.
- ***Step 10*** : Virion maturation.

## CLASSIFICATION OF ANTIRETROVIRAL DRUGS :

- ***Nucleoside reverse transcriptase inhibitors (NRTI) :*** Zidovudine, Stavudine, Lamivudine, Abacavir, Zalcitabine, Emtricitabine and Didanosine.
- ***Non-nucleoside reverse transcriptase inhibitors (NNRTI) :*** Efavirenz, Nevirapine, Delaviridine.
- ***Nucleotide reverse transcriptase inhibitors (NtRTI) :*** Tenofovir.
- ***Protease inhibitors (PI) :*** Ritonavir, Saquinavir, Indinavir.
- ***Entry / Fusion inhibitors (EI) :*** Enfuvirtide.
- ***Integrase inhibitors (II) :*** Raltegravir.
- ***CCR-5 inhibitors (CCRI) :*** Maraviroc.

### Mechanism of action :

- ***NRTI :*** Inhibition of reverse transcriptase enzyme.
- ***NNRTI :*** Inhibition of reverse transcriptase enzyme.
- ***NtRTI :*** Inhibition of reverse transcriptase enzyme.
- ***PI :*** Inhibition of Protease enzyme.
- ***EI :*** Inhibition of entry and fusion of virus in host $CD_4$ + cells.
- ***Integrase inhibitors :*** Inhibition of Integrase enzyme.
- ***CCRI :*** Inhibition of Chemokine co-receptor 5.

### Uses :

- ***HIV 1 and 2 :*** The therapy with anti-retroviral drugs is called as HAART (highly active anti-retroviral therapy). One of the following combinations can be used :

  *NRTI (2) + NNRTI (1) or NRTI (2) + PI (1) or NRTI (1) + NNRTI (1) + PI (1).*
- ***Other uses :*** HTLV 1 and HTLV 2 (zidovudine), Hepatitis-B (Lamivudine), Post exposure prophylaxis.

### Adverse effects :

- ***NRTI :*** Lactic acidosis, Severe hepatomegaly, Hepatic steatosis, Peripheral neuropathy.
- ***NNRTI :*** Steven Johnson syndrome, Elevated liver enzymes.
- ***PI :*** Hyperglycemia, Hyperlipidemia.
- ***EI :*** As it is given by injectable route it causes local reactions at injection site like nodule, rash etc.
- ***CCRI :*** Hepatotoxicity.

❑❑❑❑❑

# 71 ANTI-MALARIAL DRUGS

Malaria is caused by plasmodium and transmitted by the bite of female Anopheles mosquito.

**Types of plasmodium :**

- Plasmodium vivax, Plasmodium ovale, Plasmodium falciparum, Plasmodium malariae.

**Clinical features :**

- Fever with chills and rigors, headache, bodyache, fatigue, lethargy, nausea and, vomiting, splenomegaly.

**Lifecycle of plasmodium :**

- Lifecycle of malarial parasite is divided into sexual cycle, which occurs in mosquito (definitive host) and asexual cycle which occurs in man (intermediate host).
  - ☞ ***Step 1*** : The female anopheles mosquito is first infected by biting a malaria patient, from which male and female gametes are sucked in mosquito.
  - ☞ ***Step 2*** : The male and female gametes form zygote in the gut of mosquito which is then differentiated to oocyst.
  - ☞ ***Step 3*** : The oocyst form sporozoites which migrate in the salivary glands of the mosquito.
  - ☞ ***Step 4*** : When this infected mosquito bites a normal person, the sporozoites are released in his blood to begin the asexual cycle.
  - ☞ ***Step 5*** : The sporozoites cannot survive in the circulation; therefore they take shelter in the liver where they get transformed into schizonts (Tissue schizonts). This is called as *pre-erythrocytic stage*.
  - ☞ ***Step 6*** : The tissue schizonts in the liver mature in 1-3 weeks to form merozoites which are then released in the circulation.
  - ☞ ***Step 7*** : Now starts the eryhthrocytic cycle where, the merozoites enter the RBCs (erythrocytes) to form trophozoites.
  - ☞ ***Step 8*** : These trophozoites undergo schizogony to form blood schizonts, which then form more merozoites. The RBCs infected with merozoites eventually rupture causing release of

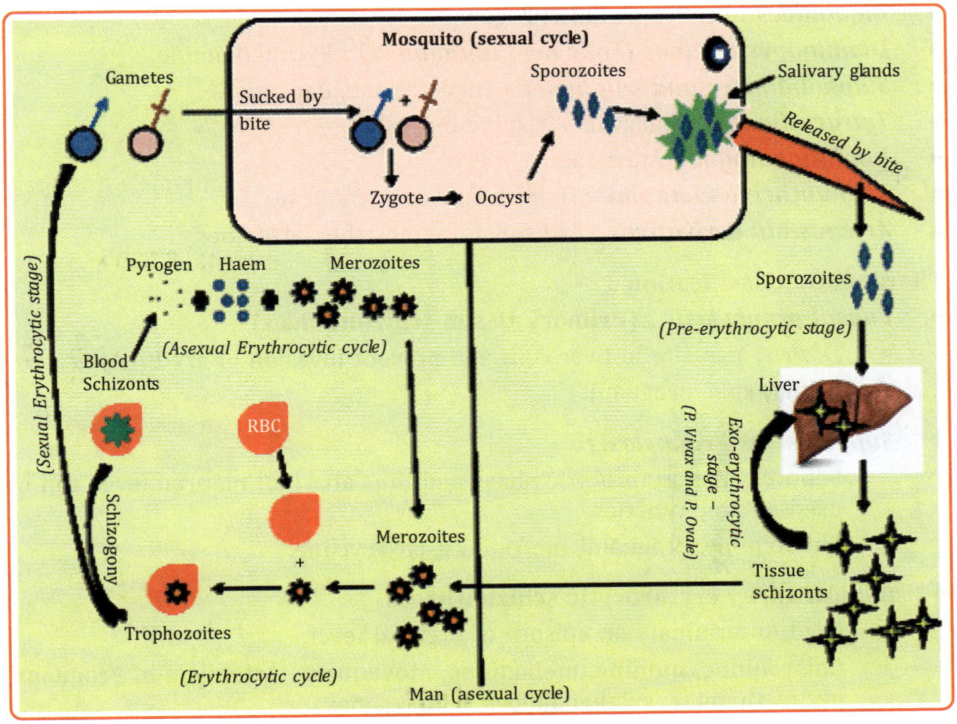


merozoites, along with hem and pyrogens in the circulation, which causes the symptoms of malaria.

- ☞ ***Step 9*** : The released merozoites then invade fresh RBCs and the cycle continues. This is called as *asexual erythrocytic cycle.*
- ☞ ***Step 10*** : Merozoites from the trophozoites also undergo *sexual erythrocytic phase*, in which there is formation of male and female gametes, which are then sucked by mosquito during the bite to a malaria patient.
- ☞ ***Step 11*** : In patients of P. vivax and P. ovale, some of the schizonts after release from the liver, re-enter another liver cells and form dormant forms which are called as hypnozoites (sleeping plasmodia). This is called as *exo-erythrocytic stage.* These hypnozoites can get released in the circulation after some days of malaria treatment and can cause relapse of malaria.

## CLASSIFICATION OF ANTIMALARIAL DRUGS :

### Chemical classification :

- ***4-aminoquinolines :*** Chloroquine, Amodiaquine, Pyronaridine, Piperaquine.
- ***8-aminoquinolines :*** Primaquine, Tafenoquine, Bulaquine.
- ***Cinchona alkaloid :*** Quinine, Quinidine.
- ***Quinoline-methanol :*** Mefloquine.

- ***Biguanides :*** Proguanil, Chlorproguanil.
- ***Diaminopyrimidines (Folic acid antagonist) :*** Pyrimethamine.
- ***Sulphonamides and sulphones :*** Sulphadoxine, dapsone.
- ***Tetracyclines :*** Tetracycline, doxycycline.
- ***Naphthoquinone :*** Atovaquone.
- ***Phenanthrine-methanol :*** Halofantrine, Lumefantrine.
- ***Artemisinin derivatives :*** Artesunate, artemether, arteether.

**Therapeutic classification :**

- ***Causal prophylaxis :* (Primary tissue schizonticides)**
  - Destroy parasite in liver cells and prevent invasion of erythrocytes.
  - Primaquine, proguanil.
- ***Suppressives Prophylaxis :***
  - Suppress the erythrocytic phase and thus attack of malarial fever, can be used as prophylactics.
  - Chloroquine, proguanil, mefloquine, doxycycline.
- ***Clinical cure :* erythrocytic schizonticides**
  - Used to terminate an episode of malarial fever.
  - Chloroquine, quinine, mefloquine, atovaquone, artemisinin, Proguanil, pyrimethamine, sulphonamides, tetracyclines.
- ***Radical cure :***
  - Eradicate all forms of P. vivax & P. ovale from the body including hypnozoites.
  - Suppressive drugs + hypnozoitocidal drugs.
- ***Gametocidal :***
  - Destroy gametocytes and prevent transmission.
  - Primaquine, Chloroquine, quinine.

## 4-aminoquinolines :

### Chloroquine :

- ***Mechanism of action :*** Chloroquine enters the lysosome of plasmodium (malarial parasite) and gets trapped inside and inhibits peptide formation. It also inhibits the parasite enzyme hem polymerase and thus protects the host's hem from being converted to hemozoin. The free hem is toxic to the malarial parasite.
- ***Pharmacokinetics :*** Well absorbed, plasma half life is 3-10 days, 60% protein bound, Concentrated in liver, spleen, kidney, lungs, leucocytes. Shows selective accumulation in retina : ocular toxicity.
- ***Uses :***
  - *Hepatic amebiasis.*

- *Giardiasis.*
- *Rheumatoid arthritis (Hydroxychloroquine).*
- *Discoid Lupus Erythematosus.*
- *Lepra reaction.*
- *Infectious mononucleosis.*

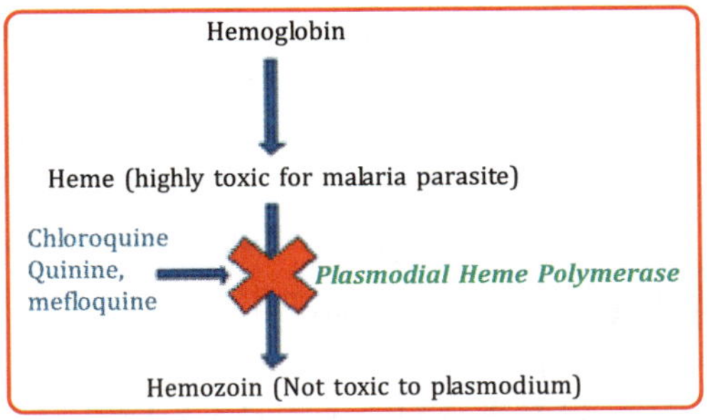


- ***Dose :*** 600 mg of base stat, 300 mg base after 8 hours, 300 mg base on 2nd day and 300 mg base on 3rd day (250 mg oral tablet of chloroquine phosphate consists of 150 mg base).
- ***Adverse effects :*** Nausea, vomiting, anorexia, skin rashes, angioneurotic edema, photosensitivity, pigmentation, exfoliative dermatititis, Ocular toxicity (High dose prolonged therapy), temporary loss of accommodation, Lenticular opacities, subcapsular cataract, retinopathy : constriction of arteries, edema, blue black pigmentation, constricted field of vision, ST & T wave abnormalities, abrupt fall in BP.

**Amodiaquine :**

- Pharmacological actions similar to Chloroquine.
- ***Mechanism of action :*** Similar to Chloroquine.
- Chloroquine resistant strains may be effective.
- ***Adverse effects :*** GIT intolerance, headache, photosensitivity and rarely agranulocytosis.

**Pyronaridine and piperaquine :**

- These are Chloroquine analogues having similar pharmacological profile like Chloroquine.
- They are most commonly used in artemisinin based combination therapy (ACTs).

## 8-aminoquinolones :

**Primaquine :**

- ***Mechanism of action :*** It is converted to quinine metabolite which inhibits coenzyme-Q (Interferes with oxygen transport system) of malarial parasite
- ***Activity :*** Active against liver hypnozoites. Weak action against erythrocytic stage of vivax, so used with suppressives in radical cure. No action against erythrocytic stage of falciparum. Has gametocidal action and is most effective antimalarial to prevent transmission of disease against all 4 species.
- ***Dose :*** 15 mg daily for 14 days.

- ***Use :*** Primary use is radical cure of relapsing malaria along with Chloroquine.
- ***Adverse effects :*** Epigastric distress, abdominal cramps, Hemolytic anemia in G6PD deficiency patients.
- *Tafenoquine and Bulaquine* are newer congeners of primaquine.

## Cinchona alkaloids :

**Quinine :**

- Isolated from cinchona bark.
- ***Mechanism of action :*** Similar to Chloroquine.
- ***Uses :***
    - *Uncomplicated resistant falciparum malaria* (dose is 600 mg orally TDS for 7 days alone or with pyrimethamine 75 mg + sulphadoxine 1500 mg as single dose or with doxycycline 100 mg orally OD for 7 days).
    - *Cerebral malaria* (dose quinine dihydrochloride 600 mg is diluted in 500 ml of 5% dextrose and infused slowly over 4 hours. 300 mg is then repeated every 8 hourly till the patient can take orally).
    - *Nocturnal muscle cramps* : 200–300 mg before sleeping.
- ***Adverse effects :*** Cinchonism (Tinnitus, nausea, vomiting, headache, mental confusion, vertigo, difficulty in hearing, visual disturbances, diarrhea, flushing, marked perspiration, still higher doses cause exaggerated symptoms with delirium, fever, tachypnea, respiratory depression and cyanosis), cardiovascular toxicity : cardiac arrest, hypotension, fatal arrhythmias and hypoglycemia.

## Quinoline-methanol :

**Mefloquine :**

- Developed to deal with chloroquine resistant malaria.
- ***Mechanism of action :*** Similar to Chloroquine.
- Rapidly acting erythrocytic schizonticide, slower than chloroquine & quinine.
- ***Use :*** Treatment of uncomplicated falciparum in MDR malaria; should be used along with artesunate (Astemisinin based combination therapy).
- ***Adverse effects :*** Bitter in taste, nausea, vomiting, abdominal pain, diarrhea, anxiety, hallucinations, sleep disturbances, psychosis, errors in operating machinery, convulsions, bradycardia, sinus arrhythmia, QT prolongation and Teratogenicity (Avoid in first trimester).

## Biguanides :

**Proguanil :**

- Biguanide converted to cycloguanil active compound.

- ***Mechanism of action :*** It inhibits plasmodial dihydrofolate reductase enzyme. As a result dihydrofolic acid (active form of folic acid) is not formed. Non-availability of dihydrofolic acid prevents synthesis of purines and pyrimidines which are essential for plasmodial nucleic acid synthesis.
- Act slowly on erythrocytic stage of vivax & falciparum. Prevents development of gametes.
- ***Use :*** Not a drug for acute attack. Used for causal prophylaxis : 100–200 mg daily.
- ***Adverse effects :*** Stomatitis, mouth ulcers, larger doses depression of myocardium, megaloblastic anemia.

## Folic acid antagonists :

**Pyrimethamine :**

- Diaminopyrimidine more potent than proguanil & effective against erythrocytic forms of all species of plasmodia.
- ***Mechanism of action :*** Similar to proguanil.
- ***Use :*** Used for clinical cure of falciparum malaria. Sulphadoxine + pyrimethamine can also be used as adjunct with quinine for Chloroquine resistant falciparum malaria. Other use is toxoplasmosis.
- ***Adverse effects :*** Megaloblastic anemia, thrombocytopenia, agranulocytosis.

## Sulphadoxine + Pyrimethamine :

- Causes sequential blockade (refer chapter on sulphonamides).
- Not recommended for prophylaxis.
- ***Use :*** Single dose treatment of uncomplicated chloroquine resistant falciparum malaria, patients intolerant to Chloroquine. First choice treatment for toxoplasmosis.
- ***Dose :*** Sulphadoxine 500 mg + pyrimethamine 25 mg, 3 tablets once for acute attack.

## Tetracyclines :

- ***Mechanism of action :*** Refer chapter on tetracyclines (Broad spectrum antibiotics).
- Slow but potent action on erythrocytic stage of all plasmodia & pre-erythrocytic stage of falciparum.
- Always used in combination with quinine or Sulphadoxine + Pyrimethamine for treatment of chloroquine resistant malaria.

## Naphthoquinone :

**Atovaquone :**

- ***Mechanism of action :*** It disrupts the plasmodial mitochondrial electron transport of the respiratory process.

- Proguanil potentiates the action of atovaquone, therefore used as a fixed dose combination of atovaquone + proguanil.
- ***Uses :*** Chemoprophylaxis and treatment of falciparum malaria (combination of atovaquone + proguanil), pneumocystis carinii pneumonia as a second choice to co-trimoxazole and toxoplasmosis.
- ***Adverse effects :*** Nausea, vomiting, abdominal pain, allergic rash.

## Phenanthrine-methanol :

### Halofantrine and Lumefantrine :

- They have potent schizonticidal properties against plasmodium of all 4 types.
- It has no gametocidal property and also doesn't work against hepatic forms of malarial parasite.
- ***Mechanism of action :*** They inhibit plasmodial proton pump.
- Bioavailability is not consistent and is enhanced by food.
- Halofantrine causes potential cardiotoxicity, hence not used much.
- Lumefantrine is a newer congener of this group which is devoid of cardiotoxicity and is mostly used in combination with artemether because the combination have synergistic effect against multidrug resistant falciparum malaria.

## Artemisinin derivatives :

- ***E.g.* Artesunate, Artemether, Arteether, Artelinate, Arterolane.**
- Artemisinin is the active principle of the plant artimisnia annua (Chinese herb). The active metabolite is *dihydroartemisnin*.
- ***Mechanism of action :*** These compounds have presence of endoperoxide bridge in their structure. The plasmodial heme iron cleaves this endoperoxide bridge. This results is generation of highly reactive free

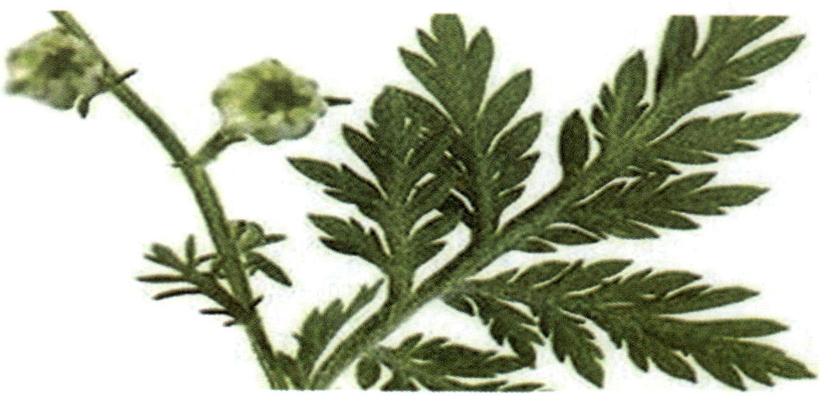

*Artemisnia annua*

radicals which damage plasmodial membrane by covalently binding to membrane proteins.

- Most potent and rapid acting blood schizonticides. They do not have effect on erythrocytic or exo-erythrocytic hypnozoites) phase.
- They have short duration of action.
- Artesunate is water soluble. It can be given orally, IV or IM.
- Artemether is oil soluble. It can be given orally or IM.
- Arteether is oil soluble. It can be given IM only.
- ***Uses :*** Cerebral malaria, chloroquine resistant malaria, multidrug resistant malaria.
- ***Adverse effects :*** They are well tolerated. Nausea, vomiting, abdominal pain and temporary QT prolongation can occur.

## ARTEMISNIN BASED COMBINATION THERAPY (ACT) :

| Sr. No. | Combination used (Act) | Dose |
|---|---|---|
| 1 | Artemether + Lumefantrine (1:6) | Artemether 80 mg BD for 3 days + Lumefantrine 480 mg BD for 3 days. |
| 2 | Artesunate + Mefloquine | Artesunate 100 mg BD for 3 days + Mefloquine 750 mg on 2nd day and 500 mg on 3rd day. |
| 3 | Artesunate + Pyrimethamine & | Artesunate 100 mg BD for 3 days + Pyrimethamine 75 mg & Sulphadoxine 1500 mg on day 1. |
| 4 | Artesunate + Amodiaquine (1:3) | Artesunate 100 mg BD for 3 days + Amodiaquine 300 mg BD for 3 days. |
| 5 | Artesybate + Pyronaridine (1:3) | Artesunate 100 mg BD for 3 days + Pyronaridine 300 mg BD for 3 days. |
| 6 | Dihydroartemisnin + Piperaquine (1:8) | Dihydroartemisnin 120 mg OD for 3 days + Piperaquine 960 mg OD for 3 days. |
| 7 | Arterolane + Piperaquine | Arterolane 150 mg OD for 3 days + Piperaquine 750 mg OD for 3 days. |

- It is a combination therapy involving artemisnin derivatives along with other anti-malarial drugs.
- ***Uses :*** Cerebral malaria, chloroquine resistant malaria, multidrug resistant malaria.
- ACTs are not recommended for pregnant (1st trimester) patients and children below 5 kg.
- WHO has recommended 5 ACTs to be used, the last 2 are recommended by National drug policy on malaria (NDPM), Ministry of health and family welfare, government of India.

## MANAGEMENT OF MALARIA :

### Chemoprophylaxis of malaria :

- It is given for prevention of malaria, especially to those people who are travelling to a malaria endemic area.
- ***Chloroquine sensitive malaria :*** Chloroquine 600 mg base on 1st and last day orally and in between 300 mg / week, followed by primaquine 0.5 mg/kg orally.
- ***Chloroquine resistant falciparum malaria :*** Mefloquine 200 mg once a week starting 1 week before and ending 4 weeks after leaving or Doxycycline 100 mg daily one day before travel and till a month after return from the endemic area.
- ***Multidrug resistant falciparum malaria :*** Atovaquone 250 mg + Proguanil 100 mg orally 2 days prior till 7 days after return.

### Clinical cure of malaria : (Acute attack of malaria)

- The asexual schizogony phase is responsible for clinical symptoms of malaria, therefore blood schizontocides can be used to terminate acute attack of malaria.
- Since, falciparum doesn't exhibit exo-erythrocytic stage, the clinical cure itself provides radical cure of malaria, whereas in vivax and ovale, exo-eryhthrocytic stage should also be treated with primaquine for radical or complete cure of malaria.
- ***Chloroquine sensitive malaria :*** Chloroquine 600 mg base stat (2 tablets of 300 mg each) followed by 300 mg base after 8 hours and 300 mg base on 2nd day and 300 mg base on 3rd day (250 mg oral tablet of chloroquine phosphate consists of 150 mg base). This is followed by Primaquine 15 mg daily orally for 15 days in case of vivax and ovale. The second option is Pyrimethamine 75 mg + Sulphadoxine 1500 mg single dose in choloroquine intolerance.
- ***Chloroquine resistant falciparum malaria :*** Quinine 600 mg orally TDS for 7 days alone or with pyrimethamine 75 mg + sulphadoxine 1500 mg as single dose or with doxycycline 100 mg orally OD for 7 days. Another option is Mefloquine 750 mg orally stat followed by 500 mg 12 hours later. Alternatively, we can give Artesunate 100 mg orally BD on 1st day followed by 100 mg OD for another 5 days. Lastly, we can also give Arteether 150 mg IM once daily for 3 days as an alternative.
- ***Multidrug resistant falciparum malaria :*** Atovaquone 1000 mg + Proguanil 400 mg orally OD for 3 days.
- ***Complicated falciparum malaria / Cerebral malaria :*** Quinine dihydrochloride 600 mg is diluted in 500 ml of 5% dextrose and infused slowly over 4 hours. 300 mg is then repeated every 8 hourly till the patient can take orally.

### Radical cure :

- Since, falciparum doesn't exhibit exo-erythrocytic stage, the clinical cure itself provides radical cure of malaria, whereas in vivax and ovale, exo-eryhthrocytic stage should also be treated with primaquine (15 mg OD orally for 15 days) for radical or complete cure of malaria.

### Acute malaria in pregnant women :

- Chloroquine is given in usual doses.
- Mefloquine is contraindicated in first trimester.
- Primaquine and tetracycline avoided due to Teratogenicity.
- Pregnant women usually have anemia, therefore iron and folic acid supplementation should be given along with antimalarials.

# 72 ANTI-AMEBIC AND ANTI-PROTOZOAL DRUGS

**Different types of protozoal infections are :**

- Amebiasis, Giardiasis, Trichomoniasis, Trypanosomiasis, Toxoplasmosis, Leishmaniasis, Cryptosporidiosis, Pneumocystis carinii (jiroveci) infection.

## AMEBIASIS :

- Caused by *Entameba Histolytica.*
- Mode of transmission is by feco-oral route.
- **Clinical features :** Asymptomatic, amebic diarrhea, amebic dysentery and liver abscess.

## LIFE CYCLE OF E. HISTOLYTICA :

Entameba histolytica exists in **two forms** :

***1. Cysts (infective) :***

- They can survive outside the human body.

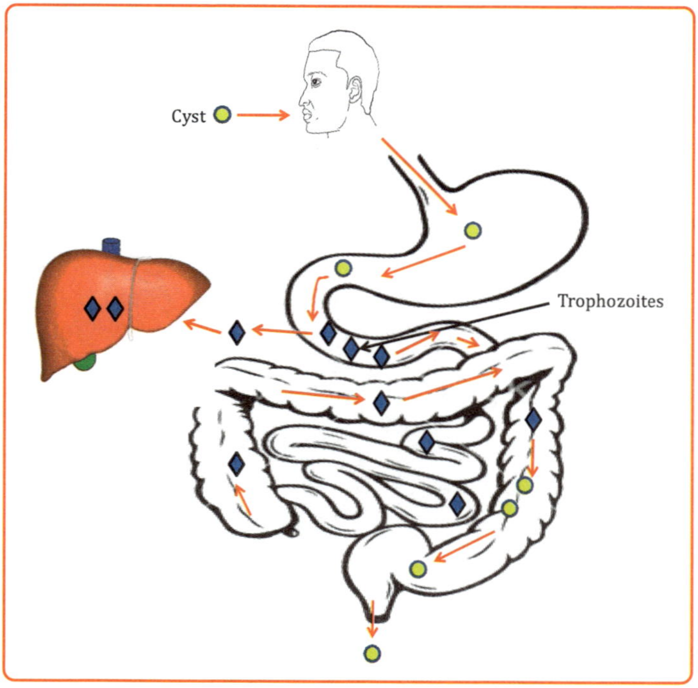

- They are ingested through food and water.
- They transform to trophozoites in the intestine.

2. *Trophozoites (non-infective; invasive) :*
   - Can reproduce.
   - They may feed on intestinal bacteria or invade and ulcerate wall of large intestine, and may migrate to liver or other tissues.
   - Finally, transform to cysts which are excreted in feces.

## CLASSIFICATION OF ANTI-AMEBIC DRUGS :

### Tissue Amebicidal drugs :

- ***For intestinal & extraintestinal amebiasis :***
  - **Nitroimidazoles :** Metronidazole, Tinidazole, Ornidazole, Secnidazole and Satranidazole.
  - **Alkaloids :** Emetine and Dehydroemetine.
- ***For extraintestinal amebiasis :*** Choloroquine.

### Luminal (Intestinal) amebicidal drugs :

- ***Amides :*** Diloxanide furoate, Nitazoxanide.
- ***8-Hydroxyquinolines :*** Iodoquinol.
- ***Antibiotics :*** Tetracyclines and paramomycin (Aminoglycoside).

### Nitroimidazoles :

**Metronidazole (prototype of this group) :**

- They have broad specrum cidal activity against protozoa, including *Giardia lamblia.*
- ***Spectrum :*** E. Histolytica, G. Lamblia, T. Vaginalis, H. Pylori, Cl. perfringens, Cl. difficile, Anaerobic streptococci and Guineaworm.
- ***Mechanism of Action :*** It enters the cell by diffusion then its nitro group is reduced by redox proteins to highly reactive nitro radical which exerts cytotoxicity by damaging DNA & other important components of the Entameba and protozoa.
- ***Pharmacokinetics :***
  - Completely absorbed from intestine.
  - Widely distributed in the body.
  - Metabolised in liver & excreted in urine.
  - Plasma half life is 8 hrs.
- ***Uses :***
  - *Amebiasis :* For intestinal amebiasis, the dose of Metronidazole is 400 mg TDS for 7 days and for amebic dysentery and amebic liver abscess, the dose is 800 mg TDS for 7 days. Metronidazole is drug of choice for extraintestinal amebiasis as it kills the trophozoites, but

the cysts are not killed, hence in intestinal amebiasis, it should be used with luminal amebicidal like Diloxanide furoate.

- *Giardiasis* (Metronidazole 200 mg orally TDS for 7 days).
- *Trichomonas vaginalis* (400 mg TDS orally for 7 days. Male partner should be treated simultaneously).
- *Oral ulcers.*
- *Pseudomembranous enterocolitis.*
- *Anaerobic bacterial infections.*
- *Helicobacter pylori gastritis/peptic ulcer.*
- *Guinea worm infestations.*

☞ ***Adverse effects :*** Anorexia, nausea, metallic taste, abdominal cramps, headache, dryness of mouth, dizziness, rashes, peripheral neuropathy and thrombophlebitis on IV infusion.

☞ ***Drug interactions :*** A disulfiram like intolerance to alcohol occurs (inhibits Aldehyde dehydrogenase enzyme); patients should avoid drinking alcohol when they are taking metronidazole.

**Tinidazole :**

☞ Second generation congener. Longer acting - once daily dose. Short course - 2 g daily, single dose for 3 days. Actions similar to Metronidazole. Better tolerated. Effective against cysts of E. histolytica.

☞ ***Uses :*** Amebiasis, Trichomoniasis, Giardiasis, H pylori.

**Secnidazole, Ornidazole :**

☞ Longer acting. Plasma half life is 17-29 hours.

☞ Single 2 gm dose is given.

☞ ***Uses :*** Amebiasis, Trichomoniasis, Giardiasis, Non specific vaginosis.

**Satranidazole :**

☞ Longer acting. Plasma half life is 14 hours.

☞ Better tolerability.

☞ No nausea, vomiting and metallic taste.

☞ No neurological effects or disulfiram like reaction.

☞ Does not produce acetamide metabolite which is a weak carcinogen.

## Alkaloids (Emetine and Dehydroemetine) :

☞ **Source :** Cephaelis Ipecacuanha. They are potent & directly acting amebicide.

☞ **Mechanism of action :** Inhibits protein synthesis.

☞ Not given orally as it is vomited out. Was also used for scorpion bite.

☞ **Adverse effects :** Toxicity is high (Cardiotoxicity). Therefore, withdrawn from market and no longer used.

## Chloroquine :

- Antimalarial drug. Tissue Amebicide especially against Amebic Hepatitis & Liver Abscess. Concentrated in liver; kills trophozoites of E. histolytica. Not effective for amebic colitis or luminal amebae because absorbed in upper part of intestine.
- ***Use :*** Hepatic amebiasis/abscess; not responding to Metronidazole.

## Luminal amebicide :

**Diloxanide Furoate :**

- Highly effective against cysts.
- ***Pharmacokinetics :*** Given orally, in gut splits into Diloxanide & furoic acid. 90% Diloxanide is absorbed & conjugated to form glucuronide : excreted in urine.
- ***Mechanism of action :*** Directly kill trophozoite responsible for production of cyst.
- ***Single course :*** High cure rate in mild intestinal amebiasis and asymptomatic cyst passers.
- Given after tissue amebicidal drug to eradicate cysts.
- ***Dose :*** 500 mg TDS for 10 days.
- ***Adverse effects :*** Flatulence, nausea, itching, urticaria.

**Nitazoxanide :**

- It's a Prodrug.
- With oral administration, it is rapidly hydrolysed to active metabolite, tizoxanide.
- ***Mechanism :*** Interference with PFOR enzyme dependent electron transfer reaction.
- ***Uses :*** Giardiasis, Cryptosporidiasis, Amebic dysentery.
- ***Adverse effects :*** Abdominal pain, nausea, vomiting, diarrhea, headache.

**8-Hydroxyquinolines (Iodoquinol) :**

- Luminal amebicide used with metronidazole to treat amebic infections. Only effective against trophozoites in lumen. 90% unabsorbed → amebicide, 10% absorbed → metabolised to glucuronides, excreted in urine. Half life 11-14 hrs.
- ***Adverse effects :*** Iodism (Dermatitis, urticaria, pruritus, fever), Diarrhea, anorexia, nausea, vomiting, abdominal pain, Headache, severe neurotoxicity, SMON (Subacute myelo-optic neuropathy).

**Paramomycin sulphate :**

- Aminoglycoside antibiotic. Not significantly absorbed. Less toxic. Superior to Diloxanide furoate in clearing asyptomatic infections. No effect on extra-intestinal amebic infections. Also used in visceral leishmaniasis parenterally.

- ***Adverse effects :*** Abdominal Distress & diarrhea.

**Tetracycline :**

- Disturbs the symbiosis between normal intestinal flora & E. Histolytica; amebae grow at expense of normal intestinal flora. Tetracyclines are broad spectrum antibiotics & kill these floras leading to death of E. histolytica also.
- Used in resistant and chronic cases.

## GIARDIASIS :

- Caused by Giardia lamblia.
- Characterised by watery diarrhea and malabsorption.
- **Treatment :** Metronidazole is 200 mg TDS for 7 days or Tinidazole 600 mg TDS orally for 7 days or 2 gm as single dose or Furazolidone 100 mg QID orally for 7 days. Furazolidone is a nitrofuran derivative which is also effective against trichomonas, shigella and other gram negative bacteria, and is used in food poisoning, diarrhea and bacillary desentery.

## TRICHOMONIASIS :

- Caused by Trichomonas vaginalis.
- It is a genital infection which can result in vulvovaginitis, frothy yellow foul smelling discharge. Males might be asymptomatic.
- Both partners should be treated at the same time, otherwise it may result in relapses.
- **Treatment :** Metronidazole 400 mg TDS for 7 days or Tinidazole 600 mg TDS orally for 7 days or 2 gm as single dose.

## LEISHMANIASIS (KALA-AZAR) :

- Caused by Leishmania donovani which causes visceral leishmaniasis (Kala-azar), Leishmania tropica and major cause cutaneous leishmaniasis and leishmania brazilensis cause mucocutaneous leishmaniasis.
- Transmitted by sandfly.
- **Kala-azar (visceral leishmaniasis) :** enlargement of lymph nodes, liver and spleen.
- Cutaneous and mucocutaneous leishmaniasis : elevated ulcerative lesions.
- **Treatment :**
  - ***Sodium stibogluconate :***
    - Pentavalent antimonial compound.
    - **Mechanism :** causes rapid efflux of glutathione from the protozoa.
    - Causes severe gastritis, therefore given IV or IM.

- ***Miltefosine :***
  - It is an oral drug used for kala-azar.
  - It inhibits key enzyme involved in the metabolism of protozoa.
  - 100 mg OD is given orally for 28 days.
- ***Other agents used :***
  - Amphotericin-B (antifungal).
  - Pentamidine.

## CRYPTOSPORIDIOSIS :

- **Treatment :**
  - Paramomycin 500 mg TDS orally for 10 days or
  - Nitazoxanide 500 mg BD orally for 3 days or
  - Azithromycin 500 mg OD orally for 21 days.

## TOXOPLASMOSIS :

- Caused by toxoplasma gondii.
- Transmitted through cats.
- Causes higher occurrence of infertility and miscarriages.
- **Treatment :**
  - Pyrimethamine along with clindamycin and folinic acid or
  - Pyrimethamine along with sulphadiazine and folinic acid or
  - Atovaquone.
  - Spiramycin which is a macrolide (if the patient is pregnant).

## PNEUMOCYSTIS CARINII / JIROVECI INFECTION :

- **Treatment :**
  - Co-trimoxazole *i.e.* trimethoprim + sulphamethoxazole (already covered) or
  - Dapsone or
  - Clindamycin or
  - Atovaquone.

# 73 ANTI-HELMINTHIC DRUGS

- Helminthes; means worms.
- Helminthiasis is a global problem but, more common in developing countries with poorer personal and surrounding hygiene.
- They are commonly transmitted through feco-oral route thus gastrointestinal tract becomes the common site of lodgement.

## Clinical features :

- Acute or chronic blood loss leading to anemia, dysentery, diarrhea, abdominal pain, malabsorption, subcutaneous nodules, allergic reactions, urticaria, injury to the visceral organs, intestinal or lymphatic obstruction, conjunctivitis, retinitis, blindness, hepatosplenomegaly and various nutrient deficiency.

## Types of Worms :

| Nematodes | Trematodes (Flukes) | Cestodes (Tape worms) |
|---|---|---|
| • **Roundworm**<br>*Ascariasis*<br>• **Hook worm**<br>*A. duodenale,*<br>*N. Americans*<br>• **Pinworm**<br>*Enterobiasis*<br>• **Threadworm**<br>*Strongyloides*<br>• **Whipworm**<br>*Trichuris trichuria*<br>• **Guinea worm**<br>*D. medinensis*<br>• **Filariasis**<br>*Wucheria bancrofti*<br>• **Trichinosis**<br>*Trichinella spiralis* | • **Blood flukes**<br>• **Liver flukes**<br>• **Lung flukes**<br>• **Intestinal flukes**<br>• **Schistosomiasis**<br>*Schistosoma sp* | • **Beef-tapeworm**<br>*Tenia saginata*<br>• **Pork-tapeworm**<br>*Tenia solium*<br>• **Fish tapeworm**<br>*D. latum*<br>• **Dwarf tapeworm**<br>*H. nana*<br>• **Dog tapeworm or hydatid worm**<br>*Echinococcus granulosus* |

## ANTI HELMINTHIC DRUGS :

- **Benzimidazoles : Albendazole, Mebendazole, Thiabendazole.**

- **Pyrantel pamoate.**
- **Piperazine.**
- **Levamisole, Tetramisole.**
- **Diethyl carbamazine.**
- **Ivermectin.**
- **Niclosamide.**
- **Praziquantel.**

## BENZIMIDAZOLES :

### Mebendazole :

- Congener of thiabendazole. Became popular because of it retained broad spectrum antihelminthic activity but not the toxicity of its predecessors. Action of mebendazole is slow, takes 2-3 days to develop. No fasting or purging is required.
- ***Mechanism of action :*** It binds to β-tubulin of worms and inhibits its polymerisation. It acts probably by blocking glucose uptake by parasites and depletion of its glycogen stores. Microtubules in the worms are gradually lost.
- ***Uses :*** It is a broad spectrum anti-helminthic drug and is used for various helminthic infestations such as :

| As $1^{st}$ choice | |
|---|---|
| *Roundworm, Hookworm, Whipworm* | 100 mg BD for 3 days |
| *Pinworm* | 100 mg single dose (repeated after 2-3 weeks) |
| **As $2^{nd}$ choice** | |
| *Trichinosis* | 200 mg BD for 4 days |
| *Dog tapeworm (hydatid cyst)* | 200-400 mg BD for 3-4 weeks |

- ***Adverse effects :*** Usually, well tolerated. Diarrhea, nausea and abdominal pain Expulsion of *Ascaris* from mouth and nose has occurred. Allergic reactions, loss of hairs, and granulocytopenia at high dose.

### Albendazole :

- Congener of mebendazole with retained broad spectrum anti helminthic activity and tolerability.
- ***Advantages :*** Single dose is enough in many cases. ***E.g. :*** Ascariasis, Hookworm and Enterobiasis (3 day treatment with mebendazole). Superior to Mebendazole in Strongyloidosis, Hookworm, Hydatid disease. No fasting or purging is required.
- It is given as a part of national de-worming programme as single dose of 400 mg to all school going children.
- ***Mechanism of action :*** Similar to that of Mebendazole.

- ***Uses :***

| As 1st choice | |
|---|---|
| *Roundworm, Hookworm, Pinworm, Whipworm* | 400 mg single dose (adults and children above 2 years), 200 mg single dose (children of 1-2 years) |
| *Neurocysticercosis* | 400 mg BD for 8-15 days. For children the dose is 15 mg/kg/day |
| *Dog tapeworm (hydatid disease)* | 400 mg BD for 4 weeks. Repeat after 2 weeks if required. |
| **As 2nd choice** | |
| *Tapeworm and Threadworm* | 400 mg BD for 3 days |

- ***Adverse effects :*** GI side effects (abdominal pain, diarrhea, bowel upset, nausea and vomiting), dizziness in few cases, headache, fever, alopecia, jaundice, neutropenia in prolonged use. Inflammation and allergic reaction can occur due to dying organisms (corticosteroids are given to prevent this adverse effect).
- ***Note :*** It should be given on empty stomach for intestinal worms but for cysticercosis, hydatid disease and cutaneous larva margins it should be given with fatty meal.

**Thiabendazole :**

- First benzimidazole introduced, polyantihelminthic, practically covers all species of nematodes. Also inhibits development of egg and kills the worm.
- ***Mechanism of action :*** as same of mebendazole.
- Also exerts antipyretic, analgesic and anti-inflammatory effect. Contributes in cutaneous larva margin and larva or worm induced inflammation.
- ***Adverse effects :*** Nausea, vomiting, loss of appetite, headache, impaired alertness, interferes with normal activities, Itching, abdominal pain, diarrhea.
- ***Uses :*** Practically against all nematodes infesting the GIT but, because of frequent side effects and poor patient acceptability it isn't used regularly these days. Only reserved for resistant cases or where other drugs are not tolerated.

## PYRANTEL PAMOATE :

- High and comparable efficacy to that of mebendazole against Ascaris, hookworm, Enterobius. But less active against Strongyloides and inactive against Trichuris.
- ***Mechanism of action :*** It causes activation of nicotinic cholinergic receptors in worms resulting in persistent depolarisation thus spastic

paralysis but, have very low affinity to human nicotinic cholinergic receptors.

- ***Uses :*** For Ascaris, Ancylostoma, and Enterobius, a single dose of 11 mg/kg is used. For Nector and Strongyloides, 3 day course is used with same dose.
- ***Adverse effects :*** Almost free of side effects. Occasional GI symptoms, headache, dizziness has been reported. It is safe during pregnancy.

## PIPERAZINE :

- Highly active drug against Ascaris and Enterobius with 90-100% cure rates but, second choice of drugs these days.
- ***Mechanism of action :*** Causes hyperpolarization by GABA agonistic action opening $Cl^-$ channels resulting in relaxation, decreased responsiveness of worm muscles to Ach and causes flaccid paralysis but, doesn't cause this effect in humans. Often a purgative is required along with it.
- ***Uses :*** Ascaris and Enterobius infestations. In pregnancy when other anti-helmintics are contraindicated. The dose is 4 gm per day for 2 days.
- ***Adverse effects :*** Safe and well tolerated. Nausea and vomiting, abdominal discomfort, urticaria, dizziness and excitement at high doses. Toxic dose produces convulsions and death due to respiratory failure. Safe during pregnancy.
- ***Contraindications :*** Renal failure and in epileptic patients.

## LEVAMISOLE, TETRAMISOLE :

- Tetramisole (D) and levamisole (L) are optical isomers. Levamisole is more active and more preferred.
- They are active against large number of nematodes but their use is restricted to only ascariasis and ankylostomiasis because of poor action against other worms.
- ***Mechanism of action :*** Stimulate ganglia in worms and cause tonic paralysis which causes explusion of worms. Also interfere with carbohydrate metabolism.
- ***Uses :*** Ascariasis, second line in A. duodenale infestations. It was used as *immuno-modulators* as adjuvants in malignancies, aphthus ulcers.
- ***Dose :*** Single dose of 150 mg for ascariasis and 2 doses 12 hr apart for A. duodenale.
- ***Adverse effects :*** Nausea, abdominal pain, fatigue, drowsiness or insomnia is low.

## DIETHYL CARBAMAZINE CITRATE (DEC) :

- First drug for filariasis (*Wucheria bancrofti*). Highly selective effects on microfilariae.

- ***Mechanism of action :*** Alters the microfilarial membrane so that they are readily phagocytosed by tissue fixed monocytes but not by circulating monocytes. Muscular activity of MF is also affected causing hyperpolarisation due to piperazine moiety.
- ***Uses :*** Filariasis, tropical pulmonary eosinophilia and Loa Loa and Onchocerca volvulus infections.
- ***Dose :*** 2-4 mg/kg TDS for 2-3 weeks.
- ***Adverse effects :*** Well tolerated usually. Nausea, loss of appetite, headache, weakness and dizziness. Rash, pruritus, lymphadenopathy, hypotension may occur due to mass microfilarial destruction (If it occurs DEC is temporarily witheld and antihistamine and/or corticosteroids are given).

## IVERMECTIN :

- Extremely potent semisynthetic derivative of antinematodal principle obtained from *Streptomyces avermitilis.*
- ***Mechanism of action :*** It acts through special type of glutamate gated $Cl^-$ channel found only in invertebrates. Potentiates GABAergic transmission in the worms. The ultimate effect is tonic paralysis in worms.
- ***Uses :*** Used for Onchocerca volvulus, strongyloides and cutaneous larva migrans. Other uses : Lice infestation (shampoo), Scabies.
- ***Dose :*** 10 mcg/kg orally single dose.
- ***Adverse effects :*** Mild side effects; Nausea, abdominal pain, constipation, pruritus, lethargy and transient ECG changes. These effects are significantly due to degradation products of microfilaria as seen with DEC (*Mazotti reaction).*

## NICLOSAMIDE :

- Highly effective against cestodes infecting humans.
- ***Mechanism of action :*** It acts by inhibiting oxidative phosphorylation in mitochondria and interfering with anaerobic generation of ATP in tapeworm. Injured by niclosamide, they are digested in intestine but the degradation products are more hazardous.
- ***Adverse effects :*** Tastless and nonirritant, minimal absorption from GIT so minimal systemic toxicity. Minor GI symptoms are produced. Malaise, pruritus, light headedness
- It is safe during pregnancy.

## PRAZIQUANTEL :

- Broad range of activity against trematodes, cestodes but not nematodes.
- ***Mechanism of action :*** Causes leakage of intracellular calcium which leads to contracture and paralysis which further leads to loss of intestinal mucosal grip of the worms and thus, are expelled from GIT.

- *Uses :* Tapeworm infestations like T. Saginata, T. Solium, H. Nana, D. Latum (10-15 mg/kg single dose), Neurocysticercosis (50 mg/kg in 3 divided doses for 2-4 weeks is used as second choice to Albendazole), Schistosomes (75 mg/kg single dose). Drug of choice for all flukes except liver fluke (75 mg/kg single dose).
- *Adverse effects :* Bitter taste, nausea, abdominal pain. Headache, dizziness.

## TREATMENT OF NEUROCYSTICERCOSIS :

- Cysticercosis is due to tapeworm Tenia solium and can occur in various organs especially brain (neurocysticercosis). It is due to migration of larvae from GIT to various organs through blood circulation. The problems occur when the larvae in the cysticercosis die and can cause meningeal inflammation, seizures, raised intracranial pressure and other neurological symptoms. But, treatment is given to prevent spontaneous reactions due to sudden deaths of larvae and also for cysticercosis causing symptoms or neurological problems.
- **Treatment :**
  - ***Albendazole*** (1$^{st}$ choice) 400 mg BD for 8-15 days. For children the dose is 15 mg/kg/day.
  - ***Praziquantel*** (second choice to Albendazole) 50 mg/kg in 3 divided doses for 2-4 weeks.
  - ***Prednisolone*** (corticosteroid) 40-60 mg/day started 2 days prior and continued till 2 weeks after completing treatment to prevent inflammatory response to killed larvae.
  - **Phenytoin and carabamazepine** - for convulsions.

❑❑❑❑❑

# CANCER CHEMOTHERAPY

# 74 ANTI-CANCER DRUGS

## CANCER :

Uncontrolled multiplication of abnormal forms of body's own cells and spread within the body.

### Treatment of cancer :

- Surgery
- Radiotherapy
- Chemotherapy (drugs)

### Adjuvant chemotherapy :

Chemotherapy given after surgery or irradiation to destroy micrometastasis & prevent development of secondary neoplasm.

### *Neo-adjuvant chemotherapy :*

Chemotherapy given before surgery or radiotherapy in order to diminish the volume of large primary neoplasm.

### Adverse effects of anticancer drugs :

- Nausea & Vomiting (Treatment discussed in chapter on antiemetic drugs).
- ***Bone marrow depression :*** agranulocytosis, thrombocytopenia and aplastic anemia, which can lead to infections and bleeding.
- Alopecia.
- ***Gonads :*** Oligospermia, impotence, unovulation.
- ***Fetus :*** Abortion, fetal death, teratogenicity.
- Carcinogenicity.
- Hyperuricemia.
- Immunosuppression.
- Stomatitis, diarrhea.
- Hazards to staff.
- Neuropathy, myopathy, cystitis.

### Phases of cell cycle :

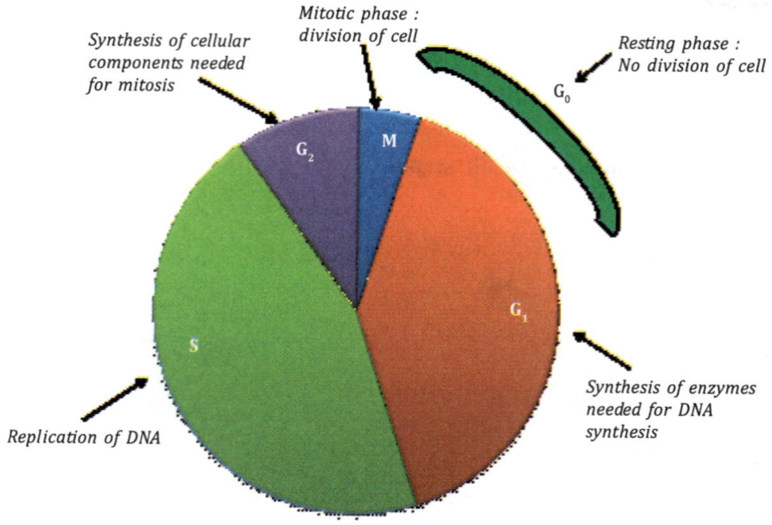


## CLASSIFICATION OF ANTICANCER DRUGS :

### Directly acting cytotoxic drugs (act on cells) :

- ***Alkylating agents :*** Mechlorethamine (Mustine), Melphalan, Cyclophosphamide, Ifosfamide, Chlorambucil, Busulfan, Carmustine, Lomustine, Dacarbazine.
- ***Antimetabolites :***
  - *Folate Antagonists* : Methotrexate.
  - *Purine Antagonists* : 6 Mercaptopurine, Azathioprine.
  - *Pyrimidine antagonists* : 5 Fluorouracil (5-FC), Gemcitabine.
- ***Anticancer Antibiotics :*** Actinomycin-D, Doxorubicin, Daunorubicin, Bleomycin, Mitomycin C.
- ***Vinca alkaloids :*** Vincristine (Oncovin), Vinblastine, Vinorelbine.
- ***Taxanes :*** Paclitaxel, Docetaxel.
- ***Enzymes :*** L-Asparginase.
- ***Epipodophyllotoxins :*** Etoposide, Tenoposide.
- ***Camptothecin analogues :*** Topotecan, irinotecan.
- ***Others :*** Cisplatin, Carboplatin, Hydroxurea, Procarbazine, Mitotane.

### Hormones & related drugs :

- ***Corticosteroids :*** Prednisolone.
- ***Estrogens :*** Ethinyl Estradiol.
- ***SERM (Selective Estrogen Receptor Modulator) :*** Tamoxifene, Toremifene.
- ***SERD (Selective Etrogen Receptor Down regulator) :*** Fulvestrant.

- ***Aromatase Inhibitors :*** Letrozole, Anastrazole, Exemestane.
- ***Progestins :*** Hydroxyprogesterone.
- ***Anti-androgens :*** Flutamide, Bicalutamide.
- ***5-α reductase Inhibitors :*** Finasteride, Dutasteride.
- ***GnRH analogues :*** Naferelin, Goserelin, Leuoprolide.

**Cell cycle specific actions :**

- **$G_1$ :** Vinblastine.
- **S :** Methotrexate, 6-Mercaptopurine 5-Fluorouracil.
- **$G_2$ :** Bleomycin, Etoposide, Topotecan Daunorubicin.
- **M :** Vincristine, Vinblastine, Paclitaxel, Docetaxel.

## Alkylating agents :

**Mechanism of action :**

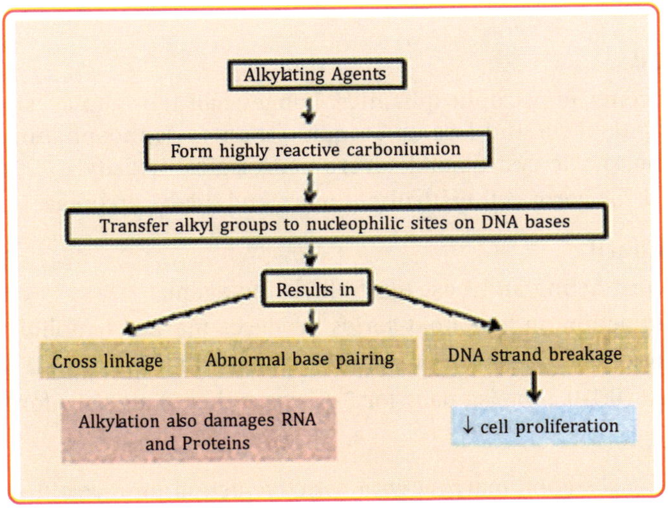


**Mechlorethamine (Mustine) :**

- Very irritant drug.
- ***Uses*** : Hematological cancers, lymphomas, solid tumors, Hodgkin's as part of MOPP, CML, CLL.
- ***Adverse effects :*** Anorexia, nausea, vomiting, bone marrow depression, aplasia, menstrual irregularities.

**Melphalan :**

- Very effective in *Multiple Myeloma.*
- Less irritant locally, less alopecia.
- ***Dose :*** 0.25 mg/kg daily for 4 days every 4-6 weeks.
- ***Adverse Effects :*** Bone marrow depression, infections, diarrhea and pancreatitis.

**Cyclophosphamide :**

- It is a prodrug which is converted to active metabolite Aldophosphamide.
- It is also a potent immunosuppressant.
- ***Uses : Neoplastic conditions*** : Hodgkin's and non Hodgkin's lymphoma, ALL, CLL, Multiple myeloma, Burkit's lymphoma, Neuroblastoma, Retinoblastoma, Carcinoma of breast, Adenocarcinoma of ovaries. ***Non neoplastic condition*** : graft versus host reaction in transplants, Rheumatoid arthritis, Nephrotic syndrome.
- ***Dose :*** 2-3 mg/kg/day oral, 10-15 mg/kg IV every 7-10 days. It can be administered IV, IM, IP, intrapleurally, Intraarterialy, directly into tumor.
- ***Adverse effects :*** Hemorrhagic cystitis, alopecia, nausea & vomiting, SIADH and hepatic damage. The most prominent adverse effect caused by it is hemorrhagic cystitis which is due to production of one metabolite called *Acrolein.* This can be prevented by a drug called as *Mesna.*

**Ifosfamide :**

- Congener of cyclophosphamide. Longer half life than cyclophosphamide. Less alopecia and less emetogenic than cyclophosphamide. Can cause hemorrhagic cystitis and severe neurological toxicity.
- Used for germ cell testicular tumors and adult sarcomas.

**Chlorambucil :**

- Slowest acting and least toxic alkylating agent.
- Main action on lymphoid series produces marked lympholytic action.
- Drug of choice for long term maintenance therapy of CLL.
- ***Dose :*** 0.1-0.2 mg/kg daily for 3-6 weeks then 2 mg daily for maintenance.

**Busulfan :**

- Depresses bone marrow with selective action on myeloid series.
- ***Use :*** Primarily used in Chronic myelogenous leukaemia (2-6 mg/day).
- ***Adverse effect :*** Interstitial pulmonary fibrosis, Veno-occlusive disease of liver, Hyperuricemia, Sterility.

**Carmustine, Lomustine (Nitrosoureas) :**

- Highly lipid soluble, Cross BBB.
- ***Uses :*** Meningeal / Brain tumors.
- ***Dose :*** 150-200 mg/m$^2$ BSA every 6 weeks (Carmustine).
- ***Adverse Effects :*** Delayed bone marrow suppression, Visceral fibrosis, renal damage.

**Dacarbazine :**

- Primary inhibitory action on RNA & protein synthesis.
- Used in malignant melanoma.

**Temozolamide :**

- New alkylating agent. Approved for malignant glioma.

## Antimetabolites :

**General Characteristics :**

- Antimetabolites are S phase specific drugs that are structural analogues of essential metabolites and that interfere with DNA synthesis.
- Myelosuppression is the dose limiting toxicity for all drugs in this class.

**Folate Antagonist : Methotrexate (MTX) :**

- ***Mechanism of action :*** The structures of MTX and folic acid are similar. MTX is actively transported into mammalian cells and inhibits dihydrofolate reductase, the enzyme that normally converts dietary folate to the tetrahydrofolate (active form needed for purine synthesis and DNA).
- ***Uses : Antineoplastic :*** Choriocarcinoma and trophoblast tumor, Remission of ALL in children, Ca breast, head & neck, bladder, ovarian cancer. ***Immuno-suppressive agent*** : Rheumatoid arthritis, Crohn's disease, wagener's granulomatosis, Prevention of graft versus host reaction, Psoriasis. Medical termination of pregnancy.
- ***Adverse effects :*** Low doses – bone marrow toxicity, megaloblastic anemia; high doses – pancytopenia, oral ulcers, diarrhea and desquamation and bleeding.
- MTX toxicity cannot be overcome with folic acid, therefore folinic acid (Leucovorin) is used to reverse the adverse effects. Leucovorin (Folinic acid) is directly converted to tetrahydrofolic acid.

**Purine antagonists : 6 Mercaptopurine, Azathioprine**

- ***Highly effective :*** antineoplastic – also primarily used as immunosuppressant.
- ***Mechanism of action :*** 6-MP is converted to corresponding monoribonucleotides which inhibits conversion of inosine monophosphate to adenine and guanine nucleotides. Gets incorporated to RNA and DNA.
- 6-MP also metabolised by methylation by thiopurine methyl transferase (TPMT) and genetic deficiency of TPMT results in toxicity.
- Toxicity of Azathioprine – enhanced due to TPMT deficiency.
- ***Uses :*** Childhood acute leukaemia, choriocarcinoma, solid tumors, both to induce remission and 6-MP to maintain Azathioprine : prodrug – converts to 6-MP (prominent immunosuppressant action) used in organ transplant and rheumatoid arthritis.
- ***Adverse effects :*** All cause BM depression, nausea vomiting with 6-MP, reversible jaundice and hyperuricemia (can be treated with allopurinol).

**Pyrimidine antagonists :** ***5 Fluorouracil (5-FC), Gemcitabine***

- ***5-FU :***
  - ***Mechanism of action :***

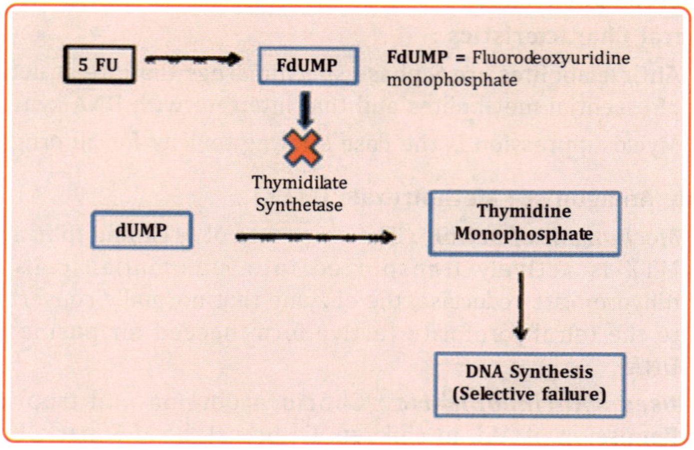


  - ***Uses :*** Solid malignancies – especially colon, rectum, stomach, pancreas, liver, urinary bladder and Head & Neck.
  - ***Adverse effects :*** Bone Marrow and GIT myelosuppression - mucositis, diarrhea, nausea, vomiting and peripheral neuropathy.
- ***Gemcitabine :*** Drug of choice in adenocarcinoma of pancreas.

## Anticancer antibiotics :

- Cell cycle non specific drugs. Derived from streptomyces species.
- ***Mechanism of action :*** Intercalation in the DNA between adjoining nucleotide pairs which blocks DNA & RNA synthesis. Generation of oxygen radicals which mediate single strand scission of DNA. Action on Topoisomerase II.

**Actinomycin-D :**

- ***Uses :*** Wilm's tumor, gestational choriocarcinoma.
- ***Adverse effects :*** Bone marrow suppression, Irritant like meclorethamine. Sensitizes to radiation, and inflammation at sites of prior radiation therapy may occur, gastrointestinal adverse effects.

**Doxorubicin :**

- Also effective in many solid tumors – breast, lung, sarcoma, thyroid, ovary, bladder.
- ***Mechanism of action :*** Intercalate between DNA strands – block DNA and RNA synthesis; also strand breakage of DNA.
- ***Adverse effects :*** Cardiotoxicity – arrhythmia and hypotension – ECG; also CHF.
- Also mutagenic and carcinogenic.

**Daunorubicin :**

- ***Uses :*** Limited to acute myeloid and lymphoblastic leukaemia.
- ***Adverse effects :*** Cardiotoxicity (cardiomyopathy), Marrow Depression, Alopecia.

**Bleomycin :**

- ***Uses :*** Epidermoid cancers of skin, oral cavity, genitourinary tract, esophagus, Testicular tumors, Hodgkin's lymphoma.
- ***Adverse effects :*** Pneumonitis, Fatal pulmonary fibrosis, Hyperpigmentation.

**Mitomycin C :**

- Highly toxic used only in resistant cancers of stomach, colon, rectum.
- Transformed to form which acts like alkylating agent.

## Vinca alkaloids :

**Vincristine (oncovin), vinblastine, vinorelbine :**

- Obtained from Madagascar periwinkle plant also known as catharanthus roseus (Vinca Rosea), popularly known as sadabahar or sadaphuli.
- ***Mechanism of action :*** They bind to microtubular protein tubulin and prevents its polymerisation which cause disruption of mitotic spindle and interfere with cytoskeletal function. Chromosomes fail to move apart during mitosis leading to metaphase arrest.
- ***Uses : Vincristine :*** ALL, Hodgkin's, lymphosarcoma, Wilm's tumor, Ewing's sarcoma. ***Vinblastine :*** Hodgkin's disease, breast cancer, testicular cancer.
- ***Adverse effects :*** Neuropathy and alopecia; also paralytic ileus, postural hypotension, urinary retention, nausea, vomiting.

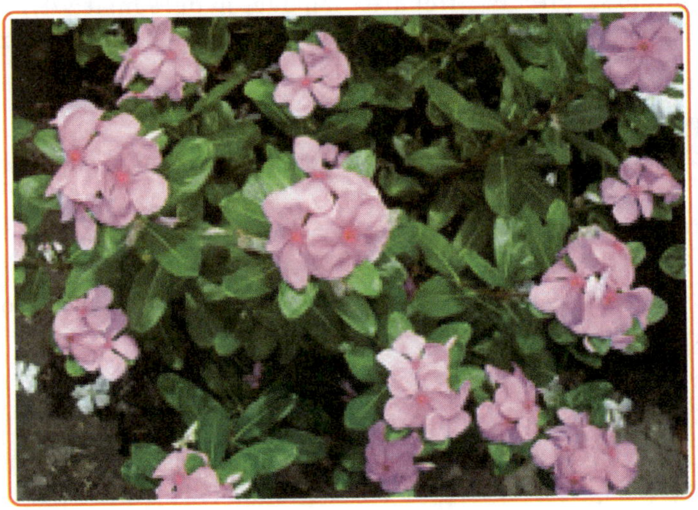

## Taxanes :

- Plant product obtained from bark of Pacific Yew tree.
- ***Mechanism of action :*** Binds to β-tubulin and enhances its polymerisation; action opposite to that of vinca alkaloids. They ultimately fail to depolymerise. Abnormal microtubules are formed.

**Paclitaxel :**

- Administered IV.
- ***Use :*** Advanced breast & ovarian cancer also lungs, esophagus, prostate cancer.
- ***Adverse effects :*** Anaphylactoid reaction because of solvent cremaphor, Myalgia, myelosuppression, peripheral neuropathy.

**Docetaxel :**

- Oral use.
- ***Use :*** Used in refractory breast & ovarian cancer.
- ***Adverse effects :*** Major toxicity neutropenia may cause arrhythmias, hypotension.

## Enzymes :

**L-asparginase :**

- Isolated from E.coli.
- ***Mechanism of action :*** Leukaemic cells are deficient in L-aspargine synthase enzyme and takes L-aspargine from surrounding medium. L-Asparginase obtained from E. coli degrades L-aspargine to L-aspartic acid. This deprives leukaemic cells and cause cell death.
- ***Use :*** Acute Lymphocytic Leukaemia (ALL).
- ***Dose :*** 6000 to 10000 U/kg IV daily for 3-4 weeks.
- ***Adverse effects :*** Hepatic damage, hypersensitivity, hemorrhage, Hyperglycemia, headache, hallucinations, confusion and coma.

## Epipodophyllotoxins :

**Etoposide & tenoposide :**

- Semisynthetic derivatives of podophyllotoxins podophyllum peltatum (plant glycoside).
- ***Mechanism of action :*** Act in S & G2 phase. Inhibit topoisomerase II which results in breakage of DNA strands & cell death.
- ***Uses :*** Testicular tumors, squamous cell cancer of lungs.

## Camptothecin analogues :

**Topotecan, Irinotecan :**

- Derived from camptotheca accuminata.
- ***Mechanism of action :*** Inhibit Topoisomerase I, as a result there is no resealing of DNA after strand has untwisted.

**Topotecan :**

- ***Uses :*** Used in metastatic ovarian cancer.
- ***Adverse effects :*** Major toxicity is bone marrow depression.

**Irinotecan :**

- ***Uses :*** Used in metastatic cancer of colon/rectum.
- ***Adverse effects :*** Diarrhea, neutropenia, thrombocytopenia, cholinergic side effects.

## Other drugs :

**Cisplatin :**

- Non cell cycle specific killing. Administered IV.
- Highly bound to plasma proteins, gets concentrated in kidney, intestine, testes.
- ***Mechanism of action :*** Cisplatin enters cells and forms highly reactive platinum complexes which cause DNA damage and inhibits cell proliferation.
- ***Uses :*** Testicular cancer (85% - 95% curative), Ovarian cancer, Other solid tumors : lung, esophagus, gastric.
- ***Adverse effects :*** Emesis, Nephrotoxicity, Peripheral neuropathy, Ototoxicity.

**Carboplatin :**

- Better tolerated.
- Less plasma protein binding.
- Nephrotoxicity, ototoxicity, neurotoxicity low.
- Less emetogenic, but thrombocytopenia and leucopenia may occur.
- ***Use :*** Primarily in ovarian cancer of epithelial origin, squamous cell carcinoma of head and neck.

**Hydroxyurea :**

- ***Mechanism of action :*** It Inhibits ribonucleoside diphosphate reductase, therefore blocks conversion of ribonucleotides to deoxyribonucleotide (S specific action).
- ***Uses :*** CML, Polycythemia vera, Radiosensitiser prior to radiotherapy and 1$^{st}$ line drug in sickle cell disease in adults.
- ***Adverse effects :*** Myelosuppression, GIT disturbance and cutaneous reactions.

**Procarbazine :**

- ***Mechanism of action :*** Depolymerises DNA & causes chromosomal damage.
- ***Uses :*** Hodgkin's disease (MOPP regimen), Non Hodgkin's lymphoma.

- ***Dose :*** 100-200 mg daily orally.
- ***Adverse effects :*** MAO inhibitor action & antabuse action.

## Glucocorticoids : *Prednisolone :*

- Marked lympholytic effect so used in acute leukaemias & lymphomas.
- They also have anti-inflammatory effect, increase appetite, prevent anemia, produce sense of well being, increase body weight, suppress hypersensitivity reaction, control hypercalcemia & bleeding, has non specific antipyretic effect and increase antiemetic effect of Ondansetron.

## Estrogens :

- Physiological antagonists of androgens. Thus used to antagonize the effects of androgens in androgen dependent prostatic cancer.
- ***Fofesterol :*** Prodrug, phosphate derivative of stilbesterol.

## SERM : Selective Estrogen Receptor Modulators.

**Tamoxifen :**

- Non steroidal antiestrogen.
- ***Mechanism :*** Antagonistic action at breast, blood vessels and agonistic action at uterus, bone, liver and pituitary.
- ***Dose :*** 10-20 mg BD.
- ***Uses :*** Hormonal treatment in OR positive breast cancer.
- ***Adverse effects :*** Hot flushes, vomiting, vaginal bleeding, menstrual irregularities, venous thromboembolism, dermatitis, rarely endometrial cancer.

**Fulvestrant :**

- Pure estrogen antagonist.
- ***Mechanism of action :*** Inhibits Estrogen receptor (ER) dimerization & prevents interaction of ER with DNA. ER is down regulated resulting in more complete suppression of ER responsive gene function.
- ***Uses :*** Metastatic ER positive Breast Ca in postmenopausal women.

## Aromatase Inhibitors :

**Letrozole :**

- Orally active non steroidal compound.
- ***Mechanism of action :*** Inhibits aromatisation of testosterone & androstenedione to form estrogen.
- ***Uses :*** Breast $Ca^-$ & adj. to mastectomy.
- ***Dose :*** 2.5 mg BD orally.

**Anastrozole :**

- More potent.
- ***Uses :*** in OR +ve Breast Ca (1 mg OD).
- ***Adverse effects :*** hot flushes.

## Progestins : *Hydroxyprogesterone :*

- ***Use :*** used in metastatic endometrial Ca.
- ***Adverse effects :*** bleeding.

## Anti Androgens : *Flutamide & Bicalutamide :*

- Androgen Receptor antagonists.
- ***Use :*** Palliative effect in metastatic Prostatic Ca after orchidectomy.
- ***Dose :*** 250 mg tds.

## 5-α REDUCTASE INHIBITORS : *Finasteride, Dutasteride :*

- Orally active.
- ***Mechanism of action :*** Inhibits conversion of Testosterone to Dihydrotestosterone.
- ***Use :*** Benign prostatic hyperplasia, Ca prostate, androgenic alopecia.
- ***Dose :*** Finasteride 5 mg/day.
- ***Adverse effects :*** Loss of libido & impotence.

## GnRH ANALOGUES : *Naferelin, Goserelin, Leuoprolide :*

- Available as nasal spray / SC injection.
- ***Mechanism :*** Decreases FSH & LH release from pituitary which decreases the release of estrogen & testosterone.
- ***Use :*** Breast Ca, Prostatic Ca.

## IMPORTANT DRUG REGIMES :

| Regime | Drugs | Condition |
|---|---|---|
| MOPP | Mechlorethamine, Oncovin (vincristine), Prednisolone, Procarbazine | Hodgkin's |
| VAMP | Vincristine, Methotraxate (Amethopterine), 6MP, Prednisolone | Acute leukaemia |
| CMF | Cyclophosphamide, Methotrexate, 5-FU | Breast carcinoma |

## NEWER SPECIFIC TARGET DRUGS :

- **Tyrosine protein kinase inhibitor :** Imatinib (CML, ALL, Gastrontestinal stromal tumors), Nilotinib (CML).
- **EGFR (Epidermal growth factor receptor) inhibitors :** Geftinib (Non small cell cancer of lungs), Erlotinib (Non small cell cancer of lungs), Cetuximab (Non small cell cancer of lungs, metastatic colorectal cancer).
- **RTK (Receptor tyrosine kinase) inhibitors :** Sunitinib (Gastrontestinal stromal tumors resistant to imatinib, renal cell carcinoma).
- **Proteasome inhibitors :** Bortezomib (Multiple myeloma).
- **Monoclonal antibody :** Rituximab (non Hodgkin's lymphoma), Trastuzumab (HER2/neu positive breast cancer), Bevacizumab (metastatic colon cancer).

# MISCELLANEOUS TOPICS

# 75 IMMUNOSUPPRESANTS AND IMMUNOSTIMULANTS (Immunomodulators)

The process of stimulation or suppression of immune system of the body is called Immunomodulation and the drugs which do it are called as **Immunomodulators**. Drugs may modulate immune mechanism by either suppressing or by stimulating one or more of the following steps :

- Antigen recognition & phagocytosis.
- Lymphocyte proliferation and differentiation.
- Synthesis of antibodies.
- Antigen-Antibody interaction.
- Release of mediators due to immune response.
- Modification of target tissue response.

**Immunomodulators types :**

- Immunosuppressants.
- Immunostimulants.

**IMMUNOSUPPRESSANTS :**

**Classification :**

- ***Calcineurin inhibitors (specific T-cell inhibitors) :***
  Cyclosporine, Tacrolimus, Sirolimus and Everolimus.
- ***Antiproliferative drugs (cytotoxic drugs) :***
  Azathioprine, Cyclophosphamide, Methotrexate, Mycophenolate Mofetil (MMF).
- ***Glucocorticoids :***
  Prednisolone and others.
- ***Antibodies :***
  Muromonab (Anti-$CD_3$), Antithymocyte globulin (ATG), Rho-D immunoglobulin, Anti TNF alpha (Infliximab, Etanercept, Adalimumab).

**Calcineurin inhibitors :**

**Cyclosporin :**

- ***Mechanism of action :*** It selectively inhibits T lymphocyte proliferation, IL-2 & other cytokine production & response of inducer T cells to IL-1, without any effect on suppressor T cells. Lymphocytes are arrested at $G_0$ or $G_1$ phase. It binds to the cytosolic protein cyclophilin (immunophilin) of immunocompetent lymphocytes, especially T-lymphocytes. This complex of cyclosporine & cyclophilin inhibit **calcineurin**, which, under normal circumstances, is responsible for activating the transcription of IL-2.

- ***Uses :*** Mainly used in kidney, liver, cardiac, bone marrow transplants to prevent transplant rejection (Can be used alone, but more effective when glucocorticoids are also administered). Useful in autoimmune disease as well. Alternative to methotrexate for the treatment of severe, active Rheumatoid arthritis. 2nd line drug for uveitis, bronchial asthma.
- ***Adverse effects :*** Renal dysfunction, tremor, hirsutism, hypertension, hyperlipidemia, gum hyperplasia, hyperuricemia, calcineurin inhibitors along glucocorticoids are having diabetogenic potential.

**Tacrolimus :**

- Chemically different from cyclosporin.
- Macrolide that is isolated from soil fungus.
- ***Mechanism of action :*** Same like cyclosporin but, it binds to different cytoplasmic immunophilin protein labelled FK506 binding protein (FKBP).
- Orally as well as i.v infusion.
- Clinical efficacy as well as toxicity profile are similar to cyclosporin.

**Sirolimus :**

- Macrolide antibiotic.
- ***Mechanism of action :*** Binds to same immunoglobulin FKBP as Tacrolimus. Sirolimus-FKBP complex inhibits another kinase called 'mammalian target of rapamycin' *i.e.* mTOR (does not interact with calcineurin). Leads to proliferation & differentiation of T-cells activated by IL-2.
- ***Uses :*** Prophylaxis of organ transplant rejection along with other drugs (cyclosporin/tacrolimus).
- ***Adverse effects :*** Increase in serum cholesterol, triglycerides, anemia, thrombocytopenia, hypokalemia, fever, GI disturbances, risk of infection and tumors.

**Everolimus :**

- Similar to sirolimus in mechanism, clinical efficacy, doses & drug interactions.
- Better absorbed orally.
- Shorter half life (approx 40 hours).
- Shorter time taken to reach steady state.
- Similar uses & toxicity.

## Antiproliferative drugs (cytotoxic drugs) :

**Azathioprine :**

- It is a purine antimetabolite.

- ***Mechanism of action :*** It selectively affects differentiation & function of T-cells. It inhibits cytolytic T-lymphocytes, cell mediated immunity is primarily depressed.
- ***Uses :*** Prevention of renal & other graft rejections, Rheumatoid arthritis.
- ***Adverse effects :*** Bone marrow suppression-leucopenia, thrombocytopenia, anemia, increased susceptibility to infection, Hepatotoxicity, alopecia, GI disturbances.
- ***Drug interaction :*** Seen along with anti-gout drug Allopurinol.

**Cyclophosphamide :**

- More marked effect on B cells & humoral immunity.
- Used in BM transplantation in which short course with high dose is given.
- In other organ transplantations it is employed only as a reserve drug.
- In RA, it is rarely used.
- Low doses are occasionally employed for maintenance therapy in pemphigus, SLE & idiopathic thrombocytopenic purpura.

**Methotrexate :**

- Folate antagonist, potent immunosuppressant
- ***Mechanism of action*** : Markedly depresses cytokine production & cellular immunity & has anti-inflammatory property.
- ***Uses*** : Used as 1st line drug in many autoimmune diseases like rapidly progressing RA, severe psoriasis, pemphigus, myasthenia gravis, uveitis, chronic active hepatitis

**Mycophenolate mofetil (MMF) :**

- It is a prodrug which is converted to mycophenelic acid.
- ***Mechanism of action :*** It selectively inhibits inosine monophosphate dehydrogenase, an enzyme essential for denovo synthesis of guanosine nucleotides in the T-cells as well as B-cells. Lymphocyte proliferation, antibody production and CMI are also inhibited.
- ***Uses :*** Used as an add-on drug to Cyclosporin and glucocorticoids in renal transplantation. It is good or even superior to azathioprine, but should not be combined with it. It can help to reduce the dose of cyclosporin and thus its toxicity.
- ***Adverse effects :*** Vomiting, diarrhea, leucopenia and predisposition to CMV infection, GI bleeds.

## Glucocorticoids :

- **Mechanism of action :** They decrease peripheral lymphocyte counts (Enhance rate of destruction of lymphoid cells). They also cause down regulation of IL-1, IL-2, IL-3, IL-6. There is also Inhibition of T-cell proliferation, increased number of RBCs, platelets & neutrophils in circulation.

- **Uses :** Transplant rejection, autoimmune diseases like RA, SLE, Psoriasis, Inflammatory Bowel Disease like Crohn's and ulcerative colitis, inflammatory and allergic eye conditions.
- **Adverse effects :** Hyperglycemia, hypertension, growth retardation, avascular necrosis of femoral head, risk of infection, psychosis, poor wound healing, Cushingoid features, cataract etc.

## Antibodies :

### Muromonab (Anti-$CD_3$ Monoclonal Antibody) :

- Murine monoclonal antibody against the $CD_3$ glycoprotein expressed near to the T-cell receptor on helper T-cell.
- Binds to $CD_3$, a component of T-cell receptor complex involved in antigen recognition and cell signalling & proliferation.
- ***Use :*** Treatment of acute organ transplant rejection.
- ***Adverse effects :*** Cytokine release syndrome, aseptic meningitis, life threatening pulmonary edema.

### Anti-thymocyte Globulin (ATG) :

- It is a Polyclonal antibody purified from horse or rabbits immunised with human thymic lymphocytes.
- ***Mechanism of action :*** It binds to T-lymphocytes & depletes them. Having potent immunosuppressant action.
- ***Uses :*** Induction of immunosuppression in organ transplantation, to suppress acute allograft rejection episodes.
- ***Adverse effects :*** Hypersensitivity, risk of infection and malignancy.

### Rho-D immunoglobulin :

- Normally plasma does not have anti-$Rh^+$ antibodies. But, if an $Rh^-$ person receives $Rh^+$ blood, the body starts to make anti-$Rh^+$ antibodies which remain in circulation. Now, if a second time, the same person receives $Rh^+$ blood, these anti-$Rh^+$ antibodies will react and cause hemolysis.
- Such type of Rh incompatibility may occur during pregnancy especially when an $Rh^-$ mother is carrying $Rh^+$ baby. Some amount of the baby's $Rh^+$ blood will cross over through placenta during delivery or abortion to the mother's side and the $Rh^-$ mother will now start making anti-$Rh^+$ antibodies. The newborn baby will not be affected but, in subsequent pregnancy, the mother's anti-$Rh^+$ antibodies will cross the placenta to the fetal side and cause hemolysis (Hemolytic diasease of the newborn).
- ***Use :*** It is used for prevention of postpartum /post-abortion formation of antibodies in $Rh^-$ women who delivered or aborted an $Rh^+$ baby. It is administered within 72 hrs of delivery/abortion; such treatment prevents Rh hemolytic disease in future offspring.

### Anti-TNF Agents :

#### *Infliximab :*

- Chimeric monoclonal antibody against TNF-α.
- *Uses :* Rheumatoid arthritis, Crohn's disease, Psoriasis, Psoriatic arthritis, Ankylosing spondylosis.
- *Adverse effects :* Infusion reaction – fever, urticaria, hypotension, dyspnea and Increased chances of opportunistic infections like tuberculosis, respiratory infections and fungal infections.

#### *Etanercept :*

- It neutralises both TNF-α & TNF-β. It also prevents activation of macrophages & T-cells.
- *Uses :* Rheumatoid arthritis, also approved for severe / refractory ankylosing spondylitis, plaque psoriasis.

#### *Adalimumab :*

- It is a human monoclonal antibody against TNF-α.
- It is less antigenic than Infliximab.
- Its serum half life is 2 weeks; therefore it is taken every 14 days.
- *Uses :* Rheumatoid arthritis

## IMMUNOSTIMULANTS :

- **Levamisole**
- **Thalidomide**
- **BCG**
- **Recombinant Cytokines : Interferons, Interleukin-2**

### Levamisole :

- Levamisole is orally active levo-isomer of tetramisole which restores depressed T-cell function.
- ***Mechanism of action :*** It mainly acts by raising c-GMP levels through interaction with thymopoietin receptor sites. This leads to decrease in metabolic inactivation of c-GMP accompanied with increased breakdown of c-AMP. Increase in c-GMP level induces lymphocyte proliferation & augmentation of chemotactic responses. This results into increased antibody production, lymphokine production, increased phagocytosis.
- ***Uses :*** Used as an adjunct in malignancies, aphthus ulcers, recurrent herpes, also used as disease modifying drug in Rheumatoid Arthritis.

### Thalidomide :

- Anxiolytic, antiemetic drug with antiinflammatory, cytokine modulatory activity.
- It decreases TNF-α and produces anti-angiogenic effect.

- ***Uses :*** Multiple myeloma, ENL (Eryhthema nodosum leprosum).
- It is teratogenic (seal limbs / phacomelia).

## BCG (Bacillus Calmette Guerin) vaccine :

- It is used as immunological enhancer to stimulate intact immune system (*i.e.* a non-specific immunoenhancer) of the body.
- BCG & its methanol extracted residue (MER) contain muramyl dipeptide as an active immunostimulant ingredient.
- T-lymphocytes are principal target cells for the action of BCG vaccine.
- It causes stimulation of macrophage function, phagocytic activity, lysosomal enzyme activity & chemotaxis mechanisms.
- It induces the production of lymphocyte-activity factor resulting of phase I of immune response.
- Because of its activity against tumor antigen it is beneficial in treatment of lung & breast cancer, ALL and AML. It is also used in bladder cancer where it is instilled and held for 2 hours.

## Recombinant Cytokines :

***Interferons (Mainly Interferon alpha$_{2b}$) :***

- Low molecular weight glycoprotein cytokines produced by host cells in response to viral infections. They have immunomodulatory activity.
- ***Mechanism of action :*** They bind to cell surface receptors and initiate intracellular events. They cause inhibition of cell proliferation, affect viral replication and increased Phagocytosis.
- ***Uses :*** Hairy cell leukemia, malignant melanoma, Kaposi's sarcoma, chronic Hepatitis B.
- ***Adverse effects :*** Flu-like symptoms – fever, malaise, headache, CVS-hypotension, Arrhythmia, CNS-depression, altered behavior.

***Interleukin-2 (aldesleukin) :***

- ***Mechanism of action :*** Causes stimulation of cellular immunity which leads to Lymphocytosis, eosinophilia, release of multiple cytokines like TNF, IL-1, IFN-γ. They also promote differentiation of T-cells.
- ***Uses :*** Metastatic renal cell carcinoma, malignant Melanoma.
- ***Adverse effects :*** Flu- like symptoms- fever, headache, fatigue, Hypotension, drowsiness, confusion, loss of appetite.

# 76 CHELATING AGENTS

These are the drugs with complex metallic ions forming rings (greek word *Chele* = Crab i.e the chelating agent grabs the metal ion like a crab's claw) and are used to treat heavy metal poisonings like Lead (Pb), Mercury (Hg), Arsenic (As), Cadmium (Cd), Iron (Fe), Copper (Cu), Zinc (Zn), Manganese (Mn) etc. Heavy metals act as a protoplasmic poison by inhibiting essential enzymes. They exert toxic effects by combining functional groups of enzyme like -SH, -OH and inactivating the enzymes.

## MECHANISM OF ACTION OF CHELATING AGENTS :

**Chelating agent + Metallic ions**

↓

**Non toxic, water soluble complex**

↓

**Eliminated by the kidney**

## CHELATING AGENTS :

- **Dimercaprol (BAL)**
- **Succimer**
- **Unithiol**
- **Calcium disodium Edetate**
- **Penicillamine**
- **Trientrene**
- **Desferrioxamine, Deferiprone and Deferasirox**

### DIMERCAPROL (BAL : British anti-lewisite) :

- Developed as antidote to lewisite (arsenical war gas) during World War II.
- Oily, pungent smelling, viscous liquid.
- Can't be given orally, given by deep IM injection.
- ***Uses :*** Poisoning by arsenic, mercury. As an adjuvant to edetate calcium disodium in lead poisoning. As an adjuvant to penicillamine in Wilson's disease.
- ***Dose :*** 5 mg/kg stat followed by 2 mg/kg 8 hourly for 2 days and then 2 mg/kg OD for 10 days.

- ***Adverse effects :*** Injection is painful, allergic reaction, nausea, vomiting, headache, lacrimation, anginal pain, tachycardia and hypertension.

## SUCCIMER :

- Analogue of dimercaprol. Orally administered, less toxic, more water soluble.
- ***Uses :*** Lead poisoning. Also used in arsenic, cadmium and mercury poisoning.
- ***Dose :*** 10 mg/kg every 8 hourly for 2 weeks.
- ***Adverse Effects :*** Nausea, anorexia, vomiting, diarrhea, weakness, dizziness, rash, transient elevation of hepatic transaminase enzymes.

## UNITHIOL :

- Analogue of dimercaprol. Water soluble. Used orally as well as IV.
- ***Uses :*** Used in severe acute poisoning with arsenic and mercury. Also effective in lead poisoning.
- ***Adverse effects :*** Urticaria, allergic reaction, nausea, vomiting etc.

## CALCIUM DISODIUM EDETATE :

- The parent compound EDTA (Ethylene Diamine Tetra Acetic acid) is a strong chelator of calcium that may cause severe hypocalcemia.
- Not absorbed orally, given IM.
- IM injection is painful.
- ***Uses :*** Lead poisoning. Also used in Iron, Zinc, Manganese and Copper poisoning.
- ***Dose :*** 50 mg/kg/day for 5 days.
- ***Adverse effects :*** Thrombophlebitis, nausea, diarrhea, renal failure, febrile reaction, myalgia, rhinorrhea, lacrimation, dermatitis, hypocalcemic tetany (especially in rapid IV infusion).

## PENICILLAMINE :

- Degradation product of penicillin.
- D-isomer is more potent (D-Penicillamine).
- Well absorbed orally.
- Absorption is inhibited by foods, Iron, antacids.
- ***Uses :*** For Copper poisoning, Wilson's disease (Hepato-lenticular degeneration). It is also used in mercury and chronic lead poisoning.
- ***Other uses :*** Rheumatoid arthritis, Cystinuria, Cystiene calculi and Scleroderma.
- ***Dose :*** 500 mg BID orally.
- ***Adverse effects :*** Headache, rash, fever, lymphadenopathy, dysguesia, aplastic anemia, agranulocytosis, thrombocytopenia, fever, polyarthritis and exfoliative dermatitis.

## TRIENTINE :

- Less toxic alternative to penicillamine.
- *Use :* Wilson's disease.
- *Dose :* 1 gm BID.
- *Adverse effects :* Anemia, nausea, gastritis.

## DESFERIOXAMINE :

- It is a chelator of iron.
- Removes iron from hemosiderin and ferritin but not from hemoglobin and cytochrome.
- Poorly absorbed after oral administration therefore used parenterally.
- *Mechanism :* Bind ferric iron to form ferrioxamine (stable, water soluble).
- *Uses and dose :* Acute Iron toxicity (10-15 mg/kg/hr constant infusion), for chronic iron intoxication (0.5 to 1 gm/day, IM) and for chelation of aluminium in dialysis patient.
- *Adverse effects :* Allergic reactions, pruritus, rash, dysuria, abdominal discomfort and diarrhea.
- *Contraindictaions :* Renal diseases, pregnancy and allergy to the drug.

## DEFERIPRONE :

- It is orally effective iron chelator, but less effective than desferrioxamine.
- *Use :* Iron poisoning in patients where desferioxamine is contraindicated or not tolerated.
- *Dose :* 50-100 mg/kg daily.
- *Adverse effects :* Anorexia, vomiting, joint pain and blood dyscrasias.

## DEFERASIROX :

- It is orally effective newer iron chelating drug.
- *Use :* It is used when desferrioxamine is contraindicated or not tolerated. It is also used in iron over load states.
- *Dose :* 20-30 mg/kg.
- *Adverse effects :* Gastritis, peptic ulceration, fanconi like syndrome etc.

### TO SUM IT UP :

| Chelating Agent | Used in Toxicity |
|---|---|
| DIMERCAPROL | Hg, As, Pb (with calcium disodium edetate) |
| SUCCIMER | Hg, As, Pb, Cd |
| UNITHIOL | Hg, As, Pb |
| EDETATE CALCIUM DISODIUM | Pb, Fe, Zn, Cu, Mn |
| PENICILLAMINE | Cu |
| TRIENTRENE | Cu |
| DESFERRIOXAMINE, DEFERIPRONE, DEFERASIROX | Fe |

# 77 ANTI-SEPTICS AND DISINFECTANTS

**ANTISEPTICS :**

These are chemical substances which inhibit the growth or kill micro-organisms on living surface such as skin and mucous membrane.

**DISINFECTANTS :**

These are chemical substances which inhibit the growth or kill micro-organisms on non-living surface such as instruments.

**STERILISATION :**

The process of killing micro-organisms (including spores) is called as sterilisation.

**CHARACTERISTICS OF AN IDEAL ANTISEPTIC/ DISINFECTANT :**

- It should be cidal and should destroy spores also.
- Should be reactive against all pathogens.
- It should be non-irritating to tissues.
- It should be chemically stable.
- It should be active even in the presence of pus or blood.
- It should be fast acting.
- It should be non-staining and non-absorbable.
- It should be economical.

**CLASSIFICATION :**

- ***Agents that cause denaturation of proteins and disrupt the cell membrane :***
  Phenols, Cresol, Chloroxylenol, Chlorhexidine, Alcohols, Aldehydes.
- ***Agents that cause oxidation of protoplasm :***
  Potassium permanganate, Hydrogen peroxide, Iodines, Chlorines.
- ***Detergent like action (increase permeability of cell membrane) :***
  Cetrimide, Soaps.
- ***Others :***
  Boric acid, Metallic salts, Dyes.

**Phenol :**

- It is one of the earliest used agent.
- ***Mechanism :*** Causes denaturation of proteins and disrupt the cell membrane.

- It injures tissue at higher concentration.
- It is used for disinfection of urine, feces and pus.

## Cresol :

- It is a phenol derivative but, less damaging than phenol.
- It is 10 times more active.
- ***Mechanism :*** Causes denaturation of proteins and disrupt the cell membrane.
- It is used for disinfection of utensils and for washing hands.

## Chloroxylenol :

- It is also a phenol derivative.
- ***Mechanism :*** Causes denaturation of proteins and disrupt the cell membrane.
- Commercial use Chloroxylenol is of concentration of 4-8%.
- ***Brand name :*** Dettol.

## Chlorhexidine :

- ***Mechanism :*** Causes denaturation of proteins and disrupt the cell membrane.
- It is used in surgical scrub, mouth wash and as general skin antiseptic.
- ***Brand name :*** Savlon (chlorhexidine+cetrimide).

## Alcohol (Ethanol / Isopropanolol) :

- ***Mechanism :*** causes denaturation of proteins and disrupt the cell membrane.
- Antiseptic action is seen at concentration of 40-90%.
- It is irritant and should not be applied to mucous membrane, ulcers, wounds and denuded skin.
- It is used before injections, incisions, hand sanitisation.
- It doesn't kill spores and causes rusting of instruments.

## Aldehydes :

- ***Mechanism :*** causes denaturation of proteins and disrupt the cell membrane.

### *Formaldehyde :*

- It is a pungent gas which is used for fumigation of operation theatres, ICU etc.
- Its 37% aqueous solution is called as formalin.
- Formalin is used to preserve dead tissue.
- It can cause eczematous skin lesions.

### *Glutaraldehyde :*

- It is less pungent, less irritating, less volatile and better sterilising agent than formalin

- It has broad spectrum of activity.
- Concentration used is 2%.
- It is used for disinfection of surgical instruments and endoscopes.
- ***Brand name :*** Cidex.

## Potassium permanganate ($KMnO_4$) :

- They are purple colored crystals, highly water soluble and liberates oxygen.
- ***Mechanism :*** Cause oxidation of protoplasm.
- Action is slower and higher concentration causes burns.
- It is used for gargling, irrigating cavities and wounds. Also used for gastric lavage in organophosphate poisonings and disinfection of water in ponds.

## Hydrogen peroxide ($H_2O_2$) :

- ***Mechanism :*** Cause oxidation of protoplasm. It liberates oxygen which oxidises the necrotic material and bacteria.
- It helps in loosening and removing of slough from the wounds and also removing ear wax.

## Iodine :

- ***Mechanism :*** Cause oxidation of protoplasm.
- It is rapidly acting, broad spectrum agent.
- It is used for cuts, wounds, antisepsis of skin before surgery etc.
- ***Disadvantage :*** Irritation and staining.

### *Iodophores :*

- They are soluble complexes of iodine.

### *Povidone iodine :*

- ***Mechanism :*** Same as iodine.
- ***Advantages :*** Non-irritating, non-staining, non-toxic, prolong action.
- It is used in boils, furunculosis, skin antisepsis before surgery, surgical wounds, non-specific vaginitis, burns, disinfection of endoscopes etc.

## Chlorine :

- ***Mechanism :*** cause oxidation of protoplasm.
- It is rapidly acting agent.
- Strength used is 0.1-0.25 ppm.
- It is used for disinfection of urban water supply.

### *Chlorophores :*

- They are compounds that slowly release hypochlorous acid. Due to ease of handling, they are more preferred than chlorine.

***Chlorinated lime (bleaching powder) :***

- ***Mechanism :*** Same as chlorine.
- It is used in disinfection of drinking water, swimming pools.

***Sodium hypochlorite :***

- ***Mechanism :*** Same as chlorine.
- Used for disinfection of infant feeding bottles, dairy cans for milk.
- It is irritant, therefore not used as skin antiseptic.

## Cetrimide :

- It is having detergent action.
- ***Mechanism :*** it alters the permeability of cell membrane.
- It efficiently removes oil, dirt, grease and dried blood from the wounds.
- It is used (1-3%) as antiseptic and disinfectant for surgical instruments, utensils and bath.

## Boric acid :

- It is a weak antiseptic and has bacteriostatic action.
- It is non-irritating, therefore used in eyes also.
- It is used as mouthwash, for irrigating eyes, in prickly heat powders, cuts and abrasions etc.

## Metallic salts :

***Silver compounds (silver nitrate, silver sulphadiazine) :***

- It rapidly kills microbes and action is long standing because of slow release of silver ions.
- They are used for tonsillitis, aphthus ulcers and burns. Silver sulphadiazine is also effective against pseudomonas infection.

## Dyes :

- Dyes used as antiseptic are Gentian violet, Acriflavine and Proflavine.
- They are not commonly used nowadays due to staining.

# 78 DRUGS ACTING ON SKIN AND MUCOUS MEMBRANE

There are various drugs which are used topically on skin and mucous membrane. They are used in various dosage forms such as :

**Demulcents :**

- They are inert substances which sooth inflamed and denuded mucosa or skin by preventing contact with air or irritants in the surroundings.
- ***E.g. :*** Methylcellulose (eye drops), Propylene glycol (cosmetics), Glycerine (for moisturising).

**Emollients :**

- They are used to soften and soothe rough, dry skin and increase absorbability of topical medications.
- They are applied generally after bathing and pat drying; applied liberally to affected areas.
- ***E.g. :*** Olive oil, sesame oil, cocoa butter, liquid paraffin.

**Adsorbants and protectives :**

- They are finely powdered, inert and insoluble solids capable of binding to their surface.
- ***E.g. :*** Magnesium and zinc stearate, talc, calamine, starch (for surgical gloves), boric acid (antiseptic, prickly heat powder) and Aloe vera gel.

**Astringents :**

- Astringents are agents which precipitate surface proteins and protect the underlying tissues.
- They are best used in eczema where vesicular or draining lesions are present.
- ***E.g. :*** Potassium permanganate, 5% acetic acid, tannic acid, alcohol.

**Topical vehicles :**

***Creams :***

- They are less greasy and most acceptable to patients. It gets applied more easily; penetrates the skin well.
- Works well in intertriginous and hairy areas.
- Have a drying and cooling effect.
- They are easy to wash off.

***Lotions :***

- They have more water content and are less viscous than creams.

***Ointments :***

- They are petroleum based and reduce dryness by prevention of evaporation.
- It also helps in removing scales.
- They enable medication to penetrate skin adequately and are also water repellant.
- They also form occlusive and protective layer.
- They have soothing and lubricating effect.

**Counter-irritants :**

- They cause surface irritation of the skin, thereby counteracting underlying pain or discomfort.
- *E.g. :* Volatile oils like turpentine oil, Clove oil, eucalyptus oil, camphor, menthol, mustard, capsicum, methyl salicylate and alcohol.

**Caustics and escharotics :**

- Caustic means corrosive and escharotic means cauteriser. They are used for tissue destruction. They are especially used in moles, warts, condylomata and papillomas.
- *E.g. :* Podophyllium resin, silver nitrate, phenol, trichloro acetic acid.

**Keratolytics :**

- These are the substances that dissolve the intercellular cementing substance and cause peeling of the superficial layers of skin.
- They are used in the treatment of warts, cones, calluses, severe xerosis.
- *E.g. :* Salicylic acid, lactic acid, urea, sulphur and benzyl peroxide.

**Anti-seborrhoeics :**

- They are used in the treatment of seborrhoeic dermatitis / dandruff.
- They are available as shampoos and lotions.
- *E.g. :* Selenium sulphide, zinc pyrithione, glucocorticoids, azole antifungals like ketaconazole, sulphur and coal tar.

**Melanising agents :**

- They increase the sensitivity of skin to solar radiation and help in pigmentation (melanisation) of skin. Mainly used in hypopigmented conditions such as vitiligo.
- *E.g. :* Psoralen, methoxsalen, trioxsalen.

**Demelanising agents :**

- They help in reducing melanisation in hyperpigmented areas of skin.
- *E.g. :* Hydroquinone, monobenzene, azelaic acid.

**Sunscreens :**

- These are the agents that protect the skin from the harmful effects of UV rays.

- ***Chemical sunscreens :*** They absorb and scatter UV rays. ***E.g.*** PABA, oxybenzene, titanium dioxide and cinnamates.
- ***Physical sunscreens :*** Petroleum jelly, zinc oxide and calamine.

## Chemotherapeutic agents :

### *Antibacterial Agents :*

- Common bacterial infections affecting skin are : Furuncle, boil, folliculitis, pyoderma, impetigo, cellulitis etc.
- We can use topical antibacterials like clindamycin, neomycin, mupirocin etc.
- Systemic antibacterials like amoxycillin, azithromycin etc. can also be used in treating bacterial skin infections.

### *Antifungal agents :*

- *Common fungal infections are :* thrush, dandruff, ringworm, oral thrush, athlete's foot, tineas etc.
- Topical antifungals like clotrimazole, ketoconazole, miconazole and terbenafine are used in treating fungal infections of skin. Sometimes systemic antifungals like fluconazole and griseofulvin are also used.

### *Antiviral agents :*

- Viral infections of skin and mucous membrane like Herpes simplex, herpes zoster are very common.
- We use either a topical or systemic antiviral drug. ***E.g.*** acyclovir.

## Drugs based on symptoms or disease :

### *Antihistaminics :*

- They are used for itching associated with various skin diseases.
- Details of antihistaminics are covered in their respective chapter.

### *Corticosteroids :*

- They are used both topically and systemically.
- Have antiinflammatory and immunosuppressant action. They reduce proliferation of keratocytes, fibroblasts and lymphocytes. They also inhibit migration of inflammatory cells and substances released due to inflammation.
- ***Systemic :*** Betamethasone, Prednisolone, Methylprednisolone, Dexamethasone, Hydrocortisone and Triamcinolone.
- ***Topical :*** Betamethasone, Clobetasol, Mometasone.
- ***Use :*** Allergic conditions, infections (bacterial/viral/fungal), pigment disorders, psoriasis, eczematous disorders, drug induced disorders etc.
- ***Adverse effects :*** Infection may exacerbate, skin atrophy on long term use, local hirsutism, de-pigmentation, glaucoma, rebound exacerbation of disease after abrupt cessation. On systemic use : hypertension, diabetes, peptic ulcer etc.

## ANDROGENIC ALOPECIA (male pattern baldness) :

- Common after age of 40 and about 50% men develop alopecia.
- **Drugs used :** Topical *Minoxidil* (1-10%). Possibly acts by increasing circulation around hair follicles, stimulation of hair follicle, reduces the effect of androgen, thickens the hair shafts, and increases their number and length. Onset is delayed and takes few months. Effect is transient; baldness recurs on discontinuation of drug. ***Adverse effects :*** local itching, burning sensation
- **Finasteride** (Competitive inhibitor of 5-α-reductase. This inhibits the conversion of Testosterone to the more potent, dihydrotestosterone (DHT), which is responsible for many of the responses to testosterone including baldness) in low dose (1 mg) is also used in androgenic alopecia.
- Definitive treatment is hair transplant surgery.

## ACNE VULGARIS :

- A common skin disorder seen in adolescents due infection of pilosebaceous unit by the bacteria *Propionibacium acnes.*
- **Changes in acne :** Plugging of hair follicle, accumulation of sebum, growth of Propionibacium acnes and Inflammation.
- **Treatment :**
  - ***Topical agents :*** Retinoic acid, benzoyl peroxide, adapalene, tazarotene, azelaic acid, topical antibiotics (clindamycin, lincomycin etc.).
  - Systemic antibiotics (amoxycillin, azithromycin, doxycycline), isotretinoin.

## PSORIASIS :

- An immunological disorder which manifests as localised or widespread erythematous scaling lesions with silvery plaques.
- Increased proliferation, inflammation of epidermis and dermis.
- Drugs can decrease the lesions but cannot cure the condition.
- **Topical Agents :**
  - ***Coal tar :*** Mainly used with UVB (antimitotic effect). Used as solution, gel and shampoo. Adverse effects : folliculitis, irritation, allergic reaction.
  - ***Calcipotriol (active vitamin D) :*** By acting on keratinocytes; causes decrease in proliferation of cultured keratinocytes and by the same mechanism, it produces antipsoriatic effect. Effective orally and topically.
- **Other drugs :** Anthralin, Tazarotene.
- **Systemic Agents :** They are required in extensive and severe disease. Cytotoxic & immunosuppressants are used.
  - ***Methotrexate :*** It is a dihydrofolate reductase inhibitor and suppresses immune component cells (mainly T-cells) in Skin. Epidermal inflammation and hyper-proliferation are retarded.
  - ***Other drugs :*** Hydroxyurea, Cyclosporin, Efalizumab etc.

## ECTOPARACITICIDES :

### Scabies :

- Highly contagious disease caused by mite Sarcoptes scabiei.
- Female itch mite burrows into superficial layers of skin and lays eggs, forms papules and cause intense itching and is highly contagious.
- ***Drugs :*** Permethrin, Benzylbenzoate, Gamma benzyl hexachloride, Ivermectin (oral).
- Topical agents are applied at night below neck all over the body followed by hot scrub bath in the morning. Permethrin is used only as single application.

### Pediculosis :

- It is a lice infestation caused by pediculus capitis. Itching is a common symptom.
- ***Drugs :*** Permethrin, malathion and DDT. Permethrin is preferred drug. Malathion used in cases not responding to permethrin.
- Ivermectin is also used.

# 79 VACCINES AND ANTISERA

## VACCINES :

They are immunobiological substances designed to produce specific protection against a given disease. It stimulates active immunity by production of protective antibodies by patient himself.

### Types of vaccines :

- ***Live attenuated vaccines :*** They consist of live microorganisms and which are rendered avirulent. The immunity is usually long lasting. ***E.g.*** BCG (Bacillus Calmette Guerin), Typhoid Ty21a, OPV (Oral polio vaccine - sabin), Measles, Mumps, Rubella etc.
- ***Killed vaccines :*** They consist of killed microorganisms. Immunity is short lasting and multiple doses and boosters are needed at intervals. ***E.g.*** IPV (Injectable polio vaccine - salk), Hepatitis B, Pertussis, HiB (H. Influenza B), Rabies etc.
- ***Toxoids :*** They are bacterial toxins which have antigenicity to provide immunity but, the toxicity is lost. ***E.g.*** Tetanus toxoid, Diphtheria toxoid.
- ***Combined vaccines :*** It is combination of different vaccines. ***E.g. :***
  - **Double** : Diphtheria + Tetanus.
  - **Triple** : DPT, MMR (Measles + Mumps + Rubella).
  - **Pentavalent** : DPT (Diphtheria + Pertusis + Tetanus) + HiB + Hepatitis B.

### National immunisation schedule :

| Time | Vaccine |
|---|---|
| **At birth** | BCG + OPV + Hepatitis B |
| **6 weeks** | DPT + OPV + Hepatitis B + HiB + IPV + Rotavirus |
| **10 weeks** | DPT + OPV + HiB + Rotavirus |
| **14 weeks** | DPT + OPV + IPV + HiB + Rotavirus |
| **6 months** | Hepatitis B |
| **9-12 months** | Measles / MR (1st dose) |
| **16-24 months** | DPT (1st booster), OPV (booster), Measles / MR (2nd dose) |
| **5-6 years** | DPT (2nd booster) |
| **10 and 16 years** | TT |
| **Pregnancy** | TT : 1st dose (early pregnancy) and 2nd dose (4 weeks after 1st dose) |

## ANTISERA AND IMMUNOGLOBULINS :

They are readymade antibodies and provide passive immunity against a given disease. These readymade anibodies are produced by another person or animal and then transferred to the patient

- ***Antisera :*** These are serum obtained from horse or rabbit that are actively immunised against specific disease or antigen.
- ***Immunoglobulins :*** These are separated human gamma globulins which carry antibodies.

**Examples :**

- ***Antisera :***
  - Anti gas gangrene serum (AGGS), Anti tetanus serum (ATS), Antirabies serum (ARS), Antidiphtheritic serum (ADS) and Antisnake venom (ASV).
- ***Immunoglobulins :***
  - Anti-D immunoglobulin, Hepatitis B immunoglobulin, Tetanus immunoglobulin and Rabies immunoglobulin.

**Adverse effects :**

- ***Allergic reactions :*** Urticaria, anaphylaxis, angio-edema, respiratory distress. Always obtain history of allergy in past and perform skin sensitivity testing before administering.
- ***Serum sickness :*** Fever, joint pain, rash, lymphadenopathy etc.
- ***Local :*** Pain, swelling, redness, Thrombophlebitis etc.

# 80 VITAMINS

Vitamins are non-energy yielding organic compounds essential for human health and required in small quantities.

**Types :**

- **Fat soluble vitamins :** A, D, E and K.
- **Water soluble vitamins :** B-complex and C.

## FAT SOLUBLE VITAMINS :

### Vitamin A :

- Biologically active forms are *retinoids* : retinol, retinal and retinoid acid.
- ***Sources :*** Animal sources : milk, meat, fish, liver. Plant sources : green leafy vegetables, yellow-orange colored fruits like carrot, mango etc.
- ***Role :***
  - **Vision :** Vitamin A is an important component of retinal pigment *Rhodopsin* which is synthesised in rods during dark (helps *see* in dark light such as in night).
  - **Immunity :** Reduces susceptibility to infections, boosts immunity and also acts as antioxidant.
  - **Epithelial cells :** Maintains structural integrity of epithelial cells, promotes mucus secretion, inhibits keratinization and resists infections.
  - **Reproduction :** It helps in spermatogenesis and fetal growth.
- ***Deficiency features :*** Night blindness, dryness of eyes, Bitot's spots in eye, keratomalacia, dry and rough skin, hyperkeratinisation, diarrhea, susceptibility to infections, sterility, growth retardation etc.
- ***Daily requirememt :*** 900 mcg and 700 mcg per day for men and women.
- ***Uses :***
  - Prophylaxis of vitamin A during pregnancy, lactation etc. : 3000-5000 IU/day.
  - Vitamin A deficiency : 50000-100000 IU/day or orally for 1-3 days followed by supplemental doses.
  - Skin diseases like psoriasis, acne : retinoids like tretinoin, isotretinoin, acitriten and tazarotene are used.

- ***Interactions :*** Vitamin E promotes storage and utilisation of vitamin A. Laxatives like liquid paraffin emulsifies and reduce absorption of all fat soluble vitamins.
- ***Hypervitaminosis A :*** It occurs after ingestion of 100000 IU of vit A per day for more than 3 weeks. It is manifested as dry itchy skin, hair loss, tender bones, fissuring of lips, brittle hair and nails, hepatosplenomegaly, headache, vomiting, papilledema, peeling of skin.

**Vitamin D :**

- Vitamin D covered under chapter of Vitamin D, Parathormone, Calcitonin and drugs affecting Calcium balance.

**Vitamin E :**

- ***Sources :*** Wheat germ oil, vegetable seed oil, nuts, egg yolk and peas.
- ***Role :***
  - Acts as antioxidant and protects from free radicals.
  - Important in maintaining fertility.
  - Enhances storage and utilisation of vitamin A.
  - Protection against cardiovascular diseases, cancers and neurodegenerative diseases.
- ***Deficiency features :***
  - Sterility.
  - Peripheral neuropathy and hemolytic anemia.
  - Cardiomyopathy and muscular dystrophy.
  - Altered gait and tendon reflexes.
- ***Daily requirement and dose :*** Daily requirement is 10-20 mg.
- ***Uses :***
  - Therapeutic dose is 400 mg/day.
  - Used in coronary artery diseases, Alzheimer's disease, nocturnal muscle cramps, intermittent claudication, fibrocystic breast disease and G6PD deficiency.
- ***Interactions :*** Laxative like liquid paraffin emulsifies and reduces absorption of all fat soluble vitamins.

**Vitamin K :**

- ***Sources :*** It is normally produced by the intestinal bacteria. Liver, green leafy vegetables and pulses.
- ***Vitamin K analogues :***
  - **Phytonadione (natural vitamin K) :** obtained from leafy vegetables.
  - **Menaquinone (vitamin $K_2$) :** synthesised by the intestinal bacteria.
  - **Menadione (vitamin $K_3$) :** synthetic.

- ***Role :*** It is required for the synthesis of clotting factors II, VII, IX and X.
- ***Deficiency features :*** Deficiency is manifested as increased bleeding tendencies and hypoprothrombinemia.
- ***Daily requirement :*** 50-100 μg/day.
- ***Uses :***
  - **Prolong antibiotic use :** this leads to suppression of intestinal bacterial flora and leads to vitamin K deficiency.
  - Overdose of oral anticoagulants like Warfarin.
  - Newborn or premature babies.

## WATER SOLUBLE VITAMINS :

### Vitamin $B_1$ (Thiamine) :

- ***Sources :*** Pulses, cereals, green vegetables, peanuts, yeast, egg and meat
- ***Role :*** Important role in carbohydrate metabolism & neuromuscular transmission.
- ***Deficiency features :***
  - Deficiency leads to failure of glucose metabolism and accumulation of lactic acid and pyruvic acid (*Beri-Beri*).
  - **Dry Beri-Beri affects CNS :** neuropathy, numbness, cramps, muscle weakness.
  - **Wet Beri-Beri affects CVS :** palpitations, breathlessness, high output failure, ECG changes.
  - In alcoholics, thiamine deficiency leads to Wernicke-Korsakoff syndrome.
- ***Daily requirement :*** 1-2 mg.
- ***Uses and dose :***
  - Therapeutic dose is 100 mg/day IM or IV, followed by 5-10 mg/day orally.
  - Beri-Beri.
  - Wernicke-Korsakoff syndrome.

### Vitamin $B_2$ (Riboflavin) :

- ***Sources :*** Pulses, sprouted cereals, liver, milk, cheese, egg and meat
- ***Role :*** Active form is flavin mononucleotide (FMN) and flavin adeninine dinucleotide (FAD) which are co-enzymes used in various oxidation-reduction reactions. Important role in carbohydrate metabolism.
- ***Deficiency features :*** Stomatitis, glossitis, seborrheic dermatitis, cataract formation and vascularisation of cornea.
- ***Daily requirement :*** 1.5-2 mg.
- ***Uses and dose :***
  - Therapeutic dose is 5-20 mg/day.

- Generally used in combination with other B-complex vitamins.
- Glossitis, stomatitis, HTN, diabetes, coronary artery disease and obesity.

### Vitamin $B_3$ (Niacin) :

- ***Sources :*** Fish, pulses, cereals, liver, egg, dry nuts and meat.
- ***Role :*** Active form is nicotinamide adenine dinucleotide (NAD) and nicotinamide adenine dinucleotide phosphate (NADP) which are co-enzymes used in various oxidation-reduction reactions.
- ***Deficiency features :***
  - *Pellagra* (Dermatitis, dementia, diarrhea, stomatitis, glossitis, headache, dizziness and depression).
  - Chronic alcoholics are at more risk of deficiency and pellagra.
  - Maize, jowar and bajra eaters are more prone to develop pellagra because they lack in tryptophan (tryptophan is a provitamin for niacin).
- ***Daily requirement :*** 2-16 mg.
- ***Uses and dose :***
  - Prophylactic dose is 15-20 mg and therapeutic dose is 200-500 mg/day.
  - Generally used in combination with other B-complex vitamins.
  - Used in pellagra and hyperlipoproteinemia.

### Vitamin $B_5$ (Pantothenic acid) :

- ***Sources :*** Meat, pulses, cereals, legumes, liver, egg yolk, milk, vegetables and fruits.
- ***Role :*** It is an important component of coenzyme-A involved in the metabolism of carbohydrates, fats and proteins.
- ***Deficiency features :*** Deficiency as such is not apparent but may lead to diarrhea, flatulence, leg cramps, paraesthesias and insomnia.
- ***Daily requirement :*** 4-7 mg.
- ***Uses and dose :*** Therapeutic dose is 50-100 mg/day. Generally used in combination with other B-complex vitamins & as nutritional supplement.

### Vitamin $B_6$ (Pyridoxine) :

- ***Sources :*** Soyabean, meat, pulses, cereals, legumes, liver and vegetables.
- ***Role :*** It is an important coenzyme (pyridoxal phosphate) involved in the metabolism of carbohydrates, fats and proteins. It also plays important role in synthesis of GABA, amino acids and heme.
- ***Deficiency features :*** Stomatitis, glossitis, peripheral neuropathy, precipitation of seizures, anemia and growth retardation.
- ***Daily requirement :*** 1.5-2 mg.

- ***Uses and dose :***
  - Prophylactic dose is 2-5 mg and therapeutic dose is 10-50 mg/day.
  - Used in pyridoxine deficiency, anemia, morning sickness, neuropathy.
- ***Interactions :***
  - It converts levodopa to dopamine peripherally and thus reduces bioavailability of dopamine centrally.
  - In TB patients, use of isoniazid leads to deficiency of pyridoxine especially in slow acetylators leading to neuropathy.

### Vitamin $B_7$ (Biotin) :

- ***Sources :*** Meat, liver, legumes, avocado, fish, egg yolk, cauliflower, nuts etc.
- ***Role :*** It is an important coenzyme involved in the metabolism of carbohydrates, fats and proteins.
- ***Deficiency features :*** Nausea, vomiting, anorexia, hair loss, dry and brittle hairs, brittle nails, dermatitis.
- ***Daily requirement :*** 0.03-30 mg.
- ***Uses and dose :*** Therapeutic dose is 10-20 mg/day. Used in biotin deficiency, hair loss, dermatitis etc.

### Vitamin C (Ascorbic acid) :

- ***Sources :*** Amla, citrus fruits (lemon, orange), potatoes, cabbage etc.
- ***Role :*** It is an important co-factor involved in oxidation, hydroxylation and amidation reactions. Has an important role to play in collagen synthesis and also synthesis of adrenal hormones, oxytocin, ADH. It also helps in absorption of iron.
- ***Deficiency features :*** **Scurvy :** gum bleeding, loosening of teeth, glossitis, delayed wound healing, hemorrhages, bleeding, hematomas etc.
- ***Daily requirement :*** **children :** 10-50 mg, **adults :** 60-120 mg.
- ***Uses and dose :***
  - Prophylactic dose is 50-500 mg/day and therapeutic dose for scurvy is 1-1.5 g/day.
  - Used in scurvy, for wound healing, viral infections, as antioxidant, common cold, UTI, cancer and acidification of urine.

❑❑❑❑❑

81

# GENERAL MANAGEMENT OF POISONINGS (Also OP Poisoning, Snake bite and Scorpion bite)

## GENERAL PRINCIPLES OF MANAGEMENT OF POISONINGS :

**Principles of management consist of :**

i. Stabilisation.

ii. Gut Decontamination.

iii. Antidote administration

iv. Elimination

### i) Stabilisation :

It includes ABC of resuscitation.

- **A**–Airway, **B**–Breathing and **C**–Circulation.

***Evaluating the patient :*** It consists of the following things : History taking, Physical examination, Routine tests and Toxicological screening.

### ii) Gut Decontamination :

- ***Ipecac syrup :*** No longer recommended for poisonings.
- ***Activated charcoal :*** Binds to most medications and potentially decreases GI absorption. Potentially useful within 1 hour of ingestion but no evidence of improved clinical outcomes. Aspiration is uncommon unless given by a nasogastric tube or in patient with altered mental status.
- ***Gastric Lavage :*** Insertion of large orogastric tube into the stomach and lavaging with several litres of fluid. Potentially useful in life threatening ingestions < 1 hour. Aspiration occurs in around 5% of patients.
- ***Whole Bowel Irrigation :*** Decreases GI transit time using Polyethylene glycol. Useful in life threatening ingestions when other methods not helpful.

### iii) Antidote :

"Antidote was defined as a therapeutic substance used to counteract the toxic actions of a specific substance". Some examples of antidotes are mentioned below.

| Drug | Antidote |
|---|---|
| Paracetamol | Acetylcysteine |
| Organophosphates | Atropine, Pralidoxime (2-PAM) |

| Drug | Antidote |
|---|---|
| Benzodiazepines | Flumazenil |
| Digoxin | Digoxin immune Fab |
| Iron | Deferoxamine (Desferrioxamine) |
| Methanol | Fomepizole |
| Opioids | Naloxone |
| Beta-blockers | Glucagon |
| Warfarin | Vitamin K |
| Heparin | Protamine sulphate |

***Universal antidote :*** It is a combination of Magnesium oxide, Charcoal and Tannic acid. Not used nowadays.

**iv) Elimination :**

Drug is eliminated from the body by various methods such as :

- Forced diuresis (urinary pH manipulation), Hemodialysis & Peritoneal dialysis.

## ORGANOPHOSPHORUS POISONING (OP POISONING) :

These are the agents which irreversibly inhibit cholinesterase, protect Acetylcholine from hydrolysis and produce cholinergic effects. They are mainly used as insecticides and pesticides in farms.

They are :

- **Irreversible :** Malathion, Parathion, Diazinon
- **Carbamates :** Propoxur

**Clinical features :**

- ***Muscarinic effects :*** Bradycardia, hypotension, rhinorrhea, bronchospasm, severe respiratory distress, hypersalivation, nausea and vomiting,

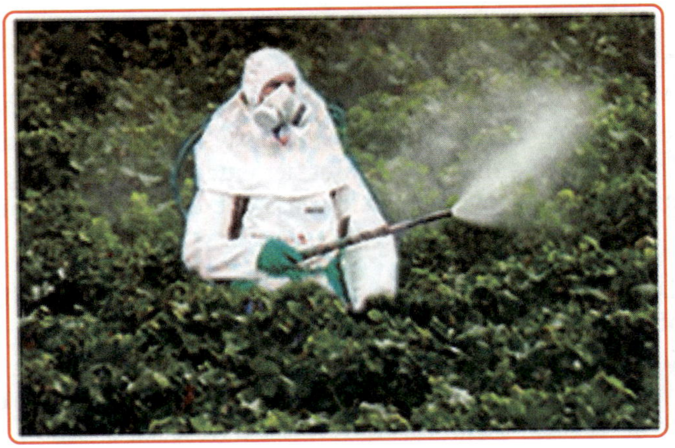

abdominal pain, diarrhea, fecal incontinence, urinary and bowel incontinence, blurred vision, miosis, increased lacrimation etc.

- ***Nicotinic effects :*** Nicotinic signs and symptoms include muscle fasciculations, cramping, weakness, and diaphragmatic failure. Autonomic nicotinic effects include hypertension, tachycardia, mydriasis and pallor.
- ***CNS effects :*** Anxiety, emotional lability, restlessness, confusion, ataxia, tremors, seizures, coma and apnea.

### Treatment :

***Primary measures :***

- Remove patient away from the site of exposure.
- Remove contaminated clothes.
- Wash body parts with soap and water.
- Check for A, B, C (airway, breathing, circulation).
- Gastric lavage with potassium permanganate.

***Pharmacotherapy :***

- Inj. Atropine 2 mg IV every 10 min till the signs of atropinisation (dilatation of pupils, tachycardia and dryness of all body secretions).
- Inj. Pralidoxime 2 gm IV slowly (should be started within 24 hours).
- Inj. Broad spectrum antibiotic can be given to prevent infection like aspiration pneumonitis.
- Inj. Furosemide 40 mg slow IV if pulmonary edema present.
- Inj. Diazepam 10 mg IV slowly if convulsions. May be repeated if needed.

## SNAKE BITE :

Snakes can be poisonous and non-poisonous. Here we will discuss only the poisonous snake bites. There are 2 types of poisonous snakes :

1) **Elapidae (Neuro Toxic)** – Naag (Cobra) & Manyar (common Krait).
2) **Viperidae (Hemotoxic)** – Ghonas (Russels viper) & Furse (Saw scaled Viper).

### Clinical features :

***Neurotoxic :*** Cobra or Krait

- **Local :** Mild burning, triple response i.e redness, swelling, inflammation.
- **Systemic :** Vomiting, giddiness, ptosis, difficulty in swallowing, staggering gait, difficult respiration, difficulty in motor activities like hand & leg movements, spreading paralysis, convulsions and death due to respiratory failure.

***Haemotoxic :*** Russell's & saw scaled Vipers

- **Local :** Local symptoms are more severe like Intense pain, swelling, cellulitis, oozing of bloody serum & formation of blisters & necrosis.
- **Systemic :** Vomiting, unconsciousness, intravascular hemolysis, epistaxis, hematuria, hematemesis, bleeding under skin like petechiae, bleeding from orifices, hypotension. Death result from cardiovascular shock or renal failure.

### Treatment :

***Primary measures :***

1) Check for vitals. Monitor CBC, platelet, PT, BT, CT for Viperidae bites.
2) To slow the absorption and spread of the poison :
   - Patient is prevented from walking. Bitten limb is immobilised in a splint.
   - Strip of cloth or handkerchief or a rubber tourniquet should be applied a few cm above the bitten area & released every 15 minutes for a period of one minute.
   - Tourniquet should not be too tight. It is just to occlude venous & lymphatic return.
3) The wound and the incision can be washed with very dilute solution of potassium permanganate.

***Definitive treatment :***

1. **Neutralise the poison by :**
   - Injection of ASV (antisnake venom). Most effective if administered within 1 to 4 hours of the bite. Sensitivity tests must be done. If the patient is not sensitive, 5cc. of the serum should be injected locally around the wound. Newer guidelines do not suggest checking for sensitivity.
   - It can be administered in 2 ways : Intravenous injections or as Infusion.
2. **For Pain :** Paracetamol. Aspirin or other NSAIDs should not be given; can exacerbate bleeding. For severe pain : opioids like Tramadol 50 mg.
3. **Neostigmine :** Is anti cholinesterase drug; prolongs the action of Acetylcholine – revert respiratory failure & Neurotoxic symptoms.
4. **Antibiotics :** Snake bites should be treated as wounds. Antibiotics are given for secondary infection.
5. **Inj. Tetanus toxoid** also given.
6. **In Respiratory Paralysis :** Endotracheal Intubation, artificial respiration.
7. **Surgery :** In Hemolytic type, when edema becomes severe, circulation of toes is diminished, and then to save the limb, emergency fasciotomy is done.
8. **Transfusion :** In cases of bleeding : Blood transfusion is given. When possible : Platelet transfusion is given, Injection Fibrinogen 300 to 600 mg IV. Injection Heparin is given if there is DIC.

## SCORPION BITE :

**Two types of scorpions are found in India :**

- Black scorpion and Brown scorpion.

### Clinical features :

- ***Local :*** More severe than snake bite; pain, edema & reddening.
- ***Systemic :*** Nausea, vomiting, restlessness, tachycardia, palpitations, hypertension, autonomic storm (increased adrenergic activity), fever, convulsions, coma.

**Treatment :**

- A tight ligature should be placed proximal to the bite.
- Ice should be applied around. $KMnO_4$ can also be applied.
- Severe pain often responds to local injection of *emetine hydrochloride* 30 mg. given through the puncture made by the sting, if this is visible.
- Injection *Fortwin or Pethidine* 10 mg IM or IV stat for pain.
- Injection Local *Lignocaine* 2% without adrenaline is infiltrated around the site of bite to reduce pain.
- *Prazosin (α–blocker)* : This drug was previously used only as Antihypertensive, but now also used in scorpion bite to prevent autonomic symptoms. This use was invented by Dr. Himmatrao Bawaskar of Mahad in Maharashtra. Dose of Prazosin is 1 mg stat followed by 0.25 to 0.5 mg every 4 to 6 hours.
- *If profuse sweating & dehydration :* Ringer lactate IV.
- *Scorpion Venom Antiserum :* made by Haffkine Bio-pharmaceuticals Mumbai. Dose is 1 vial reconstituted in 10 ml water for Injection. If symptoms persist administer another vial after 1 hour.

❑❑❑❑❑

# 82 OCULAR PHARMACOLOGY (Drugs used in Eyes)

## DRUG DELIVERY IN EYES :

A drug can be delivered to ocular tissue as :

- ***Locally :*** Eye drop, ointment, ocuserts, periocular injection and intraocular injection.
- ***Systemically :*** Orally, IV and IM.

### Eye Drops (Gutta) :

- Simplest and convenient mode. Mainly for day time use.
- ***Method :*** hold the skin below the lower eye lid, pull it forward slightly and put a drop and keep lids closed for 5 minutes after instillation.

### Eye Ointments :

- Increases the contact time of ocular medication to ocular tissue, causes long lasting effect.
- It has the disadvantage of vision blurring.
- The drug has to be high lipid soluble with some water solubility to have the maximum effect as ointment.

### Ocuserts :

- These are devices that deliver an adequate supply of medication at a steady state level
- ***Example :*** Ocusert delivering pilocarpine, ganciclovir sustained release intraocular device.

### Peri-ocular injections :

- They reach behind iris-lens diaphragm better than topical application.
- ***E.g.*** subconjunctival, peribulbar, or retrobulbar. Also steroid and local anesthetics can be applied this way.
- This route bypass the conjunctival and corneal epithelium which is good for drugs with low lipid solubility (*e.g.* penicillins).

### Intraocular injections :

- Intracameral or intravitreal.
- ***Example :*** Intracameral acetylcholine during cataract surgery, Intravitreal antibiotics in cases of endophthalmitis, Intravitreal steroid in macular edema.

## COMMON OCULAR DRUGS :

- Antibiotics, antivirals, antifungals, mydriatics and cycloplegics, antiglaucoma, anti-inflammatory agents (Glucocorticoids and NSAIDs), ocular lubricants and Local anesthetics.

### Antibiotics :

- ***Commonly Used :*** Penicillins, Cephalosporins, Sulphonamides, Tetracyclines, Chloramphenicol, Aminoglycosides, Fluoroquinolones and Macrolides.
- Used topically in prophylaxis and treatment of ocular bacterial infections like bacterial conjunctivitis.
- Used orally for the treatment of preseptal cellulitis *e.g.* amoxycillin with clavulanic acid.
- Used intravenously for the treatment of orbital cellulitis *e.g.* gentamicin, cephalosporin, vancomycin, Metronidazole.
- Can be injected intravitreally for the treatment of endophthalmitis.
- ***Amino glycosides :*** Gentamicin — 0.3% eye drop, Tobramycin- 1% eye drop.
- ***Fluoroquinolones :*** Ciprofloxacin eye drops, gatifloxacin eye drops.
- ***Chloramphenicol :*** Broad spectrum, bacteriostatic, gram positive and gram negative, Chlamydia 0.5% Eye drop, ointment.

### Antivirals :

- ***Acyclovir :*** 3% ointment 5 times 10-14 days or 800 mg oral 5 times 10-14 days intravenous for Herpes zoster retinitis.
- ***Others :*** Idoxuridine, Vidarabine, Cytarabine, Triflurothymidine and Gancyclovir.
- ***Indications :*** Herpes zoster keratitis, Viral uveitis, viral corneal ulcers.

### Antifungals :

- ***Indications :*** Fungal corneal ulcer, Fungal retinitis/Endophthalmitis.
- ***Commonly used drugs are :*** Amphotericin B, natamycin, nystatin, miconazole, ketoconazole, fluconazole.

### Mydriatics and cycloplegics :

- If we need only mydriasis : Phenylephrine or depivefrine eye drops are used.
- If we need mydriasis and cycloplegia, anticholinergics are used.
- ***Anticholinergics :*** Tropicamide or cyclopentolate are preferred.
- ***Indications :*** Fundoscopy, refraction checking.

### Antiglaucoma drugs :

- Covered in detail in chapter on drugs acting on the parasympathetic nervous system : cholinergic drugs.

### Anti-inflammatory agents :

***Glucocorticoids :***

- Dexamethasone, prednisolone, methyl prednisolone.

- Suppresses inflammation and various inflammatory cells.
- ***Uses :***
  - **Topical :** allergic conjunctivitis, scleritis, uveitis, allergic keratitis, after intraocular and extra ocular surgeries.
  - **Systemic :** Posterior uveitis, Optic neuritis, corneal graft rejection.
- ***Adverse effects :***
  - **Ocular :** Glaucoma, cataract, activation of infection, delayed wound healing.
  - **Systemic :** Peptic ulcer, hypertension, increased blood sugar, osteoporosis, mental changes, activation of tuberculosis and other infections.

***NSAIDs :***

- ***Topical use :*** flurbiprofen, indomethacin, ketorolac.
- ***Indications :*** episcleritis, scleritis, uveitis, CME.

**Ocular Lubricants :**

- ***Indication :*** ocular irritations in various diseases, dry eyes.
- Commonly used : carboxymethylcellulose, liquid paraffin, sodium hyaluronate.
- Commonly available commercial tear substitutes : Tear Plus, Moisol.

**Local anesthetics :**

***Topical :***

- ***Uses :*** Applanation tonometry, gonioscopy, removal of corneal foreign bodies, removal of sutures, examination of patients.
- ***E.g. :*** Propacaine, Tetracaine.

***Orbital infiltration :***

- Peribulbar or retrobulbar. Cause anesthesia and akinesia for intraocular surgery.
- ***E.g. :*** Lidocaine, Bupivacaine.

## COMPLICATIONS OF TOPICAL ADMINISTRATION :

- Mechanical injury from the bottle *e.g.* corneal abrasion, pigmentation : epinephrine, hypersensitivity (local anesthetics), systemic effect : phenylephrine can increase BP.

## OCULAR TOXICOLOGY :

Certain drugs given for other conditions can have an adverse effect on eyes.

- **Digitalis :** causes chromatopsia (objects appear yellow) with overdose.
- **Chloroquine :** cause retinopathy (bull's eye maculopathy).
- **Chorpromazine :** causes corneal punctate epithelial opacities.
- **Ethambutol :** causes a dose-related optic neuropathy.

□□□□□

# 83 DRUG USE DURING PREGNANCY AND LACTATION

## DRUG USE DURING PREGNANCY :

- Drug use during pregnancy and lactation needs special attention because the drug also affects the baby. Very few drugs are considered safe during this period. But, there are conditions where we need to prescribe drugs to many pregnant or lactating women. One must always be aware of the drugs used during these critical periods. There is altered pharmacokinetics during pregnancy and many drugs cross the placental barrier to affect the fetus. It is best to avoid drugs during pregnancy especially during 1st trimester.

### Pharmacokinetics in Pregnancy :

#### *Drug absorption :*

- The gastric emptying as well as gut motility is reduced resulting in slower drug absorption.
- Parenteral drug administration is preferred in order to obtain a quicker response.
- Drug compliance may be poor because of nausea, hyperemesis and fear of adverse effect.

#### *Drug metabolism :*

- Drug metabolising enzymes are induced during pregnancy probably by high concentration of circulating progesterone which can lead to more rapid metabolic degradation of drugs especially of highly lipid soluble drugs. This results in sub-therapeutic effect.

#### *Drug excretion :*

- Both, renal perfusion and GFR increases in pregnancy. Hence, the drugs which depend on the kidneys for their elimination are eliminated more rapidly than in non-pregnant state, *e.g.* Penicillin, cephalosporin and aminoglycosides.

#### *Increased total blood volume :*

- Total blood volume increases during pregnancy. This leads to change in cardiac output, BP and GFR. This results in change in volume of distribution of drug, metabolism, absorption, excretion and protein binding of drugs and also passage of drugs across placenta.

### Placental transfer of drugs :

- The placenta is not a perfect barrier to drugs and chemicals administered to mother.

- Thalidomide tragedy, showed that placenta was capable of transferring drugs ingested by mother to fetus, with potential for great harm.
- On other hand, placental transfer of drugs administered to mother has been used to treat fetal arrhythmias, congestive heart failure & other conditions.

### *Factors affecting placental drug transfer :*

- Physicochemical properties of drug.
- Rate at which drug crosses placenta & amount of drug reaching the fetus.
- Duration of exposure to drug.
- Distribution characteristics in different fetal tissues.
- Stage of placental & fetal development at time of exposure to the drug.

### Teratogenicity :

- It is the capacity of a drug to cause fetal abnormalities when administered to pregnant mother. Drugs can affect fetus at three stages : Stage of fertilisation and implantation, Stage of organogenesis & Stage of growth & development
- ***Examples :***

| Drug | Teratogenicity |
|---|---|
| **Tetracycline** | Discoloration of teeth, retarded bone growth. |
| **Phenytoin** | Craniofacial defect, cleft lip, cleft palate |
| **Fluoroquinolones** | Cartilage and bone defects |
| **Carbamazepine** | CNS defect |
| **Thalidomide** | Phacomelia |
| **Alcohol** | Fetal alcohol Syndrome |

### FDA drug risk classification :

| Category | Description |
|---|---|
| **A** | Control studies in humans show no risk to the fetus. |
| **B** | No control studies are conducted in humans, animal studies shows no risk to the fetus. |
| **C** | No control studies are conducted in animals or humans. |
| **D** | Evidence of fetal risk exists, but benefit may outweigh the risks in certain conditions. |
| **X** | Control studies in both animals and humans demonstrate fetal abnormalities, risks outweighs the benefits. |

### Drugs to be avoided in pregnancy :

- ACE inhibitors, angiotensin receptor blockers, warfarin, alcohol, barbiturates, benzodiazepines, antiepileptic drugs (phenytoin, phenobarbitone, valproic acid), anticancer drugs, antidepressants and antimaniac drugs NSAIDs, Glucocorticoids, Aminoglycosides, fluoroquinolones, thalidomide, estrogens, androgens, anti-androgens, antithyroid drugs (carbimazole, methimazole), retinoids, uterine stimulants (ergometrine, oxytocin) etc.

### Examples of preferred drugs in pregnancy :

| Category | Preferred drug(s) |
|---|---|
| **Antibiotics** | Penicillins, Cephalosporins, Erythromycin |
| **Anti-hypertensive drugs** | α-methyldopa, Labetolol, Hydralazine |
| **Anti-diabetic drugs** | Insulin (Most common), Metformin |
| **Analgesics** | Paracetamol |
| **Anti-thyroid drugs** | Propylthiouracil |
| **Anticoagulant** | Heparin |
| **Anti-epileptic drugs** | Levetiracetam, Lamotrigine, Gabapentin. Folic acid supplementation should be given to prevent neural tube defects. |

### Conclusion :

- Don't use drug unless it is absolutely necessary.
- Assess the risk-benefit ratio before prescribing a drug.
- Try to use lower doses and for short period of time.
- Use 'tried and tested' drugs whenever possible in preference to new agents;
- Remember that the fetus is most sensitive in the first trimester; consider pregnancy in all women of child bearing potential.
- Discuss the potential risks of taking or witholding therapy with the patient.
- Seek guidance on the use of drugs in pregnancy in the national formulary, drug information sources and standard textbooks.
- Warn the patient about the risks of smoking, alcohol, over the counter drugs and drugs of abuse.

## DRUG USE DURING LACTATION :

- Most drugs administered to lactating women are detectable in breast milk. Fortunately, the concentration of drugs achieved in breast milk is usually low.
- Infant would receive in a day is substantially less than what would be considered a therapeutic dose.
- If the nursing mother must take medications and the drug is a relatively safe one, she should optimally take it 30–60 minutes after nursing and 3–4 hours before the next feeding.
- **Caution :** Drugs like Sedative-Hypnotics, Lithium and Tetracyclines should be taken with caution.

❑❑❑❑❑